ABC of Medica

Department of Therapeutic Query

Proje.

Arrested to Helen Buckler

Dedicated to
Judith, Peter, Elizabeth, Gillian and Philip
who with Macbeth say:

'Throw physic to the dogs, I'll none of it'.

ABC of Medical Treatment

D.C. Banks
M.D., F.R.C.P.
Consultant Physician and Part-time Senior Lecturer in Therapeutics, City Hospital, Nottingham

CHURCHILL LIVINGSTONE,
EDINBURGH LONDON AND NEW YORK 1979

CHURCHILL LIVINGSTONE
Medical Division of the Longman Group Limited

Distributed in the United States of America by
Churchill Livingstone Inc., 19 West 44th Street,
New York, N.Y. 10036, and by associated
companies, branches and representatives
throughout the world.

First published 1979

ISBN 0 443 01766 2

British Library Cataloguing in Publication Data
Banks, David
    An ABC of medical treatment.
    1. Therapeutics
    I. Title
    615'.5   RM121   79-40257

Printed in Great Britain by
T & A Constable Ltd

Preface

This is a pocket book of therapeutics intended to be available at all times. It is not a text on clinical pharmacology. There are three main sections; the first suggests the specific treatment for individual conditions, the second details adverse effects and drug interactions observed with these drugs, and the third is an index of proprietary and approved names. Throughout each chapter on treatment, diseases are considered alphabetically for ease of reference. Dosage intervals are suggested throughout the 24 hours, rather than the conventional 2, 3 or 4 times a day, to emphasise the need for even spread of dosage intervals. Clear instructions are also given for recommended dose increments.

In writing this book we have attempted to give a practical guide to the treatment of conditions seen clinically. We have assumed throughout that the first stage of therapeutics, the establishment of the diagnosis, has been performed. From this base we have attempted to give a reasonable treatment intended for the non-expert. We have not attempted to be comprehensive nor do we think all the treatments we have recommended are necessarily the only possible treatments. In many instances the expert who is used to dealing with these particular problems will no doubt disagree with what is recommended. This is bound to happen with such a complex subject as therapeutics. We have tried, however, only to give treatments which can be accepted as being reasonable, and which will not do the patient any harm. In some parts of the book we have suggested that expert help be obtained. Following this we have given a likely treatment regime. This is because in many places it is not easy to get expert help as quickly as one would like, and therefore, a guide to the possible treatment is given. We have limited the number of alternative treatments, and have attempted to be didactic because a non-expert needs a line of treatment laid down for him, as he may not have the information necessary to make an assessment between alternatives. All the doses used throughout the book are for adults unless otherwise stated. Although this limits the use of the book, we think it also prevents confusion which can be engendered by the wide range of dosage used for children. Errors are always possible despite efforts to avoid them. We would, therefore, be very grateful for suggestions which users think would help to make this book more valuable.

Nottingham, 1979   DAVID C. BANKS

Acknowledgments

I would like to thank my colleagues who have written chapters or parts of chapters, and have allowed me to manipulate their text into the style used throughout this book. As well as the friends who have written sections, I have had a great deal of help from others who have read the whole of the text, namely, Dr J.H.M. Morewood, Dr G.D. Bell and Dr S. Pearson. Their comments have been most helpful and have ensured that the text has relevance to clinical practice. Mrs S. French (Information Pharmacist) has given me invaluable help with proof reading, particularly in the section on drugs, side effects and interactions, as did her predecessor Mrs D. Novak. Professor A.T. Birmingham has also helped by checking the proofs.

In addition, I have had help from many experts who have read individual chapters. These include Dr D. Davies, Mr N.R. Galloway, Dr J.R. Hampton, Dr D. Henry, Dr D. Hoskings, Professor W. F. O'Grady, Mr A.E.S. Richards, Dr W.H. Roderick Smith, Dr A.J. Swannell, Dr R. Tattersall, and Dr D. Toms. I would like to thank them very much for the help that they have so freely given, but would also emphasise that any errors in the text are mine and not theirs.

I would also like to thank various people who have allowed me to quote from previously published works. Professor W.F. O'Grady who agreed to my using *A Guide to Antibiotic Therapy*, a booklet which he and I have produced in Nottingham, to form the basis for the chapter on infections, Professor G. Mawer from Manchester for providing me with details of the Gentamicin Nomogram, and Dr Cecily Saunders for agreeing to my using an article she wrote for World Medicine as a basis for the chapter on 'Care of the Dying'.

I am indebted to Miss L.J. Sears for the typing of my manuscript and to my wife and family for tolerating me during its production. Finally, I would like to thank Mrs G. Evershed who was responsible for producing the proprietary to non-proprietary name index, and Professor M.J.S. Langman for the encouragement he has given me right from the inception of this project.

DAVID C. BANKS

Contributors

B.R. ALLEN, M.B.Ch.B., M.R.C.P.
Consultant Dermatologist, Nottingham City and University Hospitals.

G.D. BELL, M.Sc., M.D., M.R.C.P.
Senior Lecturer in Therapeutics, University of Nottingham.

R.P. BURDEN, M.B. B.S., M.R.C.P.
Consultant Physician, Nottingham City Hospital.

J. FLETCHER, M.A., M.D., F.R.C.P.
Consultant Physician, Nottingham City Hospital.

R.B. GODWIN-AUSTEN, M.D., F.R.C.P.
Consultant Neurologist, Nottingham and Derby Hospitals.

A.M. JEQUIER, F.R.C.S., M.R.C.O.G.
Senior Lecturer in Obstetrics and Gynaecology, University of Nottingham.

M.J.S. LANGMAN, B.Sc., M.D., F.R.C.P.
Boots Professor of Therapeutics, University of Nottingham.

M. B. McILLMURRAY, D.M., M.R.C.P.
Consultant Physician, Royal Lancaster Infirmary.

Contents

Note

Our knowledge in clinical medicine and related biological sciences is constantly changing. As new information obtained from clinical experience and research becomes available, changes in treatment and in the use of drugs become necessary. The author, the contributors and the publisher of this volume have, as far as it is possible to do so, taken care to make certain that the doses of drugs and schedules of treatment are accurate and compatible with the standards generally accepted at the time of publication. The readers are advised, however, to consult carefully the instruction and information material included in the package insert of each drug or therapeutic agent that they plan to administer in order to make certain that there have been no changes in the recommended dose of the drug or the indications or contraindications for its administration. This precaution is especially important when using new or infrequently used drugs.

Section 1

Infection

In this initial chapter I outline the treatment of many infections. It is obviously important that the diagnosis is fully established, if possible, before therapy is instituted. To do this requires the help of a microbiological laboratory in many instances. The better the material sent to the laboratory the more effective can the microbiologist be in identifying the infecting organism and thus indicating the correct therapy. In all cases samples should be taken to the laboratory as fresh as possible and without contamination. If there are doubts as to the diagnosis or the correct therapy, discussion between the clinician and the microbiologist, especially over the use of antibiotics, is particularly helpful.

AMOEBAE

Mild/moderate dysentery
either Metronidazole
      Adult 800 mg 8 hourly for 5 days
      Child 17 mg/kg 8 hourly for 7 days
  and Tetracycline 250 mg 6 hourly for 5 days
or Tinidazole 600 mg 12 hourly for 5 days
    or 2 g daily for 3 days
  and Tetracycline 250 mg 6 hourly for 5 days

Severe disease
Maintain fluid and electrolyte balance
and either Metronidazole
      Adult 800 mg 8 hourly i.v. orally or rectally for 5 days
      Child 17 mg/kg 8 hourly for 7 days
  and Chloroquine 600 mg stat
    then 6 hours later· 300 mg
    then 150 mg 12 hourly for 14 days
or Tetracycline 250 mg 6 hourly tor 10 days
  and Diloxanide 500 mg 8 hourly for 10 days
    or Di-iodohydroxyquinoline 600 mg 8 hourly for 20 days

Fulminant
Maintain fluid and electrolyte balance

and Metronidazole
        Adult 800 mg 8 hourly i.v., orally or rectally for 5 days
        Child 17 mg/kg 8 hourly for 7 days
and Emetine 60 mg i.m. daily for 10 days
  or Dihydroemetine 60 mg i.m. daily for 10 days
and Chloroquine 600 mg stat
      then 6 hours later 300 mg
      then 150 mg 12 hourly for 14 days
and Diloxanide 500 mg 8 hourly for 10 days
  or Di-iodohydroxyquinoline 600 mg 8 hourly for 20 days
and i.v. antibiotics as appropriate
and Surgery if indicated

Asymptomatic colonic amoebiasis
as for mild/moderate infection

Asymptomatic carriers – cysts found in faeces
either Diloxanide 500 mg 8 hourly for 10 days
  or Di-iodohydroxyquinoline 600 mg 8 hourly for 20 days
and Tetracycline 250 mg 6 hourly for 10 days

Hepatic abscess

Mild
Metronidazole 800 mg 8 hourly for 10 days
and Diloxanide 500 mg 8 hourly for 10 days
  or Di-iodohydroxyquinoline 600 mg 8 hourly for 20 days

Severe
Add Chloroquine 600 mg stat (to 'mild' treatment)
      then 6 hours later 300 mg
      then 150 mg 12 hourly for 14 days
  or Dihydroemetine 60 mg i.m. daily for 10 days
  and Tetracycline 250 mg 6 hourly for 10 days
  and Surgery

With clinical dysentery
Metronidazole 800 mg 8 hourly for 5 days
and Tetracycline 250 mg 6 hourly for 5 days

ANTHRAX

Attack
Benzyl Penicillin 1 mega unit i.m. or i.v. 6 hourly for 2 days
      then Phenoxymethyl Penicillin 500 mg 6 hourly for 5 days
If patient Penicillin sensitive – Tetracycline 500 mg 6 hourly for 7
days
Occasionally need tracheostomy
Rarely (in the U.K.) need treatment for pulmonary oedema
and/or shock.

Prophylaxis

At risk in job
Vaccination 0.5 ml of vaccine
    then 0.5 ml 3 and 6 weeks later
    then 0.5 ml 6 months later
    then annually to maintain immunity

Exposure
Phenoxymethyl Penicillin 250 mg 6 hourly for 5 days

BRUCELLOSIS

Attack
Tetracycline 500 mg 6 hourly for 3 weeks
    and Streptomycin 1 g daily i.m. for 3 weeks
    then Tetracycline 500 mg 6 hourly for 3 weeks
  or Co-Trimoxazole 3 tablets 12 hourly for 3-4 weeks

Prophylaxis
Eradicate from animal sources
Pasteurise milk before ingestion

CANDIDIASIS

Vaginal
Nystatin pessaries 1 twice a day for 14 days
    and Nystatin 500000 units orally 8 hourly for 14 days
    and Nystatin Cream to vulva and surrounding area 12
        hourly for 14 days.
  or Miconazole pessaries 100 mg daily for 14 days
    and Miconazole 2% cream daily for 14 days
  or Clotrimazol pessaries 100 mg nocte for 6 days
and treat consort

Oral
Nystatin pessaries to suck 8 hourly
  or Nystatin suspension 100000 u/ml 6 hourly to be held in
    the mouth and then swallowed
  or Miconazole gel 5-10 ml 6 hourly (palatable)
  or Amphotericin B lozenges to suck 8 hourly
Continue treatment until infection and symptoms controlled

CHICKEN POX

Prophylaxis
Herpes Zoster immunoglobulin given within 72 hours of exposure

Lesions
1% Gentian Violet
or Calamine

General
Sedate with Promethazine (HCL) 10 mg 8 hourly if necessary
Treat superinfection as appropriate with antibiotic

Debilitated or immunosuppressed patients
Cytarabine 3 mg/kg i.v. daily for 3 days

CHOLERA

Maintain fluid and electrolyte balance
and Tetracycline 10 mg/kg 6 hourly for 7 days
    or Co-Trimoxazole 3 tablets 12 hourly for 1 day
        then Co-Trimoxazole 2 tablets 12 hourly for 7 days

COLDS

No specific therapy
Only use antibiotics for secondary infections

DIPHTHERIA

Previously immunised
Toxoid

Not previously immunised
Anti-toxin according to following schedule:

	Mild/moderate disease seen early	Moderate/severe disease seen after 3 days
No history of allergy	15000 u i.m.	20000 u i.m.
No previous serum	15000 u i.v. ½-hour later	80000 u i.v. ½-1 hour later
Previous serum	0.2 ml of serum s/c	0.2 ml of serum s/c
	– no reaction	– no reaction
	– continue as above	– continue as above

If reaction
Prednisone 20 mg orally and Promethazine HCL 50 mg i.m.
Adrenaline 1:1000 available and drawn up
    then 0.2 ml of 1:1000 dilution of serum
If no reaction proceed as outlined *below:**

If reaction
Double Prednisone dose and repeat from beginning
0.2 ml of 1:1000 dilution of serum

Previous serum sickness	0.2 ml of 1:10 dilution of serum s/c – if no reaction in 30 minutes – proceed as above.	0.2 ml of 1:10 dilution of serum s/c – if no reaction in 30 minutes – proceed as above.

If reaction
Prednisone 20 mg orally and Promethazine HCL 50 mg i.m.
Adrenaline 1:1000 available and drawn up
   then 0.2 ml of 1:1000 dilution of serum
If no reaction proceed as outlined *below:**

If reaction
Double Prednisone dose and repeat from beginning
0.2 ml of 1:1000 dilution of serum

Asthma, eczema, hay fever, previous accelerated or anaphalactic reaction	Prednisone 20 mg orally and Promethazine 50 mg i.m. Adrenaline 1-1000 available and drawn up then 0.2 ml of 1-1000 dilution of serum – if no reaction ½ hr later 0.2 ml of 1-10 dilution of serum – if no reaction ½ hr later 0.2 ml of undiluted serum – if no reaction ½ hr later double dose and continue to double dose every ½ hr until total dose as outlined above given **If reaction** Double Prednisone dose and repeat from beginning

and Benzyl Penicillin 500000 units 6 hourly for 7 days
  or Erythromycin 500 mg 6 hourly for 7 days

When recovered ensure active immunity against TETANUS – patient unable to have further toxoid because of sensitivity

Laryngeal disease

Mild
Humidify air and treat as above

Moderate/severe
Dexamethasone 4 mg i.v.
    then Dexamethasone 0.5 mg orally 6 hourly
and Tracheostomy – best early rather than late

Contacts and carriers
Take cultures as appropriate
   then Erythromycin 500 mg 6 hourly for 7 days

ECHINOCOCCUS

Surgery
No specific drug therapy

ERYSIPELAS

Benzyl Penicillin 1 mega unit 6 hourly for 7 days
      Change to Phenoxymethyl Penicillin 500 mg 6 hourly when
        disease under control.
      Tablets taken ½ – 1 hour before meals.
or if allergic to Penicillin:
      Erythromycin 500 mg 6 hourly for 10 days

GAS GANGRENE

Surgical debridement – EARLY
and Penicillin 2 mega units 6 hourly i.m. or i.v. for 7 days
   or if allergic to Penicillin:
      Erythromycin 500 mg 6 hourly i.v. for 7 days
and Anti gas gangrene serum – initially mixed and then monovalent
   antitoxin when organism known.

     Prophylactic soon after wound
      25000 units i.v. or i.m. (healthy muscle)

     Therapeutic
      at least 75000 units i.v. repeated 4-6 hourly depending on
response and ? Hyperbaric oxygen

GONORRHOEA

Uncomplicated
either Probenecid 1 g orally stat
      then 30 minutes later: Benzyl Penicillin 2.4 mega units i.m.
   or Amoxycillin 3 g orally
If Penicillin allergy or after 'Penicillin failure' to cure
      Spectinomycin 2 g i.m.
        or Tetracycline 1.5 g orally stat
          then Tetracycline 0.5 g 6 hourly for 4 days
If pregnant and Penicillin allergy:
      Erythromycin 0.5 g i.v. 6 hourly for 3 days

Complicated
either Probenecid 1 g orally stat
      then Benzyl Penicillin 2.4 mega units i.m. stat
      then Amoxycillin 0.5 g 8 hourly for 10 days
      and Probenecid 0.5 g 8 hourly for 10 days

or Tetracycline 1.5 g orally stat
> then Tetracycline 0.5 g 6 hourly for 10 days
If pregnant and Penicillin allergy:
> Erythromycin 0.5 g i.v. 6 hourly for 3 days

Arthritis
either Benzyl Penicillin 10-20 mega units/day i.v. for 3 days
> then Amoxycillin 0.5 g 8 hourly for 5 days
or Tetracycline 1.5 g orally stat
> then Tetracycline 0.5 g 6 hourly for 7 days
if Pregnant and Penicillin allergy:
> Erythromycin 0.5 g i.v. 6 hourly for 3 days
IN ALL CASES: OBTAIN EXPERT HELP
> – CONTACTS SHOULD BE SOUGHT AND TREATED,
> – TEST FOR CURE ONE WEEK AFTER STOPPING THERAPY,
> – TEST FOR SYPHILIS

Neonatal

Prevention
Regular ante-natal checks in patients at high risk

Attack
Benzyl Penicillin 50000 units/kg/day i.v. x 2 days

Septicaemia
Benzyl Penicillin 50000 units/kg/day i.v. x 2 days
and Gentamicin 3.0 mg/kg i.m. 12 hourly for 2 days

Ophthalmia
Penicillin 50000 units/kg/day i.m. for 7 days
and saline irrigation to the eye
and Chloramphenicol eye drops, initially every 15 minutes until response and then less frequently

---

IMPETIGO

Remove crusts with Cetrimide 1%
then either Neomycin ointment
> or Chlortetracycline 3% ointment

If severe
Penicillin 1 mega unit 6 hourly for 7 days
If staphylococcal infection:
Flucloxacillin 500 mg 6 hourly taken ½-1 hr before food.

INFECTIOUS MONONUCLEOSIS

Symptomatic treatment only
AVOID Ampicillin and Amoxycillin

Respiratory obstruction
Hydrocortisone 100 mg i.v.
　　　then Prednisone 10 mg 6 hourly for 3-4 days

Jaundice
Avoid alcohol for six months

LEPTOSPIROSIS

Attack
Maintain water and electrolyte balance
and Benzyl Penicillin 500000 units i.m. or i.v. 4 hourly x 6
　　　then Benzyl Penicillin 500000 units i.m. 6 hourly for 6 days
HERXHEIMER REACTION COMMON WITH EARLY TREATMENT
　but usually no specific therapy required
Occasionally use Prednisone 60 mg just before initial dose of
Penicillin to prevent reaction
May need peritoneal dialysis to control anuria

Prevention
Avoid contact with infected animals
Use Protective clothing
Clean all wounds carefully

MALARIA

Prophylaxis
Start 1 week BEFORE ENTERING and continue for 8 WEEKS AFTER
LEAVING endemic area.

either Chloroquine 300 mg of base ⎫
　and Primaquine 45 mg ⎭ Once a week

or Amodiaquine 400 mg ⎫
　and Primaquine 45 mg ⎭ Weekly

or Pyrimethamine 12.5 mg ⎫
　and Dapsone 100 mg ⎭ Weekly

or Proquanil 100 mg daily
or Sulphadoxine 1 g ⎫ every 2 weeks—when Chloroquine
　and Pyrimethamine 50 mg ⎭ resistance anticipated

Uncomplicated attack
Quinine sulphate 650 mg of salt three times a day for 14 days
　or Chloroquine 600 mg of base
　　　then 300 mg 6 hours later
　　　then 300 mg daily for 2 days
　or Amodiaquine 600 mg of base
　　　then 400 mg daily for 2 days

Emergency treatment
Quinine hydrochloride 650 mg of salt in glucose solution injected
i.v. very slowly;
6 hours later repeat if necessary.
No more than 3 injections in 24 hours.
   or Quinine hydrochloride 2 g slowly as i.v. infusion over 24 hours
      Change to oral route as soon as possible.
   or Chloroquine hydrochloride 200 mg i.m.
         then 200 mg i.m. 6 hours later
      Change to oral route as soon as possible.
      DO NOT USE THIS THERAPY when 4 Aminoquinoline resistant
      P. falciparum known to exist in that area.

Drug resistant P. Falciparum
Quinine sulphate 650 mg of salt 8 hourly for 14 days
and if from South East Asia add:
Pyrimethamine 25 mg 12 hourly for 3 days
and Sulphadiazine 0.5 g 6 hourly for 5 days

Radical cure of Vivax, Ovale and Malariae
Primaquine diphosphate 15 mg of base daily for 14 days
(to eradicate Hepatic cycle).
BEWARE G.6.P.D. deficiency

MEASLES

No specific therapy

MUMPS

Control pain with either: Aspirin 300-600 mg 6 hourly
   or Paracetamol 0.5-1 g 6 hourly
and maintain fluid intake

Orchitis
Analgesia as above
May need Morphine 10–15 mg i.m. 6 hourly
and Occasionally Prednisone 60 mg per day
        then Prednisone 40 mg for 1 day
        then Prednisone 20 mg for 1 day
        then STOP
        This helps to relieve pain but not the infection

NON-SPECIFIC URETHRITIS

Initial attack
Exclude Gonorrhoea or Trichomoniasis
        then Tetracycline 250 mg 6 hourly for 2-3 weeks
Avoid alcohol and sexual intercourse during therapy

Recurrent attacks
Investigate for structural abnormalities
  If present, treat as appropriate
  If absent, treat as above
and treat regular consort
Get expert help.

PSITTACOSIS

Attack
Tetracycline 1 g 6 hourly for 2 days
then Tetracycline 0.5 g 6 hourly for 5 days

Prevention
Isolate infected birds

QUINSY

Benzyl Penicillin 1 mega unit 6 hourly for 7 days

RICKETTSIAL INFECTIONS including Q fever

Tetracycline 500 mg 6 hourly for 10 days

RUBELLA

No specific therapy
If local irritation:
  Calamine lotion
AVOID drugs, especially if pregnant

Pregnant
Check for antibodies
  if present – reassure
  if not present – check again in 10 days
  if still absent – not rubella
  if present – rubella confirmed
Consider termination depending on risks

> *Risks*
> 1st month 50-60% affected
> 4th month 4-5% affected

SALMONELLA

Diarrhoea
Replace fluids and electrolytes
and either Kaolin et Morph. 5 ml as necessary
  or Diphenoxylate with Atropine 1-2 tablets 8 hourly
  or Codeine Phosphate 15-30 mg every time bowels open
  or Loperamide 4 mg stat then 2 mg when bowels open to
  maximum of 16 mg/day.
NO ANTIBIOTICS UNLESS SYSTEMIC SPREAD OF INFECTION
Prevent spread of disease by attention to general hygiene

Systemic infection (Salmonella typhimurium etc.)
Chloramphenicol 500 mg 6 hourly for 7 days
  or Amoxycillin 500 mg 8 hourly for 7 days
  or Co-Trimoxazole 3 tablets 12 hourly for 7 days
Prevent spread of disease by attention to general hygiene

Typhoid fever (Salmonella typhi)

Attack
Maintain fluid and electrolyte balance and
Maintain calorie intake with milky drinks until
normal diet is resumed.
and Chloramphenicol 500 mg 4 hourly for 2-3 days
          then Chloramphenicol 500 mg 6 hourly for 12 days
  or Ampicillin 1 g 4 hourly for 2 weeks
  or Co-Trimoxazole 3 tablets 12 hourly for 2 weeks
Occasionally in severe toxaemias:
Prednisone 5 mg 6 hourly for 1 week

Carriers
Cholecystogram normal:
  Amoxycillin 500 mg 8 hourly for 3 months
Cholecystogram abnormal:
  Cholecystectomy and Amoxycillin 500 mg 8 hourly for
  3 months

Urinary carriers
Look for anatomical abnormalities and treat as appropriate.
and Amoxycillin 500 mg 8 hourly
Instruct patient in general hygiene
Prevent patient from handling food etc. to prevent spread of disease.

Para-typhoid fever
Treat as for typhoid fever.

SCARLET FEVER

Benzyl Penicillin 1 mega unit 6 hourly for 2 days
        then Phenoxymethyl Penicillin 500 mg 6 hourly for 8 days
           taken ½-1 hour before food.
If allergic to Penicillin:
        Erythromycin 500 mg 6 hourly for 10 days

SCHISTOSOMIASIS

Prevention
Reduce contamination at water supply
   with education and provision of sanitation
and separate clean water supply to reduce infection rate
and use molluscicides to remove secondary host

Cure
REFER TO SPECIALIST CENTRE
  S. Japonicum
Stibocaptate 3-5 mg/kg i.m. weekly x 10 (not more than 2.5 g total)
  or Niridazole 25 mg/kg/day orally for 7 days
  S. Haematobium
Stibocaptate 3-5 mg/kg i.m. weekly x 10
  or Niridazole 25 mg/kg/day orally for 7 days
  or Lucanthone 0.5-1 g 12 hourly for 3 days (total dose at least 70 mg/kg)
  or Hycanthone 2.5-3.0 mg/kg i.m. x 1 (maximum 200 mg)
  or Metriphonate 7 5 mg/kg i.m. at 2 weekly intervals x 3
  S. Mansoni
Stibocaptate 3-5 mg/kg i.m. weekly x 10 (not more than 2.5 g total)
  or Niridazole 25 mg/kg/day orally for 7 days
  or Lucanthone 0.5-1 g 12 hourly for 3 days (total dose at least 70 mg/kg)
  or Hycanthone 2.5-3.0 mg/kg i.m. x 1 (Maximum 200 mg)

SEPTICAEMIA

Organism known or suspected
Take adequate specimens then treat immediately with antibiotic according to sensitivity of previous isolates.

Organism not known

After abdominal or thoracic surgery
Gentamicin – dose according to Mawer Nomogram (see p. 323)
and Cloxacillin 0.5-1 g i.m. or i.v. 6 hourly
and Metronidazole 400 mg 8 hourly orally or rectally

Leukaemic or immunosuppressed patient
Gentamicin – dose according to Mawer Nomogram (see p. 323)
and Cloxacillin 0.5-1 g i.m. or i.v. 6 hourly

Infected intravenous catheters
Flucloxacillin 250-500 mg orally 6 hourly ½ an hour before food
   or Cephalothin 500 mg i.v. 6 hourly

Ascending cholangitis
Ampicillin 500 mg i.m. 6 hourly
   or Amoxycillin 250-500 mg 8 hourly
   or Co-Trimoxazole 2-6 tablets 12 hourly

   If jaundice
add Gentamicin – dose according to Mawer Nomogram (see p. 323)

SHIGELLA

Maintain fluid and electrolyte intake
No antibiotic indicated

SHINGLES

Pain
Either Aspirin 300-600 mg 6-8 hourly
   or Paracetamol 0.5-1 g 6-8 hourly
Occasionally:
Chlorpromazine 25-100 mg 6-8 hourly
and either
   Pethidine 25-50 mg 6-8 hourly
   or Morphine 10-15 mg 6-8 hourly
   or Amantadine 100 mg 12 hourly for 14-28 days

Rash
Idoxuridine 40% in Dimethylsulphoxide applied continuously for 3-4
days.
   or Idoxuridine 5% in Dimethylsulphoxide 6-8 hourly to lesions
   for 1 week.
THE EARLIER THE TREATMENT THE MORE EFFECTIVE

Eye
Get expert help
1-2% Atropine eye drops
and Antibiotic/Steroid eye ointment
and Idoxuridine eye drops 0.1%, 1 drop hourly – stop when lesions
healed
   or Idoxuridine eye ointment 0.5% (less well absorbed than drops).

Post herpetic pain
Chlorprothixene 50 mg 6 hourly for 2 weeks
  or Amitriptyline 10-50 mg 8 hourly
and/or Amantadine 100 mg 12 hourly for 14-28 days
Occasionally:
local infiltration with local anaesthetics
  or electrical stimulation may help.

Encephalitis
Get Expert Help
Cytarabine 2-4 mg/kg i.v. daily for 5 days

SMALLPOX

Prophylaxis

General
Vaccination

Specific
Contacts and during epidemic
Methisazone 3 g orally (after food)
      then Methisazone 3 g 8-12 hours later (after food)

Established disease
General nursing care
Isolation

Vaccinia
General nursing care
and Dexamethasone; either 4-10 mg i.v. daily
  or 4-10 mg i.m. 6 hourly to reduce cerebral oedema
and Methisazone 200 mg/kg stat
      then Methisazone 50 mg/kg 6 hourly for 48 hours
Repeat after 7 days if necessary

SYPHILIS
Primary and Secondary
Procaine Penicillin 600 0000 units daily for 8 days
  or PAM (Procaine Penicillin Aluminium Monosterate)
      2-4 mega units stat
      1-2 mega units – 3 days later.
      1-2 mega units – 3 days later
  or Benzathine Penicillin 2.4 mega units stat
If Penicillin allergy:
Erythromycin 1 g 6 hourly for 10 days
  or Tetracycline 1 g 6 hourly for 10 days

Tertiary
Either Procaine Penicillin 1 mega units daily i.m. for 21 days
   or Benzathine Penicillin 3 mega units weekly i.m. x 3
If Penicillin allergy:
Tetracycline 1 g 6 hourly for 20 days

Congenital syphilis

CSF normal
Benzathine Penicillin 500000 units/kg i.m. x 1

CSF abnormal
Benzyl Penicillin 20000 units/kg 12 hourly i.m. or i.v. for 10 days
   or Procaine Penicillin 50000 units/kg i.m. for 10 days
IN ALL CASES: OBTAIN EXPERT HELP
                CONTACTS SHOULD BE SOUGHT AND TREATED
                TESTS OF CURE SHOULD BE CARRIED OUT AFTER
                COMPLETING THERAPY

TOXOPLASMA

Congenital
Either Spiramycin 500 mg orally 6 hourly for 2-6 weeks ⎤ May
   or Pyrimethamine 25 mg orally daily for 2-6weeks ⎬ induce
and Sulphadimidine 1 g orally 6 hourly for 2-6 weeks ⎦ folate
                                                      deficiency

With eye involvement
Anti-Protozoal treatment as given above
and Prednisone 60 mg daily
        then reduce after 4 weeks
Continue anti-protozoal treatment for 2 weeks after stopping
prednisone

Acquired disease
Either Spiramycin 500 mg orally 6 hourly for 2-6 weeks ⎤ May
   or Pyrimethamine 25 mg orally daily for 2-6 weeks ⎬ induce
and Sulphadimidine 1 g orally 6 hourly for 2-6 weeks ⎦ folate
                                                      deficiency

---

TRACHOMA

Sulphatriad 3 g – stat.
        then Sulphatriad 1 g 4 hourly for 10 days
    or Tetracycline 250 mg 6 hourly for 3-6 weeks.
and Sulphacetamide eye ointment 10% 6-8 hourly
    or Tetracycline eye ointment 1% 6-8 hourly

TRICHOMONIASIS

1st trimester of pregnancy
Either antiseptics, e.g.
Acetarsol pessaries 2 nocte for 2-3 weeks
   or Hydrargaphen pessaries 2 nocte for 2-3 weeks
or specific therapy with:
Clotrimazole pessaries 2 nocte for 3 nights

At any other time
Metronidazole 200 mg 8 hourly by mouth for 14 days
   or Metronidazole 2g stat
or Nifuratel 200 mg 8 hourly for 7 days
} for women

and Metronidazole 200 mg 8 hourly orally for 7 days
   or Metronizadole 2g stat
   or Nifuratel 200 mg 8 hourly for 7 days
} for men
AVOID intercourse and alcohol during treatment
NB: Disulfiram reaction

WHOOPING COUGH

During outbreak
Erythromycin 10-30 mg/kg 8 hourly
given when early symptoms in child might abort attack.

Established attack
No specific therapy
Only use antibiotics for secondary infection
NB: COUGH SUPPRESSION NOT HELPFUL

FURTHER READING

Garrod, L.P., Lambert, H.P., & O'Grady, F. (1973) *Antibiotics Chemotherapy* Edinburgh: Churchill Livingstone.
Hunter, Swartzwelder & Clyde (1976) *Tropical Medicine* London: W.B. Saunders
Noone, P. (1977) *A Clinician's Guide to Antibiotic Therapy* London: Blackwell Scientific Publications
Smith, H. (1977) *Antibiotics in Clinical Practice* Tunbridge Wells: Pitman Medical

Respiratory

ABSCESS

Obtain sputum specimen if possible

Start therapy with
Gentamicin initially according to the Mawer Nomogram (p. 323) and then according to serum levels
and Flucloxacillin 250-500 mg 6 hourly
and Postural drainage
and Bronchoscopy – to obtain specimen
                    – to exclude neoplasia
                    – to exclude foreign body

Review antibiotics when laboratory results available
a. patient improving: no change
b. patient not better: change antibiotics to one suggested by the laboratory sensitivities.
Surgery may occasionally be necessary.

ACUTE LARYNGITIS

Steam inhalation
Linctus Codeine 5 ml in warm water – to suppress cough.

ASTHMA

Prophylaxis against attacks
Avoid known precipitating factors.
If exercise induced use Salbutamol or Terbutaline inhaler before exertion.
Treat infections early with appropriate antibiotics.
and: Salbutamol tablets 2-4 mg 6-8 hourly
    or Salbutamol inhaler 200-400 μg 4-6 hourly
    or Terbutaline 2.5-5.0 mg 6-8 hourly
    or Terbutaline inhaler 250-500 μg 6-8 hourly
and Disodium Chromoglycate 1-2 spincaps 8 hourly (no use during an acute attack).
and/or Beclomethasone dipropionate inhalation 50-100 μg 8 hourly
and/or Prednisone tablets in minimal dosage
and Regular physiotherapy – breathing exercises
Look for allergic factors

Acute attack

Mild
Reassurance
and Salbutamol inhaler 200-400 μg
   or Terbutaline inhaler 250-500 μg
and increase oral therapy with Salbutamol or Terbutaline

Severe
Reassurance
and Salbutamol inhaler 200-400 μg
   or Terbutaline inhaler 250-500 μg
If ineffective
either Salbutamol 5 mg $\Big\}$ Given via a nebulizer
   or Terbutaline 5 mg
and/or Salbutamol 0.5 mg subcutaneously or i.m. repeated every 4
hours.
   or Salbutamol 0.25 mg slowly i.v. repeated if necessary
and/or Adrenaline 1 : 1000/0.2-0.5 ml subcutaneously
and/or Aminophylline 250 mg slowly i.v. repeated after ½ an hour
   if necessary to a total of 1 g. (unless given slowly may cause
   tachycardia and hypotension).
MAY BE NECESSARY TO GIVE I.V. BRONCHODILATORS BEFORE
INHALED DRUGS CAN WORK.
and Prednisone 60 mg daily
When attack controlled slowly reduce Prednisone dosage e.g.
   Prednisone 40 mg daily for 2 days
        then Prednisone 30 mg daily for 2 days
        then Prednisone 20 mg daily for 2 days
        then Prednisone 10 mg daily for 2 days
        then Prednisone 5 mg daily for 2 days
        then Prednisone 2.5 mg daily for 2 days
        then STOP
ONLY REDUCE CORTICOSTEROIDS DOSE IF NO RELAPSE.

Status asthmaticus (Severe attack which has lasted for several
hours or has not responded to the treatment as outlined above).
Corticosteroid mandatory
Initially Hydrocortisone 4 mg/kg i.v. followed after 3 hours by
       3 mg/kg i.v. 3 hourly
       or 3 mg/kg infusion over 6 hours
and Prednisone 100 mg/day continued until attack controlled
       then Reduce dose slowly using a similar regime to that
         described above.
and either Salbutamol 5 mg $\Big\}$ given via nebulizer
or Terbutaline 5 mg
and/or Salbutamol 0.5 mg subcutaneously or i.m. repeated every 4
hours.
   or Salbutamol 0.25 mg slowly i.v. repeated as necessary

and/or Aminophylline 250 mg slowly i.v. followed after ½ an hour
by infusion of 500 mg 8 hourly
and 0.9% Sodium Chloride i.v. to rehydrate
(Aminophylline 250 mg or Salbutamol 5 mg may be added to the
infusion fluid).
and humidified 35% Oxygen unless hypercapnic when Oxygen
concentration should be reduced to 28% or 24%
and Amoxycillin 250 mg 8 hourly
   or Co-Trimoxazole 2 tablets 8-12 hourly.
If patient is exhausted or the pCO_2 rises intermittent positive
pressure respiration may be necessary – depending on the patient's
original state.
THE EFFECTIVENESS OF THERAPY IS MONITORED WHENEVER
PRACTICAL BY THE MEASUREMENT OF PEAK FLOW OR FEV[1].

BRONCHIECTASIS

Acute exacerbation
Intensive physiotherapy to increase bronchial drainage
Antibiotics as appropriate
Initially Amoxycillin 250-500 mg 8 hourly
   or Co-Trimoxazole 2-3 tablets 12 hourly
When bacterial culture results are available:
   a. patient improving: no change
   b. patient not better: change antibiotic to one suggested by
      laboratory sensitivities.

Prevention of attacks
Daily postural drainage – preferably twice daily for a set time as
measured on a clock.
Surgical treatment of infection of nasal sinuses if indicated.
Early treatment of respiratory infections
with initially Amoxycillin 250-500 mg 8 hourly
   or Co-Trimoxazole 2-3 tablets 12 hourly
When bacterial culture results are available:
change antibiotic if necessary as appropriate.
   a. patient better: no change
   b. patient not better: change to antibiotic as suggested by the
      laboratory sensitivities.
Immunisation against influenza.
If due to fibrocystic disease with pancreatic insufficiency then
Pancreatin and supplements of Vitamins A and D should also be
given.
Occasionally surgery which may be curative if the disease is
localised.

BRONCHITIS

Acute
Steam inhalation

Mucoid sputum
No antibiotics, unless sensitive organisms isolated

Muco purulent sputum
Amoxycillin 250 mg 8 hourly
   or Co-Trimoxazole 2-3 tablets 8-12 hourly
   or Tetracycline 250-500 mg 6 hourly
(NB: Pneumococci resistant to tetracycline are becoming
increasingly common).
When bacteriology result available:
   a. patient improving: no change
   b. patient not better: change to antibiotic as suggested by
      laboratory sensitivities.

Chronic
Stop smoking
Bronchodilators, if evidence of REVERSIBLE airways obstruction
Physiotherapy to aid bronchial drainage
Linctus Codeine 5 ml in hot water – for cough

Acute exacerbation
Physiotherapy to aid bronchial drainage
and steam inhalation to help expectoration
and Amoxycillin 250 mg 8 hourly
                  or Co-Trimoxazole 2-3 tablets 8-12 hourly
   or Tetracycline 250-500 mg 6 hourly
(NB: Pneumococci resistant to tetracycline are becoming
increasingly common).
When bacteriological results are available:
   a. patient improving: no change
   b. patient not better: change to antibiotic as suggested by the
      laboratory sensitivities.

CARCINOMA OF THE LUNG

Localised with good respiratory function
a. Squamous Cell – surgery
b. Oat Cell – radiotherapy/surgery
c. Bronchiolar Cell – surgery
d. Adenocarcinoma – surgery

Not localised and/or poor respiratory function

Asymptomatic
Probably none
Possibly: either chemotherapy
with Cyclophosphamide 0.5-1 g daily to a total of 7g , given into fast
running i.v. infusion of Sodium Chloride 0.9%

Monitor white count daily
Stop if count falls below 2000
? continue with oral therapy at 50-200 mg daily
　　or Mustine 0.4 mg/kg body weight given into a fast
　　running i.v. infusion of Sodium Chloride 0.9%
　　or Combination chemotherapy (see p. 138)
　　Sedation is usually needed because of nausea.
　　　　or Radiotherapy

Symptomatic
PAIN-local radiotherapy
RECURRENT PAIN: analgesia as necessary including Dipipanone,
Methadone, Diamophine, with or without an antiemetic.
　　or Brompton Cocktail (see chapter on Care of the Dying)
Occasionally nerve blockade or destruction may be useful.
NB: Analgesia should be given REGULARLY and in sufficient dosage
to STOP PAIN. Additional analgesia on demand may be useful, but
should not be used alone.

BREATHLESSNESS
1. Pleural effusion
Drain and instil Mepacrine 100-200 mg on 3 consecutive days
　　or Thiotepa 60 mg on 3 consecutive days
　　or Mustine 20 mg in 20 ml 0.9% Sodium chloride on 3
consecutive days.
2. Wheeze
Salbutamol 2-4 mg 8 hourly
　　or Terbutaline 5 mg 8 hourly
If no effect on symptoms or peak flow STOP
3. Other causes
No effective treatment

SUPERIOR VENA CAVA OR TRACHEAL OBSTRUCTION
Chemotherapy as outlined above
and Prednisone 60 mg daily
followed immediately by radiotherapy.
Prednisone MAY prevent further obstruction caused by swelling due
to the treatment with radiotherapy.
NB: Other symptoms should be treated on conventional lines, e.g.
DEPRESSION – Amitriptyline
ANXIETY – Diazepam or Chlorpromazine
CEREBRAL SECONDARIES – Dexamethasone or Anticonvulsants.

COUGH

Find cause and treat as appropriate
Occasionally: Linctus Codeine 5 ml in hot water, as symptomatic
therapy.

EMPHYSEMA

Stop smoking
No specific treatment apart from physiotherapy
Treat associated bronchitis as outlined on page 19.

EMPYEMA

Aspirate fluid and culture
Treat with appropriate antibiotic
Whilst waiting for laboratory results aspirate as much pus as
possible and instil Penicillin 600 mg in 10 ml of sterile water.
Repeat aspiration and instillation every other day until improved
If the pus becomes inspissated, instil Streptokinase 200 000 units.
Leave for several hours, then re-aspirate.
Occasionally rib-resection and formal surgical drainage will be
necessary.
Look for the underlying cause and treat as appropriate.

EXTRINSIC ALLERGIC ALVEOLITIS

Exclude possible causes, e.g. Farmers Lung
                                Bird Fanciers Lung
                                Mushroom growers Lung
If one of these is found, remove from exposure to antigen.
Otherwise Prednisone 40 mg initially with reducing dosage may
help.
Occasionally Azathioprine 50 mg daily may allow a lower dose of
Prednisone to be used with a reduction in the untoward side
effects.

FIBROSING ALVEOLITIS

Exclude possible causes, e.g. Sulphafurazole or Busulphan
If one of these is found, remove from exposure to antigen.
Otherwise Prednisone 40 mg initially with reducing dosage may
help.
Occasionally Azathioprine 50 mg daily may allow a lower dose of
Prednisone to be used with a reduction in the untoward side
effects.

HAEMOPTYSIS

Find cause and treat as appropriate.

MEDIASTINAL MASSES

Find cause and treat as appropriate.

MUCO-VISCIDOSIS

Treat bronchiectasis with postural drainage, 10 minutes by the clock daily and antibiotics for infections.
Treat associated pancreatic dysfunction with a low fat diet
   and Pancreatin 6 g daily
   and Vitamins A and D supplements.

PLEURAL EFFUSION

Unless diagnosis obvious, aspirate and do pleural biopsy.
NB: TOO RAPID REMOVAL OF FLUID CAUSES CHEST DISCOMFORT, COUGH AND PULMONARY OEDEMA. ASPIRATION SHOULD BE STOPPED IF ANY OF THESE OCCUR.

Transudate

Congestive cardiac failure
Digoxin and diuretics (see p. 34)

Hepatic disease
Diuretics (see pp. 39 and 44)
NB: Spironolactone is often particularly useful

Renal disease
Diuretics (see pp. 39 and 121)

Meig's syndrome
Remove ovarian tumour

Exudate

Pneumonia
Antibiotics as appropriate (see p. 25)
Repeated aspiration may be needed and occasionally antibiotic instillation will be necessary. See Empyema on p. 22

Tuberculosis
Triple therapy for 6 weeks, then maintenance therapy, (see p. 29)

Carcinoma
Drain and instil Thiotepa 60 mg on 3 consecutive days
   or Mustine 20 mg in 20 ml of 0.9% sodium chloride
        on 3 consecutive days
   or Mepacrine 100-200 mg on 3 consecutive days
   or Radio Gold
   or Yttrium
Occasionally Prednisone will slow the recurrence rate.

Haemothorax
Aspirate to dryness
Find cause and treat as appropriate

B

Chylous effusion
Do not aspirate repeatedly unless causing significant symptoms
(Because of loss of calories as fat)
Find cause and treat as appropriate (e.g. traumatic rupture of the
thoracic duct or malignant obstruction).

PLEURAL TUMOURS

Relieve pain with Pethidine 25-50 mg 4-6 hourly
   or Morphine 5-15 mg 4-6 hourly
   or Diamorphine 2.5-5.0 mg 4-6 hourly
Aspirate any effusion as often as necessary
Possibly Chemotherapy

Mesothelioma
Once diagnosis established the less interference the better.
Relieve pain but aspirate only if significant symptoms.

PLEURISY

Find cause and treat as appropriate
Stop pain with: Pethidine 25-50 mg 4-6 hourly
   or Morphine 5-15 mg 4-6 hourly
   or Diamorphine 2.5-5.0 mg 4-6 hourly
Some patients obtain pain relief from chest strapping

PNEUMOCONIOSIS

Prophylaxis
Keep exposure to minimum
NB some dusts are harmless: barium – iron – tin
    some are fairly harmless: coal dust
      but serious if complicated: pulmonary massive fibrosis
    some are always harmful: silica – asbestos

Established
No specific treatment
Remove from environment which induced lung damage
NB: this depends on:
1. material – see above
2. age of patient, e.g. simple coal miners disease
   and young patient: take out of mine.
   Age 55 or more: leave until retires.

PNEUMONIA

In all patients
Stop pain with adequate analgesia
Encourage coughing with physiotherapy

24% Oxygen unless normocapnic
If normocapnic or no rise in pCO_2 increase Oxygen concentration.
Obtain sputum specimen if possible and start antibiotic according to
the following schedule.
1. *In a previously fit adult*
   a. Lobar Pneumonia
      Benzyl Penicillin 1-2 mega units 6 hourly
      or Cephaloridine 500 mg 6 hourly
   b. Associated with influenza
      Amoxycillin 250-500 mg 8 hourly
         and Flucloxacillin 250-500 mg 6 hourly
      or Co-Trimoxazole 2-3 tablets 12 hourly
   c. Post operatively + others
      Amoxycillin 250-500 mg 8 hourly
      or Co-Trimoxazole 2-3 tablets 12 hourly
2. *In immunologically depressed or debilitated patients whilst
   on antibiotic therapy or whilst on a ventilator*
Gentamicin initially according to the Mawer Nomogram (p. 323)
   and then monitored by serum levels.
and Flucloxacillin 250-500 mg 6 hourly.
IN ALL CASES THERAPY SHOULD BE REVIEWED WHEN
BACTERIAL RESULTS ARE AVAILABLE.

If patient not improving consider change of antibiotic, e.g.
1. if due to mycoplasma pneumoniae
   Tetracycline 500 mg 6 hourly
2. if due to Coxiella burnetti (Q fever)
   Tetracycline 500 mg 6 hourly
3. if due to Chlamydia psittaci (Psittacosis)
   Tetracycline 500 mg 6 hourly
4. if due to Klebsiella pneumoniae
   Gentamicin according to the Mawer Nomogram (p. 323) and then
   following serum levels
   and Flucloxacillin 250-500 mg 6 hourly
NB: USE LABORATORY SENSITIVITIES AS A GUIDE

PNEUMOTHORAX

Tension
Insert needle immediately, when pressure fallen insert intercostal
drain and treat as described below.

Non-tension

Lung one third collapsed or less
Observe with no limitation on activities
Check progress with repeat X-rays

More than one third collapsed
Insert intercostal tube and connect to underwater drainage to allow
air to escape.
X-ray daily.

When fluid no longer 'swings' on respiration
Check if lung expanded with X-ray

   If fully expanded
   Wait 24 hours then remove tube.

   If not expanded
   Unblock tube or replace

If lung does not expand at all or only expands very slowly
Add a suction pump to the underwater seal and continue to
aspirate until fully expanded and then continue as outlined above.

Recurrent
either instil either Mepacrine 100-200 mg on 3 consecutive days.
   or Thiotepa 60 mg on 3 consecutive days
   or Lung decortication

PULMONARY COLLAPSE

Prophylactic
Pre-operative physiotherapy
Stop smoking
and Avoid anaesthetics when patient has upper respiratory infection.

When established
Physiotherapy to induce coughing and to dislodge mucous plugs
and/or bronchoscopy to aspirate mucous plugs and exclude growth
   or foreign bodies.

PULMONARY EMBOLUS

Prophylactic
Heparin 5000 units 12 hourly sub-cutaneously
or Regular calf compression during period of risk, e.g. during operation.

Large
Oxygen in high concentration

Critically ill
Hydrocortisone 100 mg i.v. to prevent reactions
        then Streptokinase 600000 units over ½ an hour, then
           100000 units an hour for 72 hours.
Liaise with haematologists so that therapy can be monitored.

Less Critically ill
Heparin 10000 units 6 hourly i.v.

In either case after 48 hours start anticoagulation with
Warfarin 30 mg initially
then 6 mg on the 2nd day
then check prothrombin time and adjust dose as necessary.
Continue Warfarin for 3-6 months.

Small
Heparin 10000 6 hourly i.v. for 48 hours
and Warfarin as above, continued for 3-6 months

Recurrent
Warfarin as above
or Inferior vena cava plication (rarely used in the U.K.)

PULMONARY OEDEMA

Reassurance
and Diamorphine slowly i.v., the dose (2.5-5.0 mg) being titrated
against the patient.
or Morphine slowly i.v., the dose (5-15 mg) being titrated against
the patient
(Both of these reduce vaso-constriction).
and Frusemide 40 mg i.v.
or Bumetanide 1 mg i.v.
and Aminophylline 250 mg i.v. repeated ½ an hour later if
necessary
(Reduces vaso-constriction, increases myocardial contractility and
increases diuresis).
and if not on Digoxin, Digitalise with Digoxin 0.5 mg 6 hourly x 2
then 0.25 mg 6 hourly x 4
then 0.25 mg 12 hourly as maintenance.
Adjust dose according to size, age and renal function.
and 50% Oxygen – by mask to increase oxygen to the tissues.
NB: CHECK EFFECT ON BLOOD GASES
Occasionally venous tourniquets or venesection may be needed to
rapidly reduce blood volume.
Very rarely intermittent positive pressure ventilation may be
required.

RESPIRATORY FAILURE

Hypoxaemia normocapnia
Find cause and treat
Use highest concentration of inspired Oxygen, which does not
cause a rise in pCO_2

Hypoxaemic hypercapnia

24% oxygen continuously. The concentration may be increased if the pCO_2 does not rise.
Physiotherapy to remove bronchial secretion
and Amoxycillin 250 mg 8 hourly
   or Co-Trimoxazole two tablets 12 hourly
When bacterial culture results available:
a.   patient improving: no change
b.   patient not better: change to antibiotic as suggested by the laboratory sensitivities.
and rarely (Respiratory Stimulants) Nikethamide 0.5-2 g i.v.
   or Doxapram 0.5-1.0 mg/kg i.v., repeated in 5 minutes to a total of 2 mg/kg
   or as infusion at 5 mg/minute reducing to 1-3 mg/minute with a maximum total dosage of 4 mg/kg.
Positive pressure ventilation: only if the preceding respiratory state was reasonable.
NB: NO SEDATIVES SHOULD BE GIVEN AS ALL ARE RESPIRATORY DEPRESSANTS

SARCOIDOSIS

Erythema nodosum with hilar lymphadenopathy

Initially
Only symptomatic treatment is needed, e.g.:
Aspirin 300-600 mg 8 hourly
   or Phenylbutazone 100-200 mg 8 hourly
   or Indomethacin 25-50 mg 8 hourly

No sign of resolution after 1 year
Rarely Prednisone 20 mg 8 hourly reducing the dose once resolution has started.

Involvement of other organs e.g. Uveitis, Myocarditis, Lung Involvement (progressive deterioration in lung function tests).
Prednisone 20 mg 8 hourly
reducing to smallest dose able to keep disease inactive

Hypercalcaemia: Needs urgent treatment (see p. 98)
Prednisone 20 mg 8 hourly (the serum calcium falls on Prednisone and this distinguishes the hypercalcaemia of sarcoidosis from other causes of hypercalcaemia).
If needs urgent reduction:
0.9% Sodium Chloride infusion
and Frusemide 80 mg i.v.
   or Bumetanide 2 mg i.v.
and Prednisone as outlined above.

TUBERCULOSIS

The treatment of tuberculosis has changed rapidly over the last few
years, both in duration and form. It is not necessary to admit all
patients to hospital.

Initial therapy
Collect sputum specimen (6 weeks for culture result)
then start treatment with three drugs:

Isoniazid 300 mg
and Rifampicin 450 mg (less than 50 kg)
    or 600 mg (more than 50 kg)
and Streptomycin 1 g i.m.
    (0.75 g if older than 40)
  or Ethambutol 15 mg/kg

Taken as a single dose of
all drugs ½ an hour before
breakfast.

Maintenance therapy
After 2 months of initial therapy check laboratory sensitivities and
continue with either:

Isoniazid 300 mg
  and Rifampicin 450 or 600 mg
or Isoniazid 300 mg
  and Ethambutol 15 mg/kg

Taken as a single dose in
combination tablets ½ an
hour before breakfast.
For a total of 9 months.

or A combination of drugs as indicated by the sensitivities, when
  the therapy may be needed for 18 months.
NB: 1. At least 2 drugs should be used all the time.
    2. Regular urine testing helps to assess patient compliance.
    3. Once treatment is established the patient does not need to
      be isolated.

Contacts
Contacts: should have a Heaf test performed and those with
POSITIVE results should have a chest X-ray and full investigation.
Those with a negative Heaf and recent contact, should have a
repeat test in six weeks. If in doubt treat with:

Isoniazid 300 mg
  and Rifampicin 450 or 600 mg
or Isoniazid 300 mg
  and Ethambutol 15 mg/kg

Taken as combination
½ an hour before breakfast
for 9 months.

FURTHER READING

Avery G. (1976) *Drug Treatment* Edinburgh: Churchill Livingstone
Crofton J. & Douglas A. (1975) *Respiratory Disease* London:
  Blackwell Scientific Publications.
Medical Education (International) Ltd. (1975) *Medicine* Volumes 22-
  23

Cardiovascular

ANGINA PECTORIS

General
Reduce to ideal body weight
Stop smoking
Remain as active as possible

For each attack
Trinitrin 0.5 mg sublingually
a. prophylactically to allow necessary activity which is known to induce pain.
b. to reduce duration of pain in conjunction with rest.
NB: There is no limit to the number of tablets which can be used or the frequency of their use.
Discarding the tablet as soon as the pain has gone reduces the headache.
Chewing the tablets induces a quicker effect.
Long acting Trinitrins are of doubtful use.

To prevent attacks
Beta blocking drugs

either non-selective:
Propranolol 40-160 mg 8 hourly

or selective:
Metoprolol 50-150 mg 12 hourly
(causes less bronchoconstriction)
Bronchoconstriction if induced can be reversed by either
Terbutaline or
Salbutamol
(see asthma on page 17)

NB: BOTH MAY INDUCE LEFT VENTRICULAR FAILURE
USE WITH CARE IN ASTHMA AND HEART FAILURE

ARRHYTHMIAS

Multiple ectopic beats

Supraventricular: ignore

Ventricular: ignore, unless large numbers or symptoms
then Procainamide 250-500 mg 6 hourly

or Mexiletine 200-250 mg 8-12 hourly
or Phenytoin 50-150 mg 12 hourly
or Disopyramide 100-200 mg 6 hourly

After myocardial infarction
Supraventricular: ignore
Ventricular: ignore, unless more than 6/minute or multifocal
Lignocaine 100 mg i.v. repeated as a bolus as necessary. When
controlled, infuse Lignocaine 1-3 mg/minute to abolish
ectopics.
> or Lignocaine 100 mg i.v. and 100 mg i.m. when infusion
> impractical, e.g. when transferring to hospital.
> or Procainamide 250-500 mg slowly i.v. under ECG
> control. Then a slow infusion to control.
> *NB:* MAY PRODUCE PROFOUND HYPOTENSION
> or Procainamide 250-500 mg 6 hourly by mouth.
> or Propranolol 1 mg/minute i.v. repeated if necessary
> every 2 minutes, to a total of 10 mg.
> or Disopyramide 2 mg/kg/5 minutes i.v. to a maximum of
> 150 mg.

Associated with sinus bradycardia
Atropine 0.6 mg i.v. repeated after 5 minutes to a total
of 2.4 mg.

Tachycardia

Sinus
Look for cause, e.g. bleeding, anxiety, incipient LVF and treat as
appropriate.

Supraventricular
Vagal stimulation: carotid sinus pressure
                 valsalva manoeuvre
                 eye ball pressure

Not on digoxin: Digitalise with:
Digoxin 0.5 mg 6 hourly x 2
     then 0.25 mg 6 hourly x 4
     then 0.25 mg 12 hourly for maintenance
(Adjust maintenance dose according to size and age).
> or Propranolol 40 mg 8 hourly increasing to 80 mg 8 hourly if
> necessary.
> or Phenytoin 50 mg 12 hourly increasing to 100 mg 8 hourly
On digoxin: STOP. Check serum potassium level and supplement
as necessary.
    and/or Propranolol 40-80 mg 8 hourly
       or Phenytoin 50-100 mg 8 hourly
With hypotension: Propranolol 1-10 mg i.v. slowly

or Phenytoin 250-500 mg i.v. slowly

If converts, continue with oral dosage as outlined above.
If fails to convert, DC shock as described on p. 35.

Atrial fibrillation
Digitalise with Digoxin 0.5 mg 6 hourly x 2
       then 0.25 mg 6 hourly x 4
       then 0.25 mg 12 hourly as maintenance.

Atrial flutter
Vagal stimulation: carotid sinus pressure
                   Valsalva manoeuvre
                   eyeball pressure
Digitalise with Digoxin 0.5 mg 6 hourly x 2
       then 0.25 mg 6 hourly x 4
       then 0.25 mg 12 hourly as maintenance.
  or Propranolol 40 mg 8 hourly
D.C. shock (see page 35) if causing haemodynamic changes, and
of recent onset.

Wolff-Parkinson-White syndrome

Regular ventricular rhythm
Vagal stimulation: carotid sinus pressure
                   Valsalva manoeuvre
                   eyeball pressure
Digitalise with Digoxin 0.5 mg 6 hourly x 2
       then 0.25 mg 6 hourly x 4
       then 0.25 mg 12 hourly as maintenance.
  or Propranolol 1-10 mg slowly i.v.   ⎫
  or Verapamil 5-10 mg slowly i.v. – under ECG control⎰ NOT BOTH

Irregular ventricular response
Vagal stimulation and digitalis are CONTRA-INDICATED In this
situation.
Propranolol 1-10 mg slowly i.v.   ⎫
  or Verapamil 5–10 mg slowly i.v. – under ECG control⎰ NOT BOTH
  or Procainamide 250 mg slowly i.v. – under ECG control
Further attacks may be prevented by the oral administration of
these drugs.
NB: PATIENTS WHO HAVE HAD BOTH VERAPAMIL AND BETA
BLOCKERS MAY DEVELOP ASYSTOLE.

Ventricular tachycardia
  Rate over 100 per minute:
    Lignocaine 100 mg i.v., repeated as a bolus as necessary, to a
    maximum of 300 mg. When controlled infuse Lignocaine 1-3
    mg/minute to maintain sinus rhythm.
      or Procainamide 250-500 mg slowly i.v. – under ECG control
      or Phenytoin 50-250 mg slowly i.v. – under ECG control
      or Disopyramide 2 mg/kg/5 minutes to a maximum of 150 mg
      or D.C. shock as described on p. 35.

Continue treatment for 36 hours and then reduce dose to see if tachycardia still persists.
If tachycardia still present – Oral Procainamide 250-500 mg 6 hourly
Rate under 100 per minute: Ignore.

Ventricular fibrillation
External cardiac massage
Ventilation
D.C. shock as soon as possible – start at maximum e.g. 400 watt second
If initial shocks not effective 100 ml of 8.4% Sodium Bicarbonate (100 mmol) i.v. to correct acidaemia.
Then shock again
If fails: Practolol 5-20 mg i.v.
   or Lignocaine 100 mg i.v. followed by further D.C. shocks may help.
If fails: then
Isoprenaline 1-2 mg
   or Adrenaline 1 ml of 1:1000 into heart via 4th left intercostal space one inch from the sternum to coarsen the fibrillation. when a further shock may succeed.

Bradycardia

Sinus
Look for cause, e.g. myxoedema, raised intercranial pressure and treat as necessary.
If in acute situation and is associated with multiple ectopic beats:
Atropine 0.6 mg i.v. repeated in 5 minutes to a total of 2.4 mg

Heart block

   First degree: Ignore

   Second degree: Wenchebach – ignore
   2:1 etc. – Atropine 0.6 mg i.v. repeated after 5 minutes up to a total of 2.4 mg
         then – if fails: Pacemaker
   Mobitz 2 block – Pacemaker
   Complete heart block:
      After myocardial infarction – temporary pacemaker (see p. 39)
      Others, if stable and no symptoms – no treatment
      If stable, with rare or doubtful symptoms and elderly –
      Sustained action Isoprenaline (Saventrine) 30-60 mg 8 hourly
      If unstable and/or symptoms – Pacemaker
   Right bundle branch block and left anterior hemiblock –
   After myocardial infarction – temporary pacemaker (see p. 39).

Asystole (usually less successful than ventricular fibrillation)
Bang on the chest, and then
External cardiac massage and ventilation

Isoprenaline 2 mg
   or Adrenaline 1 ml of 1:1000 into the heart via the 4th left
   interspace one inch from the sternum.
and/or Calcium Gluconate 10 ml of 10% i.v. or intracardially in an
attempt to induce V.F.
If successful D.C. shock – (see V.F).
If unable to induce V.F.: pacemaker (if possible).

CARDIAC FAILURE

Congestive cardiac failure
Digoxin 0.5 mg 6 hourly × 2 (increases myocardial contratility)
         then 0.25 mg 6 hourly x 4
         then 0.25 mg 12 hourly as maintenance (adjust dose
         according to age, size and renal function)
   Indications of overdose are,
         loss of appetite
         nausea and vomiting
         and excess bradycardia
   Reduce dose in elderly, e.g. 0.25 mg 8 hourly to digitalise over a
few days, and then 0.25 mg or less daily as maintenance.
and, if necessary, either
Bendrofluazide 5-10 mg daily: slow action
   or Frusemide 40-160 mg daily: acts over a few hours
   or Bumetanide 1-4 mg daily: acts over a few hours
   (To reduct salt and water retention)
and Maintain a high potassium intake with Citrus fruits, etc.
   or add a Potassium supplement.
Then, if needed, add either
Spironolactone 25-50 mg 6 hourly – takes several days to act
   or Amiloride 10-40 mg daily – acts in 2-3 hours
These drugs are potassium sparing and therefore no supplements
are needed.

Left heart failure
Sit the patient up – reduces pulmonary venous pressure
and reassure – reduces vasoconstriction
and Diamorphine 5 mg i.v. relieves pain and vasoconstriction
   or Morphine 15 mg i.v. or i.m. – relieves pain and vasoconstriction
and Frusemide 40 mg i.v. – reduces blood volume
   or Bumetanide 0.5-1.0 mg i.v. – reduces blood volume.
and, if necessary,
Aminophylline 250-500 mg slowly i.v. –
   reduces bronchoconstriction
   increases myocardial contractility
   increases diuresis.
Oxygen by face mask to increase tissue oxygen.
Rarely venous tourniquets or venesection of 1 pint (500 ml) to
reduce blood volume.
Remove cause if possible, e.g. severe hypertension

Then, Digoxin – to increase myocardial contractility
If not already on Digoxin 0.5 mg 6 hourly x 2
then 0.25 mg 6 hourly x 4
then 0.25 mg 12 hourly as maintenance.
If on Digoxin: Review dose

D.C. SHOCK (ELECTIVE)

Treat as for a general anaesthetic.
Use i.v. Diazepam to sedate
Be prepared to intubate if necessary
Start at the lowest voltage setting on the machine
Trigger on the R wave
Ensure that discharge occurs with each QRS complex
Apply conducting jelly to paddles
Place paddles along the axis of the heart and press discharge button
If unsuccessful after 2 discharges, increase discharge strength and repeat
Try 2 discharges at 50, 100 and 200 Joules
If still unsuccessful try a third shock at 200 Joules
If this fails inject 5-20 mg of Practolol i.v. and repeat shock at 200 Joules
If fails try 400 Joules, once.

HYPERLIPO-PROTEINAEMIA

Type I (Children with abdominal pain)
Diet with a low fat content

Type IIa – high serum cholesterol, normal triglyceride, raised ß lipo-protein
Diet reducing to ideal body weight.
Then reduce fat intake to 30% of calories.
Reduce cholesterol intake, especially eggs.
Increase percentage of polyunsaturated fats.
AND, if not normal on diet:
    Cholestyramine 16-36 g/daily in divided doses
plus Clofibrate 1.5-2 g/daily in divided doses (if necessary).
    or Nicotinic Acid 25 mg 8 hourly increasing over 2-6 weeks to 3-6 g/day.

Type IIb – mixed IIa and IV
Treat as for Type IV

Type III – serum cholesterol high, serum triglyceride high,
        broad ß lipo-protein
Diet reducing to ideal body weight.
Then reduce carbohydrate intake and fat intake to 45% of calories.
AND, if not normal on diet:

Clofibrate 1.5-2 g/daily in divided doses (if necessary)
or Nicotinic Acid 25 mg 8 hourly increasing over 2-5 weeks to
   3-6 g/daily.

Type IV – high serum triglyceride, variable cholesterol,
            raised pre ß lipo-protein
Diet reducing to ideal body weight.
Then reduce carbohydrate intake and reduce cholesterol intake.
Increase percentage of polyunsaturated fats.
AND, if not normal on diet:
   Clofibrate 1.5-2 g daily in divided doses (if necessary)
   or Nicotinic Acid 25 mg 8 hourly increasing over 2-6 weeks to
      3-6 g/day.

Type V – serum cholesterol high, serum triglyceride high
Diet reducing to ideal body weight
Then reduce fat to 30% of calories
Reduce carbohydrate intake
Increase percentage of polyunsaturated fats
AND, if not normal on diet:
   Nicotinic Acid 25 mg 8 hourly increasing over 2-6 weeks to 3-6
   g/day.

HYPERTENSION (raised blood pressure for age, measured on at

least two occasions)

Find cause and treat as appropriate

Essential

Benign
either Bendrofluazide 5 mg daily
         and if necessary
      Propranolol 40-160 mg 8 hourly
      or Metoprolol 50-200 mg 12 hourly
      or Atenolol 50-100 mg daily,
         and if necessary
         Hydrallazine 25-50 mg 8 hourly
or if fails:
either Methyldopa 250-500 mg 6-12 hourly
      or Bethanidine 10-60 mg 8 hourly
      or Guanethidine 20-40 mg daily as a single dose
      or Other beta blockers
         With or without Bendrofluazide 5 mg daily.
In ALL cases start with low dose and increase according to the
blood pressure response.

Malignant or accelerated (Grade III or IV fundi):
Hydrallazine 10-20 mg slowly i.v.
   or Pentolinium tartrate 2 mg s/c with the patient sitting up.

May be repeated after 15 minutes to increase or maintain drop in blood pressure.
or Diazoxide 300 mg rapidly i.v. with patient lying, response in 15 minutes.
May be repeated after 2-3 hours. No more than 1200 mg/24 hrs.
or Bethanidine 10 mg oral, repeated in 2-4 hours as necessary
Then establish conventional treatment.

In pregnancy
Methyldopa 250-500 mg 6-12 hourly
  or Clonidine 0.05-0.1 mg 8 hourly
  or Hydrallazine 25-50 mg 8 hourly

INFECTIVE ENDOCARDITIS

Prophylaxis (as recommended by American Heart Association)

Adult & child
Either Benzyl Penicillin 1 mega unit i.m.
  Child 30000 units/kg i.m.
                                              ½ an hour before
  and Procaine Penicillin 600000 units i.m.   manipulation
  Child 600000 units

or Phenoxymethyl Penicillin 2 g orally   ½-1 hour before
  Child less than 60 lbs 1 g orally   manipulation
or Benzyl Penicillin 1 mega unit i.m.
  Child 30000 u/kg
  and Procaine Penicillin 600000 units i.m.
  Child 600000 units   ½-1 hour before
  and Streptomycin 1 g   manipulation
  Child 20 mg/kg
Then
IN ALL CASES Phenoxymethyl Penicillin 500 mg   6 hourly
Child 250 mg   for 2 days

if Penicillin allergy
  Vancomycin infusion 1 g i.v.   over ½-1 hour, starting ½-1 hour
  Child 20 mg/kg   before manipulation

  then Erythromycin 500 mg
  Child 10 mg/kg   6hourly for 2 days
Alternative regimes:
either Benzyl Penicillin 1 mega unit
      and Procaine Penicillin 300 mg   ½ an hour before manipulation
  then Procaine Penicillin 300 mg 24 hours later
or if already on Penicillin or hypersensitive to Penicillin:
Cephaloridine 1 g i.m. ½ hour before manipulation
  then Cephaloridine 500 mg 12 hourly for 48 hours.

Curative

Base treatment on laboratory selection of optimum bacteriocidal agent or combination.

Strep. viridans

either Benzyl Penicillin 5 mega units 6 hourly i.v. as bolus
and either Streptomycin 1 g daily for a week
   or Gentamicin according to the Mawer Nomogram (p. 323) for a week.
After 1 week or when temperature settled change to oral Penicillin, providing bacteriacidal levels are known and blood levels can be measured.
Aim to keep trough level (just before next dose) at least 10 x the cidal level. Continue this therapy for 6-8 weeks.
   or Cephaloridine 600 mg 6 hourly i.v. Continue for 6-8 weeks

Enterococcus

Benzyl Penicillin 20 mega units/day as i.v. bolus
and Streptomycin 1 g/day i.m.
Changing to oral Penicillin after 1 week if satisfactory response.
Continue for 6-8 weeks.

Following cardiac surgery

Appropriate Penicillin
and appropriate aminoglycoside.
Removal of prosthesis may be necessary.

Blood culture negative (often due to previous antimicrobial therapy).

Benzyl Penicillin 20 mega units/day as i.v. boluses
and Streptomycin 1 g/day for a week.
Then continue with Penicillin alone or change to oral treatment as outlined above. Continue treatment for 6 to 8 weeks.

NB. INFECTION MAY BE DUE TO COXIELLA BURNETTI WHICH
   SHOULD BE TREATED WITH:
   TETRACYCLINE 500 mg 6 HOURLY FOR SEVERAL WEEKS.

MYOCARDIAL INFARCTION

Immediate

Relieve pain with either Diamorphine 5 mg i.v. or i.m.
   or Morphine 10-15 mg i.v. or i.m.
May need anti-emetic as well:
Cyclizine 50 mg i.m.
   or Prochlorperazine 12.5 mg i.m.
If transferring to hospital and has multiple ectopics:
Lignocaine 100 mg i.v. and 100 mg i.m.
Treat cardiac failure on conventional lines:- see section on cardiac failure.

Treat arrhythmia early: *see* section on arrhythmia.
Bed rest until patient in stable state or up to 48 hours.
Then mobilise over one week.
If complicated or severe congestive cardiac failure anticoagulate
with:
   Warfarin 30 mg stat
        then Warfarin 3 mg 12 hourly for 1 day
   Check prothrombin time on 2nd day
     and adjust dose as necessary

Late
Remove risk factors: Stop smoking
                  Reduce weight
                  Reduce blood pressure
If male aged less than 55 – anticoagulate
Return to work and full activities as soon as able to do so – usually
within one month.

OEDEMA

Establish the cause and treat the underlying disease if possible

Then
Bendrofluazide 5-10 mg daily
   or Cyclopenthiazide 0.25-1.0 mg daily

If no effect on oedema or weight, change to
Frusemide 40-160 mg daily
   or Bumetanide 1-4 mg daily
   or Ethacrynic Acid 50-200 mg daily
These all cause potassium loss and therefore need supplements
unless dietary intake is high (Citrus fruits etc.)

If there is still little or no response:
add Spironolactone 25-50 mg 6 hourly
   or Amiloride 5-20 mg daily
These conserve potassium therefore supplements are not necessary
and may cause hyperkalaemia.
Rarely it is necessary to restrict salt intake to induce a diuresis.

NB. Too rapid a diuresis – weight loss of more than 0.5 to 1 kg/day
may cause problems, especially with hepatic disease.
Review need for continuing therapy at frequent intervals.

PACING

Temporary
The tip of the pacing wire should be placed in the apex of the right
ventricle, either via the ante cubital fossa or via an infra-clavicular
vein puncture.

Pacing should be on demand
The rate should be 70-80 beats per minute
The voltage should be the threshold x 2, but not more than 4 millivolts.
The threshold should be measured at least once daily and the pacing voltage increased as necessary, to a maximum of 6 millivolts.
The position should be checked by X-ray daily
When sinus rhythm is established, turn off pacemaker but leave in place.
If not needed remove after a further 24 hours.

Permanent
Should only be done in a centre which runs a special service for patients needing pacing.

RHEUMATIC FEVER

Acute attack
Bed rest
Benzyl Penicillin to remove streptococci – 1 mega unit i.m. initially
        then Penicillin V 250 mg 6 hourly for one week.
        then Prophylaxis
and Salicylates 5-10 g or more/day to obtain plasma level of 20-30 mg/100 ml
Continued until disease no longer active.

Prophylaxis
To prevent recurrent attacks
Penicillin V 250 mg 12 hourly
The length of therapy is controversial with suggestions ranging from 5-30 years.
It is probably sufficient to continue until community living, e.g. school is finished.

THROMBOEMBOLISM

Acute massive pulmonary embolus
Oxygen in high concentration

Critically ill
Hydrocortisone 100 mg i.v. followed by
Streptokinase 250000-600000 units i.v. given over 10-30 minutes.
then 100000 units hourly. (Most effective on thrombi that are less than 3 days old).
Requires laboratory assistance.

Less critically ill
Heparin 10000 units 6 hourly

In either case maintain essential functions as necessary and after 48 hours add Warfarin and continue with oral anticoagulation for 1-6 months.

Prophylaxis

Short term risk
e.g. undergoing surgery
Heparin 5000 units subcutaenously 12 hourly before, during and until mobile after surgery.

Medium risk
e.g. established venous thrombosis
Heparin 5000 units i.v. 3 hourly or by continuous infusion
add Warfarin 30 mg stat
   then Warfarin 3 mg 12 hourly x 1 day
   then Prothrombin time and adjust daily dose as necessary.
Heparin is stopped after 48 hours when Warfarin should be effective.
Treatment with Warfarin is continued for 1-6 months.

Long term risk
e.g. mitral stenosis or valve replacement
Warfarin 30 mg stat
   then Warfarin 3 mg 12 hourly x 1 day
   then Prothrombin time and adjust daily dose as necessary.
or RARELY
Dipyridamole 100 mg 8 hourly 1 hour before food.
(Has been used during Pregnancy as Warfarin seems to be associated with a high fetal loss).

FURTHER READING

Avery, G. (1976) *Drug Treatment* Edinburgh: Churchill Livingstone
Medical Education (International) Ltd. (1975) *Medicine,* Volumes 24-27
Oram, S. (1971) *Clinical Heart Disease* London: Heinemann

Gastroenterology

M.J.S. Langman and G.D. Bell

BILIARY CIRRHOSIS

Primary

Symptomatic

Pruritus
Cholestyramine 2-4 g 6-12 hourly
Once relief, reduce dose to lowest which controls itching.
If fails: add,
Phenobarbitone 30 mg 8 hourly

Jaundice
occasionally Phenobarbitone 30 mg 8 hourly

Steatorrhoea
Diet low in fat (less than 40 g/day)
and medium chain triglycerides up to 40 g/day
and Vitamin A 100000 units i.m. monthly
and Vitamin D 100000 units i.m. monthly
and Vitamin K 10 mg i.m. monthly
And Calcium Gluconate 4 g daily

Specific treatment
Get expert help.
Occasionally:
Penicillamine – 500-750 mg daily may help
    or Azathioprine 2 mg/kg/day may help

Secondary

Early
Surgery

Late
as for Primary Biliary Cirrhosis
with Ascending Cholangitis
Ampicillin 250-500 mg 6 hourly
    or Tetracycline 250 mg 6 hourly
    or Co-Trimoxazole 2 tablets 12 hourly

or if Jaundiced
Gentamicin according to Mawer Nomogram (see p. 323)

BILIARY COLIC

Control pain with
Pethidine 75-100 mg orally or i.m. 4-6 hourly
and Propantheline 30 mg stat
   then Propantheline 15 mg 4 hourly
Rehydrate
either simple fluids orally
   or i.v. if vomiting
Consult Surgeon
If jaundice
Surgery
If rigors and/or pyrexia
No jaundice:
Ampicillin 500 mg 6 hourly
Jaundice:
Gentamicin according to Mawer Nomogram (see p. 323)
   then surgery

CHOLECYSTITIS

Acute
Rehydrate
Control pain with either Pethidine 50-100 mg 4-6 hourly
   or Dihydrocodeine 30-60 mg 6 hourly
         then if fails to resolve spontaneously within 48 hours or
         signs of deterioration –
antibiotics:
either Ampicillin 500 mg 6 hourly for 7 days
   or Tetracycline 250 mg 6 hourly for 7 days
   or Co-Trimoxazole 2tabs 12 hourly for 7 days
   and: Consider Surgery
   if resolves: Consider surgery 6 weeks later

CHRONIC HEPATITIS

Check hepatitis B status

Chronic persistent hepatitis
Exclude associated disease
Reassure patient
No active treatment

Chronic active hepatitis
exclude drugs, Wilson's disease and associated bowel disease as
cause.

then Prednisone 10 mg 8 hourly
When liver enzymes normal:
  slowly reduce dose to lowest possible to maintain liver function
  tests normal
  If a high dose:
  add Azathioprine 2 mg/kg/day to allow further dose reduction.
  Continue for 1 year
  Then slowly reduce Prednisone before Azathioprine.
  If fails:
  Increase dose, re-establish maintenance and continue for 1-2
  years
  Then try to withdraw again.

CIRRHOSIS

Establish cause and treat as appropriate

Ascites
Establish nature of fluid
Start no added salt diet
If no weight loss in 2 days:
  Bendrofluazide 5 mg-10 mg daily
  and Potassium supplements
If no weight loss after 48 hours change to:
  Frusemide 40 mg daily
  and Potassium supplements
If no weight loss after 48 hours:
  cautiously increase dose to maximum of 200 mg/day
If weight loss more than 1 kg/day – reduce dose
If no weight loss and/or urinary sodium less than 5 mmol/24 hours
  add either Spironolactone 50 mg 6 hourly
  or Amiloride 10 mg 12 hourly
  NB: STOP Potassium supplements.
Maintain normal serum potassium levels throughout

Precoma, coma
Avoid sedative drugs
Remove protein from diet
and Neomycin
  if conscious – 1 g 6 hourly orally
  if unconscious – 2 g 6 hourly as enemata
and Magnesium Sulphate 10 g 2 hourly until diarrhoea induced
then – adjust dose to cause 2 fluid stools per day
  or Lactulose 10-15 ml 8 hourly – adjust dose to cause 2 fluid
  stools/day.
and Vitamin K 10 mg i.m. daily or i.v.
and maintain blood sugar with
  oral or parenteral fluids containing glucose,
  e.g. 500 ml of 20% glucose 6 hourly
and maintain electrolyte balance, especially potassium

Then look for precipitating cause
Slowly re-introduce protein as improves.

Varices

Not bleeding
No therapy

Bleeding
Establish cause – haematemesis/melaena OFTEN NOT due to varices
If variceal bleeding:
  Pitressin 20 units in 100 ml of 5% Dextrose i.v. over 10 mins
  (care in patients with vascular disease)
If continues to bleed:
  Get Expert Help
  ? Sengstaken-Blakemore tube (only if surgical candidate)

COELIAC DISEASE

Gluten free diet
Supplement if necessary with
  Folic Acid 5 mg 8 hourly
  and Vitamin D 12.5 μg-1.25 mg daily with Calcium Gluconate
  1-5 g/daily
  and Ferrous Sulphate 200 mg 12 hourly (with food)
If fails:
  Check compliance with diet
  ? lymphoma
  ? hypolactasia
    then add Prednisone 30-40 mg daily until responds

CONSTIPATION

Establish cause and treat as appropriate.
Instruct in early response to call to stool
High residue diet
If necessary add
  Methyl Cellulose 10 ml with 200 ml of water 12 hourly
  and Magnesium Sulphate 10-30 g daily
If necessary add
  Bisacodyl 5-10 mg daily
If hard stool
  Dioctyl Sodium Sulphosuccinate forte 1-2 tablets 8 hourly

CROHN'S DISEASE

Symptomatic

Ileitis and/or segmental colitis
Prednisone 10 mg 6-8 hourly
  with or without

Sulphasalazine 1 g 8-12 hourly
and vitamin B and C daily as Vitamin Capsules BPC

Anaemia
Establish cause and treat as appropriate
? Transfuse if haemoglobin less than 10 g/100 ml

Wasting
Parenteral feeding and/or dietary supplements

Rectal disease
Proctitis or Proctosigmoiditis
Prednisolone suppositories or enemata 12-24 hourly
    and Sulphasalazine 1 g 8 hourly
When in remission treat as outlined below.

Severe diffuse disease

If proctitis
Prednisolone enemata or suppositories 12-24 hourly
    and Sulphasalazine 1 g 8 hourly
if fails
add Prednisone 10-15 mg 8 hourly orally

No proctitis:
As above, but local Prednisolone ineffective.
When remission induced, reduce oral Prednisone and then manage
as outlined below.

Occasionally
Metronidazole 200 mg 8 hourly for 1-2 months
    or Azathioprine 4 mg/kg daily for 5 days
        then Azathioprine 2.5 mg/kg daily for 6-12 months
    or Ampicillin 250 mg 6 hourly
    or Co-Trimoxazole 2 tabs, 12 hourly for 1-2 months

Maintenance treatment
Sulphasalazine 1 g 12 hourly
If fails:
add Prednisone 10-15 mg/daily on alternate days
    or Azathioprine 2.0 mg/kg/day

Complications
Get expert help.

DUODENAL ULCER

Stop smoking
Avoid excess alcohol
Small regular meals

Dyspepsia
either Magnesium Trisilicate mixture 10 ml with pain or
prophylactically
   or Aluminium Hydroxide mixture 10 ml with pain or
prophylactically (up to 50 ml/day)
or Magnesium Trisilicate Co, or Aluminium Hydroxide Antacid
tablets. (up to 50 ml/day)

If symptoms persist, specific therapy with:
either Cimetidine 200 mg t.d.s. and 400 mg at night for 6-8 weeks
   or DeNol 5 ml in 15 ml water t.d.s. ½ an hour before food and 2
     hrs after last meal for 6-8 weeks
   or Carbenoxolone 50 mg 6 hourly for 6-8 weeks (as capsules)
     15-30 minutes before meals
Then review outcome
   No symptoms – stop therapy
   Ulcer healed + symptoms – stop specific therapy, review diagnosis
   Ulcer not healed + symptoms – either change specific therapy or
   Surgery
Recurrent ulcer after initial healing
either Surgery
or Specific therapy as above
When healed:
   Consider Cimetidine 400 mg at night for 6-12 months.

DYSPEPSIA

Establish cause and treat as appropriate
or Symptomatic therapy:
Reassurance
and either Magnesium Trisilicate mixture 10 ml with pain or
prophylactically (up to 50 ml/day)
   or Aluminium Hydroxide mixture 10 ml with pain or
     prophylactically (up to 50 ml/day)
and either Propantheline 15 mg before meals and 30 mg at night
   or Dicyclomine 10-20 mg 6-8 hourly
   or Metoclopramide 10 mg before meals and at night

GALL STONES

Fat free diet
Reduce to ideal body weight
Then surgery
or if surgery contra-indicated and functioning gall bladder with non-
opaque stones:
Consider – Chenodeoxycholic Acid 15 mg/kg/day for 6-12 months
If diarrhoea, start at lower dose and slowly increase over 2-4
weeks.

GASTRIC CANCER

Treat associated anaemia as appropriate
? surgery
If inoperable treat as outlined in chapter on management of the dying.

GASTRIC ULCER

Stop smoking
Avoid excess alcohol
Small frequent meals

Dyspepsia
either Magnesium Trisilicate mixture 10 ml with pain or prophylactically (up to 50 ml/day)
    or Aluminium Hydroxide mixture 10 ml with pain or
        prophylactically (up to 50 ml/day)
    or Magnesium Trisilicate Co or Aluminium Hydroxide Antacid
        Tablets
Persistent symptoms, specific therapy with:
Carbenoxolone 100 mg 8 hourly for 1 week
        then Carbenoxolone 50 mg 8 hourly for 4 weeks
    or Cimetidine 200 mg t.d.s. and 400 mg at night for 6-8 weeks
    or DeNol 5 ml in 15 ml water t.d.s. ½ hour before food and 2
        hours after last meal for 6-8 weeks
Then review outcome:
    Ulcer healed and no symptoms – stop treatment
    Ulcer healed and symptoms – stop specific therapy and review
    diagnosis
    Ulcer unhealed, no symptoms – ? Malignant, then repeat specific
    therapy
    Ulcer unhealed, symptoms – ? Malignant, ? Surgery
Recurrent ulcer after initial healing:
either Surgery
or Further course of specific therapy.

GIARDIASIS

Metronidazole 200 mg 8 hourly for 7 days
If fails:
Mepacrine 100 mg 8 hourly for 7 days

HAEMATEMESIS AND MELAENA

Assess blood loss and treat as appropriate
Establish diagnosis
    Then if continues to bleed or rebleed and ulcer:
    Consider Surgery

If stops bleeding and chronic ulcer –
Treat as for specific symptoms
If stops bleeding and no specific lesion –
symptomatic treatment
If non ulcer bleeding treat as appropriate.

HAEMOCHROMATOSIS

Venesection of 500 ml weekly or twice weekly for 2 years.
When haemoglobin and serum iron begin to fall adjust frequency of
venesection to maintain iron in the normal range

Diabetes
Diet
and Insulin as necessary

Cardiac disease
Treat as outlined in cardiovascular system chapter.

HEPATIC FAILURE

Get Expert Help
Exclude Paracetamol overdose
    Halothane
    MAOI
    PAS
    Rifampicin
    and other drug causes
AVOID ALL UNNECESSARY drugs.

Portal systemic encephalopathy
as for precoma, coma above (p. 44)

Hypoglycaemia
Blood sugar less than 5.5 mmol/l:
    Glucose 50% 100 ml i.v. stat
    Repeated as necessary.
Blood sugar more than 5.5 mmol/l: consider
    Glucose 20% 500 ml i.v. 6 hourly
    with Potassium Chloride 2.4 g 6 hourly (if normal renal function)

Hypocalcaemia
Calcium Gluconate 10% 10 ml i.v. daily

Respiratory failure
Oxygen
Intubation
and Ventilation

Renal failure
Salt free Albumin i.v. often helpful
    then as in renal chapter

Infection
No routine antibiotics
Treat infection with appropriate antibiotic as necessary

Bleeding
No arterial punctures – they do not stop bleeding
No gastric aspiration – may induce gastrointestinal haemorrhage
Vitamin K 10 mg i.m. daily
Fresh frozen plasma ⎫   As necessary according to
Platelet rich plasma or ⎬   Laboratory data and likelihood
Plasma concentrate ⎭   of recovery

Haematemesis/Melaena
Cimetidine 200 mg i.v. or orally as preventive treatment
Repeated every 2-4 hours as necessary

HEPATITIS

Alcoholic
Stop drinking
then as for hepatic failure (if necessary)

Viral

Prevention
Type A (Infectious Hepatitis)
General hygiene
Take care with urine and faeces, etc.

Type B (Serum Hepatitis)
Avoid blood products if possible
Use disposable needles
and sterile technique
BEWARE accidents with possibly infected blood

Immunization (Passive)

Type A
If within 1-2 weeks of exposure or accident with infected blood:
    Immune Serum Globulin 0.02 ml/kg i.m.
If going to endemic area for prolonged period (more than 3 months)
    Immune Serum Globulin 5 ml i.m. 6 monthly

Type B
If punctured with *known* infected material:
    Immune Serum Globulin 10 ml i.m. might help

Acute attack

Initially
Bed rest
and a high carbohydrate, low fat, diet

Prolonged cholestasis
Pruritus:
Cholestyramine 4 g 8-12 hourly
   Occasionally Prednisone 30 mg/day for 5 days
                           25 mg/day for 5 days
                           20 mg/day for 5 days
                           15 mg/day for 5 days
                           10 mg/day for 5 days
                            5 mg/day for 5 days

In all cases: NO ALCOHOL for 6 months

Chronic
Check hepatitis B status

Chronic persistent hepatitis
Exclude associated disease
Reassure patient
No active treatment

Chronic active hepatitis
exclude drugs, Wilson's disease and associated bowel disease as
cause
   then Prednisone 10 mg 8 hourly
When liver enzymes normal:
   slowly reduce dose to lowest possible to maintain liver function
   tests normal
   If a high dose:
   add Azathioprine 2 mg/kg/day to allow further dose reduction.
   Continue for 1 year.
      then Slowly reduce Prednisone before Azathioprine.
If fails:
Increase dose, re-establish maintenance and continue for 1-2 years.
   then try to withdraw again.

HEPATOLENTICULAR DEGENERATION

Get Expert Help
D. Penicillamine 250-500 mg 6 hourly
until urinary copper excretion normal
Then maintain with:
D. Penicillamine – dose according to copper balance
Check relatives and treat homozygotes

INFECTIVE DIARRHOEA

Mild
Liberal fluid intake

Moderate
Oral fluids with glucose and saline
plus potassium supplements as necessary
    or Sodium Chloride and Dextrose compound powder (BPC) 22 g in
       500 ml of water
       plus potassium supplements as necessary

Severe
Rehydrate with i.v. fluids
and if necessary
Codeine Phosphate 30-60 mg 12 hourly
NB: ANTIBIOTICS HAVE NO PLACE IN SIMPLE INFECTIVE
DIARRHOEA

Amoebic
See Infectious Disease Chapter (p. 1)

Shigellosis
No specific therapy needed

Salmonellosis
See Infectious Disease Chapter (p. 11)

Prophylaxis
General hygiene
No other effective regime

Non-specific
Rule out other causes
then high residue diet
and Methyl Cellulose 10 ml 12 hourly without water
and if necessary:
Codeine Phosphate 30-60 mg 8 hourly
    or Diphenoxylate with Atropine 1-2 tablets 6 hourly
    or Loperamide 4 mg
      then 2 mg with each stool to a maximum of 16 mg/day

IRRITABLE BOWEL SYNDROME

High residue diet
and Methyl Cellulose 10 ml 12 hourly with 200 ml of water
    or Ispaghula husk 10 ml 12 hourly with 200 ml of water
and Propantheline 15 mg t.d.s. before meals
    or Dicyclomine 10-20 mg t.d.s. before meals

If fails:
  Consider lactose intolerance
  Consider Giardiasis
  and review diagnosis

JEJUNAL DIVERTICULOSIS

No steatorrhoea or megaloblastic anaemia:
  No treatment
Single large diverticulum:
  Surgery
Multiple diverticula:
  Tetracycline 250 mg 12 hourly indefinitely.

OESOPHAGEAL CANCER

High
Radiotherapy
then Surgery

Low

Squamous
Surgery
then ? radiotherapy

Adenocarcinoma
Surgery
(radiotherapy is ineffective)

Large and fixed
Intubate surgically or endoscopically

OESOPHAGEAL REFLUX

Reduce to ideal weight
Stop smoking
Avoid tight clothing
Block bed head

Heartburn
either liquid or tablet preparation of antacids, e.g. Gaviscon
  or Magnesium Trisilicate mixture 10 ml after meals and at night
  or Aluminium Hydroxide mixture 10 ml after meals and at night
  or Magnesium Trisilicate Co tablets after meals
  or Aluminium Hydroxide Co tablets after meals
if fails
  Metoclopramide 10 mg before meals and at night

if fails
   Cimetidine 400 mg at night
if fails
   Surgery

OESOPHAGEAL STRICTURE

Establish diagnosis with histology
then treat as for reflux
and if young:
   consider surgery.
if old:
   consider endoscopic dilatation

PANCREATITIS

Acute

Rehydrate
with i.v. fluids (often more than you think and includes blood)
Simple fluids only orally

Pain control
Pethidine 75-100 mg i.m. 4-6 hourly

Hypocalcaemia (Fat necrosis)
Calcium gluconate 10% 10 ml i.v. up to 4 hourly depending on
serum levels

Later
Find cause and treat as appropriate

Chronic
Avoid fatty foods
Avoid alcohol
Look for possible cause
   then *Pain control*
   Dihydrocodeine 30-60 mg 6 hourly
      or Paracetamol 0.5-1 g 4-6 hourly
   and either:
   Propantheline 15 mg 6 hourly
      or Dicyclomine 10 mg 6 hourly
AVOID MORE POTENT ANALGESICS IF POSSIBLE

Severe pain
Confirm diagnosis
Then look for operable duct lesion
As last resort:
   Pancreatectomy

Malabsorption and/or steatorrhoea
Low fat diet (40 g/day)
and medium chain triglycerides 40 g/day
and Pancreatin tabs strong B.P. 1 before, 2 with, and 1 after, meals
If fails:
   add Aluminium Hydroxide mixture 10 ml with meals
If fails:
   add Cimetidine 200 mg 8 hourly

Diabetes
Treat as in Endocrine Chapter

POST GASTRECTOMY SYNDROMES

Malabsorption

Iron
Ferrous Sulphate 200 mg 12 hourly

Fat
Pancreatin tablets strong 1 before, 2 with, and 1 after, meals

Vitamin D
12.5 μg-1.25 mg/day and
Calcium Gluconate 1-5 g daily

Dumping
Small frequent meals
Avoid large amounts of sugar
Reduce fluid intake with meals
If fails:
   Consider Surgical revision

General malnutrition
High protein diet
Water soluble Vitamins 1-2 capsules (BPC) daily
and Folic Acid 5 mg daily

Bilious vomiting
Surgery

Post vagotomy diarrhoea
either Ispaghula husk 5-10 ml 12-24 hourly with meals
   or Methyl Cellulose 5-10 ml 12-24 hourly with meals
   or Diphenoxylate with Atropine 1-2 tabs. 8-12 hourly as
      necessary
   or Codeine Phosphate 15-60 mg 8-24 hourly as necessary
   or Loperamide 2 mg 8 hourly
   or occasionally:
      Cholestyramine 3-4 g 6 hourly

C

PROCTALGIA FUGAX

Reassure
and Propantheline 15 mg t.d.s. before meals
  or Dicyclomine 10-20 mg t.d.s. before meals
and a high residue diet

TROPICAL SPRUE

If multiple deficiencies and steatorrhoea:
  Folic Acid 5 mg 8 hourly
  and either
    Tetracycline 250 mg 6 hourly for 1-2 months
    or Ampicillin 250 mg 6 hourly for 1-2 months
If Vitamin B12 deficiency:
  Hydroxocobalamin 200 μg weekly x 6

ULCERATIVE COLITIS

Acute episode

Proctitis or proctosigmoiditis
Prednisolone suppositories or enemata 12-24 hourly
  and Sulphasalazine 1 g 8 hourly
When in remission treat as outlined below.

More diffuse disease
Prednisolone enemata 12-24 hourly
and Sulphasalazine 1 g 6-8 hourly
If fails or symptoms moderately severe or disease proximal to
splenic flexure
  add Prednisone 10-15 mg 8 hourly orally
When remission induced, reduce oral Prednisone and then manage
as outlined below:

Severe disease (Toxic Dilatation)
GET EXPERT HELP INCLUDING SURGEON
  Exclude toxic dilatation with X-ray
  Then Prednisolone-21-Phosphate 20-40 mg 8 hourly i.m. or i.v.
  Rehydrate and maintain fluid and electrolyte balance
  Maintain haemoglobin above 10.5 g/100 ml
  Clear fluids only by mouth
  Consider parenteral feeding
  and Ampicillin 250 mg 6 hourly i.v.

After 2-3 days
  if better:
  Restart oral fluids
  Reduce Prednisolone and change to oral therapy
  Then as outlined below
  if not better:
  Surgery

Maintenance therapy
Sulphasalazine 1 g 12 hourly (occasionally 6 or 8 hourly)
occasionally:
Ispaghula husk 5-10 ml 12 hourly
  or Methyl Cellulose 5-10 ml 12 hourly
  or Codeine Phosphate 30-60 mg 12 hourly

Pan-colitis
KEEP WATCH FOR DEVELOPMENT OF MALIGNANT DISEASE

ZOLLINGER-ELLISON Syndrome

Cimetidine 1-4 g daily before surgery
Get expert help

FURTHER READING

Bouchier, I.A.D. (1977) *Gastroenterology* London: Balliere Tindall
Langman, M.J.S. (1973) *A Concise Textbook of Gastroenterology*
  Edinburgh: Churchill Livingstone
Naish, J.M. & Reed, A.E.A. (1974) *Basic Gastroenterology* Bristol:
  Wright
Schiff, L. (1976) *Diseases of the Liver* Lippincott C.
Sherlock, Sheila, (1975) *Diseases of the Liver and Biliary System*
  London: Blackwell Scientific Publications
Sleisenger M.W. & Fordtran, J.S. (1973) *Gastrointestinal Disease*
  London: W.B. Saunders

Central nervous system

With R.B. Godwin-Austen

BELLS PALSY

If seen early
Prednisone 40 mg daily for one day
   then Prednisone 30 mg daily for two days
   then Prednisone 20 mg daily for two days
   then Prednisone 10 mg daily for two days
   then STOP
Protect the cornea
and if chemosis develops:
   treat with local antibiotics
Treat pain with
   either Aspirin 300-600 mg 4-6 hourly
     or Paracetamol 500-1000 mg 6-8 hourly
Maintain facial muscle tone
   with active movements of the affected muscles performed in front
of a mirror twice daily.

BENIGN ESSENTIAL TREMOR

If disabling:
   either Alcohol (in moderation)
   or Diazepam 5 mg 8 hourly
   or Propranolol 40-80 mg 8 hourly
   or Methyl Pentynol 250 mg 8 hourly.

BENIGN POSITIONAL VERTIGO

Explain cause
Prevent sudden head movements.

BRAIN ABSCESS

IN ALL CASES EXPERT NEUROLOGICAL/NEUROSURGICAL HELP
SHOULD BE OBTAINED WHEN DIAGNOSIS IS SUSPECTED
Avoid Lumbar Puncture

Sinusitic in origin
Penicillin 4-5 mega units 6 hourly i.v.
  or if Penicillin allergy:
    Erythromycin 0.5-1 g 6 hourly i.v.

Otic in origin
  Chloramphenicol 600 mg 6 hourly i.v.
    or Gentamicin 8 hourly i.m. or i.v. – dose according to Mawer
    Nomogram (see p. 323)
  and Metronidazole either 400 mg 8 hourly orally
                        or   600 mg 8 hourly i.v.
  and Penicillin 3-4 mega units 6 hourly i.v.
    or Ampicillin 500 mg 6 hourly i.v. or orally
    or Co-Trimoxazole 2-6 tablets 12 hourly orally
    or as an injection 10-15 ml diluted to 250-375 ml
    with 0.9% Sodium Chloride given every 12 hours

Metastatic or cryptogenic
  Chloramphenicol 600 mg 6 hourly i.v.
    or Gentamicin 8 hourly i.m. or i.v. – dose according to Mawer
    Nomogram (see p. 323)
  and Metronidazole either 400 mg 8 hourly orally
                          600 mg 8 hourly i.v.
  and Penicillin 3-4 mega units 6 hourly i.v.
    or Ampicillin 500 mg 6 hourly i.v. or orally
    or Co-Trimoxazole 2-6 tablets 12 hourly orally
      or as an injection 10.15 ml diluted to 250-375 ml
      with 0.9% Sodium Chloride given every 12 hours

Post traumatic or spinal
Sodium Fusidate 500 mg 8 hourly orally or i.v.

CARPAL TUNNEL SYNDROME

Find cause and treat as appropriate e.g. Myxoedema
Frusemide 40 mg daily
and night splints
  or Hydrocortisone by local injection
  or Surgery.

EATON LAMBERT SYNDROME

See non-Metastatic Neurological Syndromes, p. 68.

ENCEPHALITIS

Herpes simplex
Analgesics as necessary for headache
Dexamethasone 4-8 mg 6 hourly

Continued for a few days and then reduced
  and if diagnosis proven
  Cytosine arabinoside 20 mg/m²/i.v. as intravenous bolus 12
hourly for 5 days

Complicating fevers, e.g. Morbilli, Varicella or Mumps
Analgesics as necessary for headaches

If fits
Anticonvulsants – *see* Epilepsy.

Non-specific
With neurological deficit
ACTH 40 units twice a day for 1 week
  then ACTH 40 units daily for 4 days
  then ACTH 20 units daily for 3 days
  then STOP.

EPILEPSY

Investigate to see if Idiopathic or Secondary
STOP driving
AVOID at risk situations

Idiopathic
One fit – no therapy
Two fits – consider therapy
Three fits – treat

Grand mal
Start with low dose and gradually increase dose until control
obtained or therapeutic plasma level exceeded. In the following lists
are given the range of maintenance dose and the plasma level.
Most drugs are best given once daily.
  Phenytoin 200-600 mg (300) per day
    Maintain plasma level between 10-20 µg/ml
    or *Sodium Valproate 250-750 mg (1200) 6-8 hourly
      Maintain plasma level between 50-100 µg/ml
    or *Phenobarbitone 60-400 mg (90) per day
      Maintain plasma level between 10-40 µg/ml
    or *Primidone 500-1000 mg (750) per day
      Maintain plasma level between 5-10 µg/ml
      *Either drug can be used alone or in combination with
      Phenytoin.*

Petit mal
  Sodium Valproate 250-750 mg (1200) 6-8 hourly
    Maintain plasma level between 50-100 µg/ml
    or Ethosuximide 500-2000 mg (750) per day
      Maintain plasma level between 40-80 µg/ml

Petit mal with grand mal
    Ethosuximide 500-2000 mg (750) per day
        Maintain plasma level between 40-100 μg/ml
            and either Phenytoin 200-600 mg (300) per day
                Maintain plasma level between 10-20 μg/ml
            or Phenobarbitone 60-400 mg (90) per day
                Maintain plasma level between 10-40 μg/ml
            or Sodium Valproate 250-750 (1200) mg 6-8 hourly
                Maintain plasma level between 50-100 μg/ml

Pregnancy
    Phenytoin 200-600 g (300) per day
    Maintain plasma level between 10-20 μg/ml
      or Phenobarbitone 60-400 mg (90) per day
        Maintain plasma level between 10-40 μg/ml.

Symptomatic
Investigate fully to find cause

Temporal lobe epilepsy
    Carbamazepine 400-1200 mg (600) per day
    Maintain plasma level between 4-10 μg/ml
      or Phenytoin 200-600 mg (300) per day
        Maintain plasma level between 10-20 μg/ml
      or Phenobarbitone 60-400 mg (90) per day
        Maintain plasma level between 10-40 μg/ml
      or Primidone 500-1000 mg (750) per day
        Maintain plasma level between 5-10 μg/ml
      or Occasionally:
        Pheneturide 600-1000 mg per day
        (Use slowly, increasing dose – change maximum of once a
        week)
      or If intractable: ? Surgery

Myoclonus
Clonazepam 0.5-2.0 mg nocte or 12 hourly
    or Sodium Valproate 200-600 mg 8 hourly

Status epilepticus
    either Diazepam 5-10 mg slowly i.v. over 2-4 minutes
        Repeating as necessary to maximum of 200 mg/24 hrs)
      or Chlormethiazole 0.8% infusion 60-100 drops/min
        adjusting drip rate to maintain fit free.
        Maximum dose 500 ml per day.
      or if fails:
        i.v. Thiopentone 1 g/litre may be necessary
    Occasionally add: Dexamethasone 4-8 mg 6 hourly
NB: RESPIRATORY DEPRESSION IS COMMONLY CAUSED AND
THEREFORE THE AIRWAY MUST BE PROTECTED AND
VENTILATION MAY BE REQUIRED.

Maintain fluid and electrolyte balance.
When the status is controlled, if the patient has not had previous therapy, start therapy with either:
    Phenytoin or Phenobarbitone
NB: CONTINUE CONTROL WITH I.V. DRUGS FOR FURTHER 24 HOURS.
If they have had previous therapy, continue with their usual drugs and dosage given by nasogastric tube.
then adjust dose as necessary to control fits.
Then investigate to find cause.

FACIAL PAIN (Specific diagnosis essential)

Trigeminal neuralgia
Carbamazepine 100-400 mg 6-8 hourly
    or Phenytoin 200-600 mg daily

Atypical facial pain
Antidepressants in full dosage
    e.g. Amitriptyline 10-50 mg 8 hourly

Post herpetic neuralgia
Chlorprothixene 50 mg 6 hourly for 2 weeks
and antidepressants
    e.g. Amitriptyline 10-50 mg 8 hourly
Occasionally:
    local infiltration with local anaesthetic
        or electrical stimulation may be helpful.

Giant cell arteritis (medical emergency)
Prednisone 60 mg daily for 3 days, gradually reducing to
            20 mg daily
then adjust dose according to clinical response and erythrocyte sedimentation rate
Continue therapy for at least 6 months.
See also Migraine and Migrainous Neuralgia

HERPES ZOSTER

See facial pain (above) and shingles in infection chapter, p. 13.

HUNTINGTONS CHOREA

Tetrabenazine   25 mg 12 hourly increasing every 3-4 days to
            200 mg daily or effective dose
if no effect in one week of maximum therapy – STOP.
    or Chlorpromazine 10-25 mg 8 hourly increasing dose as necessary.
    or Thiopropazate 5-10 mg 8 hourly

INAPPROPRIATE ANTIDIURETIC HORMONE SECRETION

See Non-Metastatic Neurological Syndromes, p. 68.

MENIERES DISEASE

Reduce endolymphatic pressure
with a low salt diet
and/or Bendrofluazide 5-10 mg daily

and/or Increase blood supply
with Betahistine 8-16 mg 8 hourly

and/or Vestibular sedatives
either Prochlorperazine 5-10 mg 4 hourly orally or as a suppository
   or Cinnarizine 15-30 mg 8 hourly orally

If fails and attacks disabling:
   Consider surgery

MENINGITIS

Collect CSF
then:

Neonate GET EXPERT HELP AT ONCE

Enterobacteria, e.g. Pseudomonas
Gentamicin 2-3 mg/kg 12 hourly i.m. – Monitor blood level.
   and Benzyl Penicillin 20-60 mg/kg 6 hourly i.m. (33000 to
100000 units)
until the laboratory results of the CSF available then continue as
appropriate.
Daily intrathecal or intraventricular injection of
Gentamicin 1-2 mg may be necessary.

Streptococcus pneumoniae
other Streptococci
Listeria monocytogenes
Benzyl Penicillin 20-60 mg/kg 6 hourly i.v. (33000 to 100000
units)
   or Ampicillin 40-50 mg/kg 6 hourly i.v.

Straphylococcus aureus
Penicillin 20-60 mg/kg 6 hourly i.v. (33000 to 100000 units)
   and Flucloxacillin 50 mg/kg 6 hourly orally; or i.m.

Organism unknown
Ampicillin 40-50 mg/kg 6 hourly i.v.
   and Gentamicin 2-3 mg/kg 12 hourly i.m. – Monitor blood level

Infants and children GET EXPERT HELP AT ONCE

Haemophilus influenzae
Ampicillin 50-100 mg/kg 6 hourly i.v.
  or Chloramphenicol 15-20 mg/kg 6 hourly i.m. or orally

Streptococcus pneumoniae
Penicillin 150 mg/kg 6 hourly i.v. (250000 units)
  or Cephaloridine 20-25 mg/kg 6 hourly i.v.

Neisseria meningitides
Penicillin 150 mg/kg 6 hourly i.v. (250000 units)
  or Ampicillin 50-100 mg/kg 6 hourly i.v.

Organism unknown
Ampicillin 50-100 mg/kg 6 hourly i.v.

Adults

Haemophilus influenzae
Ampicillin 0.5-1.5 g 6 hourly i.v.
  or Chloramphenicol 0.5-1 g 6 hourly i.m. or orally

Streptococcus pneumoniae
Penicillin 3-5 g 6 hourly i.v.
        (5-8 mega units)
  or Cephaloridine 1 g 6 hourly i.v.

Neisseria meningitides
Penicillin 3-5 g 6 hourly i.v.
        (5-8 mega units)
  or Ampicillin 0.5-1.5 g 6 hourly i.v.
  and/or Sulphadiazine 1-1.5 g 4 hourly i.v. for 2 days
        then 1 g 6 hourly orally

Tuberculosis
Isoniazid 10 mg/kg/day for two weeks
        then 300 mg daily
  and Pyridoxine 50-100 mg daily (to prevent peripheral
  neuropathy)
  and Rifampicin 450 mg if less than 50 kg
    or 600 mg if more than 50 kg
  and Streptomycin 1 g i.m. if less than 40 years
    or 0.75 g i.m. if more than 40 years
    or Ethambutol 15 mg/kg
ALL drugs taken together ½ an hour before breakfast

Organism unknown
Ampicillin 0.5-1.5 g 6 hourly i.v.

NB: INAPPROPRIATE ADH SYNDROME CAN OCCUR – *see* p. 68).

MIGRAINE

Simple or classical migraine

Symptomatic
At onset of symptoms:
either Soluble Aspirin 600 mg 4 hourly
   or Dihydrocodeine 30 mg 4-6 hourly
   or Paracetamol 1000 mg 6 hourly
Symptoms severe and/or not controlled by above:
Ergotamine tartrate 1-2mg sublingually
   or Ergotamine tartrate 2 mg rectally
Then (as early as possible) Aspirin 600-900 mg 4 hourly
NB: OVERDOSAGE with ergotamine is common and characterised
   by; headache and nausea – may be mistaken for migraine.
  with nausea or vomiting:
  Metoclopramide 10 mg 6-8 hourly
    or Prochlorperazine suppositories 25 mg 6 hourly
    or Thiethylperazine 10 mg

Prophylactic
Avoid factors that induce attacks
Treat any associated condition (e.g. hypertension or depression)
and withdraw provocative medication (e.g. oral contraceptives).
  then Clonidine 25-50 μg 12 hourly
   or Pizotifen 0.5 mg 8 hourly
Occasionally:
  Methysergide 1 mg daily increasing by 1 mg a day to a maximum
  of 2 mg 6-8 hourly.
  Continue therapy no longer than 6 months.
  Side effects are common.

Hemiplegic migraine and ophthalmoplegic migraine:
Refer for specialist advice.

Migrainous neuralgia:
Ergotamine tartrate 2 mg rectally each night for 6 nights
Repeated weekly until bout ceases
  and/or Pizotifen 0.5 mg 8 hourly
  and Medihaler Ergotamine 0.36 mg at onset of pain
  or Ergotamine tartrate 0.25 mg i.m. at onset of pain

MULTIPLE SCLEROSIS

Acute relapse
ACTH 40 units daily for one week
  then 30 units daily for one week
  then 20 units daily for one week
  then 20 units alternate days for one week
  then 10 units alternate days for one week
  then Stop   (increases rate of recovery)

Chronic state

Dietary supplements containing unsaturated fats, e.g.
  Sunflower seed oil might help.

Symptomatic

Spasticity
either Diazepam 5-15 mg daily
  or Baclofen 5 mg 8 hourly increasing by 15 mg per day until
  effective or 20 mg 8 hourly.
  or Dantrolene 25 mg 12 hourly increasing gradually to 100 mg
    6 hourly or effective dose
Occasionally intrathecal Phenol

Urgency of micturition
Ephedrine 15 mg as necessary
  or Emepromium 100 mg 8 hourly

Pressure ulcers
  see p. 174

Urinary infection
  see p. 124.

MYASTHENIA GRAVIS

Diagnosis
Edrophonium chloride 10 mg i.v.

Treatment
Neostigmine 15 mg 8 hourly to 60 mg 4 hourly x 5/day
(avoiding 4.00 am)
  or Pyridostigmine 60 mg 8 hourly to 240 mg 4 hourly x 5/day
  (avoiding 4.00 am)
    and
    Atropine 0.5 mg 8-12 hourly
    or Propantheline 15 mg 8-12 hourly
    to reduce side effects
    rarely
      Ephedrine sulphate 25 mg 8 hourly
and/or Spironolactone 25-50 mg 6 hourly
and/or Prednisone – may make patient temporarily worse, therefore
          needs to be initiated in hospital and maintain on
          alternate day regime.
and Thymectomy – if indicated

Myasthenic crisis
Endrophonium chloride 5-10 mg i.v.
Improvement:
  Myasthenic crisis –
  increase dose

Worse:
Cholingeric crisis –
STOP all therapy and observe effect –
Ventilation is usually necessary
NB: IN ALL CASES MEANS OF ARTIFICIAL VENTILATION MUST BE AVAILABLE
MANY DRUGS MAY MAKE MYASTHENIA WORSE, e.g.
AMINOGLYCOSIDES, TETRACYCLINES AND ANTI-ARRHYTHMIC AGENTS.

MYOTONIA

Phenytoin 300-400 mg per day – monitor plasma level (therapeutic range 10-20 μg/ml)
    or Procainamide 250-500 mg 8 hourly – watch for development of antinuclear factor. If found review treatment

NEUROSYPHILIS

Get expert help.

Tabes dorsalis

Lightning pains:
Aspirin 600 mg as necessary
    or Carbamazepine 200 mg orally 6-8 hourly

The infection:
Procaine Penicillin 600000 units i.m. daily for 21 days
    or Benzathine Penicillin 2.4 mega units i.m. weekly for 5 weeks
    or if Penicillin sensitive
Tetracycline 3 g daily for 4 weeks.

GPI
Admit to hospital
Then Prednisone 5 mg 6 hourly for 3 days
After 24 hours start Procaine Penicillin 600000 units daily i.m. for 21 days.
(Prednisone prevents the Jarisch Herxheimer Reaction)
    and if needed for sedation:
    Chlorpromazine 100 mg i.m.

In both cases
Repeat lumbar puncture at 6 weeks and three months
If cells fall and remain down – no therapy
If cells do not fall or fall and rise again *Get Expert Help*
Repeat as described above.

NON METASTATIC NEUROLOGICAL SYNDROMES

Remove primary tumour if possible

Inappropriate antidiuretic hormone secretion
Restrict fluid intake
Demeclocycline 300 mg 8-12 hourly
   or Frusemide 40-160 mg a day

Eaton Lambert syndrome (Myasthenic Syndrome)
Guanidine 5-20 mg/kg 8 hourly
May take several days to be effective
   and Atropine 0.5 mg 6-8 hourly
   (to counteract some of the side effects)

Myositis (and Dermatomyositis)
Prednisone

Cerebellar degeneration
No specific treatment

OPTIC NEURITIS

Find cause and treat as appropriate, e.g. Toxins including drugs, and
Infection

Due to multiple sclerosis
Rate of recovery increased by:
ACTH 40 units daily for a week
   then ACTH 30 units daily for a week
   then ACTH 20 units daily for a week
   then ACTH 20 units alternate days for one week
   then ACTH 10 units alternate days for one week
   then STOP

PARKINSONS DISEASE

Idiopathic
Levodopa and decarboxylase inhibitor given as a combined tablet
(acts mainly on bradykinesia)

Initially
Either 'Sinemet 275' ½ tablet 12 hourly ($\equiv$ 125 mg of Levodopa)
or 'Madopar 125' 1 tablet 12 hourly ($\equiv$ 100 mg of Levodopa)
Increase dose weekly by 125 mg of Levodopa until effective dose or
side effects.

Maintenance
When side effects produced reduce dose by about 20% and
continue.

The usual maintenance dose of Levodopa in combination is 250 mg 8 hourly.
    and/or anticholinergics, e.g. Benzhexol 2 mg 8-12 hourly, then increasing if necessary to 2-5 mg 6-8 hourly
    and/or Amantadine 100 mg twice a day (after the morning and midday meal.)
Effects may decline after 6 weeks treatment.

Drug induced

Stop Phenothiazine, e.g. Chlorpromazine
    or Butyrophenone, e.g. Haloperidol
If Phenothiazine or Butyrophenone *must* be continued
    Levodopa is not effective
    therefore use anticholinergics, e.g. Benzhexol,
    initially 2 mg 8-12 hourly
    then increase as necessary to 2-5 mg 6-8 hourly
    Effects may decline after 6 weeks treatment

PERIODIC PARALYSIS

Hypokalaemia

Attacks (Acute)
Potassium Chloride 5-10 g orally,
e.g. Slow K 9-18 tablets

Prophylaxis
Spironolactone 25 mg 6 hourly
    or Acetazolamide 250 mg 8-12 hourly
    or Hydrochlorthiazide 25 mg 8-12 hourly

Hyperkalaemia

Attacks (Acute)
Calcium Gluconate 1-2 g slowly i.v.

Prophylaxis
Acetazolamide 250 mg 8-12 hourly
    or Hydrochlorothiazide 25 mg 8-12 hourly

Normokalaemia

Attacks (Acute)
Sodium Chloride

Prophylaxis
Acetazolamide 250 mg 12 hourly
    and Fludrocortisone 0.1 mg daily

PERIPHERAL NEURITIS

The treatment is dependent upon the cause. Symptomatic treatment of paraesthesiae is usually unsatisfactory.

Guillain-Barre syndrome
For pain – Paracetamol 0.5-1.0 g, 4-6 hourly
   or Soluble Aspirin 300-900 mg 4-6 hourly
ACTH starting at 40 u i.m. daily
and reducing slowly according to response.

Diabetic neuropathy
Scrupulous diabetic control.

Deficiency or nutritional neuropathies
Alcoholic Neuropathy:
   Abstinence
   Thiamine injection 500 mg daily for 1 week
      then Vitamin B compound tablets 12 hourly
Sub-acute Combined Degeneration of the Cord:
(Vitamin B_{12} deficiency)
   Hydroxocobalamin injection 1000 μg daily for 1 week
      then Hydroxocobalamin injection 1000 μg weekly for 1 month
      then Hydroxocobalamin injection monthly for life.
Isoniazid Neuropathy:
(Pyridoxine Deficiency)
   Pyridoxine 50 mg 8 hourly

Collagen diseases
especially Polyarteritis nodosa or
Systemic Lupus Erythematosus
Prednisone starting at a daily dose up to 80 mg
and reducing slowly according to response.

Toxic neuropathies
e.g. Nitrofurantoin, Vincristine, disulphiram, lead, arsenic, or tri-ortho cresylphosphate.
Identify causative agent and stop.

Cryptogenic neuropathy
Refer to Neurologist

POLYMYOSITIS

Refer to Neurologist

RAISED INTRACRANIAL PRESSURE

either *Corticosteroids*
    Dexamethasone 10 mg i.m. stat then
                2-4 mg 6 hourly orally or i.m.
or occasionally *Hypertonic solutions*
    Mannitol 20% infused over 4-8 hours
or occasionally *Diuretics*
    Frusemide 40-80 mg orally daily

SPASMODIC TORTICOLLIS

either Diazepam 2-5 mg 8 hourly
    or Tetrabenazine 25 mg 12 hourly
        increasing by 25 mg every 3-4 days until effective or a dose of
        200 mg is reached
    or Haloperidol 1 mg 8-12 hourly
    or Thiopropazate 5 mg 8 hourly
and Analgesics, e.g. Aspirin 300-900 mg 6-8 hourly
    or Paracetamol 500-1000 mg 6-8 hourly

SPASTICITY

Diazepam 2-5 mg 8 hourly
    or Baclofen 5 mg 8 hourly
        increasing dose by 15 mg/day until effective or 60 mg per day.
    or Dantrolene 25 mg 12 hourly
        increasing dose gradually until effective or 100 mg 6 hourly.

STROKES

Prophylactic
Control hypertension
Anticoagulate if cause for thrombus formation present, e.g. mitral stenosis
Control cardiac dysrhythmias

Transient ischaemic attacks
Find cause and treat as appropriate
In the absence of hypertension
    In the carotid territory
    Warfarin 30 mg stat
    then Warfarin 3 mg 12 hourly for 2 days
    then Prothrombin time
    and adjust dose as necessary
    Continue treatment for one year, then stop to see effect.
        In vertebro-basilar territory
    only treat if frequent attacks affecting nuclei or long tracts.
    Then Warfarin as described above.
    Continue treatment for one year, then stop to see effect.

Completed stroke
Treat precipitating factors, e.g. hypertension
                                       polycythemia
                                       and any source of emboli
Start rehabilitation as soon as possible.

SUB-ACUTE COMBINED DEGENERATION OF THE SPINAL CORD

Hydroxycobalamin 1000 μg x 6 over 2-3 weeks
   and then 1000 μg every 3 months for life.

SUBARACHNOID HAEMORRHAGE

Establish diagnosis with lumbar puncture
Then refer to Neurosurgical Unit
(each patient is different)

SUBDURAL HAEMOTOMA

Always a difficult diagnosis
Treatment unsatisfactory in the elderly
If in doubt refer to Neurosurgical Unit

SYDENHAM'S CHOREA

Prophylactic Phenoxymethyl Penicillin 250 mg twice a day
   and if needed Tetrabenazine 25 mg 8 hourly
      increasing by 25 mg every 3-4 days
      to a maximum dose of 200 mg/day
   or Thiopropazate 5-10 mg 8 hourly

SYNCOPE

Find cause and treat as appropriate, e.g. Cardiac arrhythmia
                                          Autonomic neuropathy
                                          or anaemia
Explain mechanism
Avoid precipitating factors, e.g. suddenly getting up from a lying position.

Cough syncope
Stop smoking
Treat bronchitis etc. – *see* chapter on Respiratory Disease

Micturition syncope
Advise men to sit during micturition

TETANUS

Acute attack
Get expert help early.

To prevent toxin absorption
Either Human anti-tetanus immunoglobulin 30-300 iu/kg/im
   or if no reaction ½ hour after a test dose of 0.2 ml of a 1 in 10
   dilution s/c Equine tetanus antitoxin 10000 units i.m.
   and Surgical debridement to wound
Most patients need curarisation and positive pressure ventilation
until toxin no longer active – may be up to 3 weeks.
   and Diazepam as necessary to sedate
   and Penicillin 2 mega units 6 hourly for 5 days
     or Erythromycin 500 mg 6 hourly for 5 days
     or Tetracycline 250 mg 6 hourly for 5 days
   and control of other infections as appropriate
   and control of fluid balance
   and parenteral feeding as necessary
     then active immunisation

Prophylaxis

Active immunisation
either
   with Absorbed Toxoid (0.5 ml) x 2 at 4-6 week intervals
   then Absorbed Toxoid (0.5 ml) x 1 at 6-12 months
   then Absorbed Toxoid (0.5 ml) x 1 every 5-10 years

Or passive immunity NOT IF ACTIVELY IMMUNE
Used when tetanus prone injury
   either Human immunoglobulin 250-500 units i.m.
     plus 1 dose of tetanus toxoid (use a different syringe, needle
and site)
   or Equine antitoxin 0.1 ml s/c
If not untoward response then 1500 iu s/c
     plus first dose of toxoid (in different syringes, needles and sites)
   and either Phenoxymethyl Penicillin 250 mg 6 hourly for 5 days
   or Erythromycin 500 mg 6 hourly for 5 days
   or Tetracycline 250 mg 6 hourly for 5 days

THROMBOPHLEBITIS

Cortical

With fits
Anticonvulsants – *see* Status Epilepticus

With raised intercranial pressure
Dexamethasone 4-8 mg 6 hourly

Basal sinus
Chloramphenicol 600 mg 6 hourly i.v.
   or Gentamicin 8 hourly i.m. or i.v. – dose
     according to Mawer Nomogram (see p. 323)
and Metronidazole 400 mg 8 hourly orally
        or 500 mg 8 hourly i.v.
and Penicillin 3-4 mega units 6 hourly i.v.
   or Ampicillin 500 mg 6 hourly i.v.
   or Co-Trimoxazole 2-6 tablets 12 hourly orally
     or 10-15 ml diluted to 250-375 ml with 0.9%
     Sodium Chloride given as injection every 12 hours.

VERTIGO

Establish cause and treat as appropriate
See relevant heading for details

Symptomatic treatment
either Prochlorperazine 5-10 mg 8 hourly
   or Cyclizine 50 mg 8 hourly
   or Cinnarizine 15-30 mg 8 hourly
STOP treatment when Vertigo stops.

VESTIBULAR NEURONITIS

Symptomatic treatment only
either Prochlorperazine 5-10 mg 8 hourly
   or Cyclizine 50 mg 8 hourly
   or Cinnarizine 15-30 mg 8 hourly
Continue for 3 weeks and then gradually withdraw.

VITAMIN B. DEFICIENCY

Beriberi
Thiamine 25-100 mg daily by mouth or i.m. for one week
Then ensure regular intake of all vitamins.

Wernickes's encephalopathy
or Korsakoff's psychosis
Thiamine 25-100 mg daily by mouth or i.m. for one week
Then ensure regular intake of all vitamins.

WILSON'S DISEASE

Penicillamine 0.5-1 g 12 hourly
Dose is adjusted to maintain negative copper balance
  and Cation exchange resin
  or occasionally Dimercaprol.

FURTHER READING

Miller, H & Matthews W.B. (1975) *Textbook of Neurology* London:
Blackwell Scientific
Patten, J. (1977) *Neurological Differential Diagnosis* New York:
Springer Verlag

Psychiatry

In this chapter I describe psychiatric disorders from the physician's point of view. I have limited the therapy to a few simple remedies rather than to involve the large number of drugs that are available so that the non-expert can help the majority of patients he is likely to see. There will be patients who do not respond to these therapies and in this instance help of a professional psychiatrist should be sought.

ANOREXIA NERVOSA

Get support of family and/or friends
Bed rest
Chlorpromazine 50-500 mg daily
used in increasing dosage to allow eating to restart.
May need Orphenadrine 50-100 mg 8 hourly in addition to control side effects
GET EXPERT HELP – EARLY (Psychotherapy plays a major part in treatment).

ANXIETY

Establish cause and treat as appropriate
with either 'psychotherapy'
   or support
   or social help
If needed
Diazepam 2-5 mg 8 hourly
        and 2-20 mg at night
  or Chlordiazepoxide 5-10 mg 8 hourly
          and 10-50 mg at night
  or Diphenhydramine 10-25 mg 8 hourly
          and 25-50 mg at night
  or Amitriptyline 25-100 mg at night
In ALL cases reassess treatment after 7 days.
Best to give short repeated courses rather than prolonged therapy.

CONFUSION

Look for and treat cause
  e.g. Drugs   Anaemia
       Infections   Metabolic
       Dehydration Vascular

If this fails:
Chlorpromazine 10 to 25 mg orally 6 hourly
or
Chlorpromazine 25 to 100 mg intramuscularly
or in the elderly
Thioridazine 10 to 25 mg orally 4 to 6 hourly

DELIRIUM TREMENS

Sedate with either Diazepam 5-20 mg i.v.
then Diazepam 5 mg i.v. every 5 minutes if necessary
or Chlormethiazole 0.8% infusion 60-100 drops/minute,
adjusting drip rate as necessary to keep patient calm

When controlled
Diazepam 40 mg in 500 ml of Sodium Chloride 0.9% infused at a
rate needed to keep calm.
or Chlormethiazole 0.8% infusion to keep patient calm
or Chlorpromazine 100 mg i.m. repeated as necessary
and a Multivitamin preparation i.v.
and Maintain fluid and electrolyte balance
OBTAIN expert help.

DEPRESSION

Treat precipitating cause with either social help and/or
'pyschotherapy'

Mild
Supportive therapy only.

Moderate
Amitriptyline 25 mg 12 hourly then increasing dose every 2-3 days
by 25 mg with major dose being given at night up to 150 mg per
day.
or Imipramine (less sedative)
25 mg 12 hourly increasing every 2-3 days by 25 mg up to 150
mg per day.

If no response in 2-3 weeks:
Get Expert Help

If response:
Slowly reduce dose to maintenance level.

If first attack:
Consider stopping after a few weeks

If second or subsequent attack:
Continue therapy for months
and GET EXPERT HELP.

Severe (Suicidal)
either Amitriptyline 25 mg 12 hourly and increasing
   every 2-3 days by 25 mg with major dose being taken at night up
to 225 mg per day.
or Imipramine (less sedative)
   25 mg 12 hourly increasing every 2-3 days by
   25 mg up to 225 mg per day.
Get Expert Help AT ONCE – may need ECT

NB: WITH EITHER DRUG A DRY MOUTH INDICATES THERAPEUTIC
DOSAGE
There are many other alternatives, but it is best only to use a few
simple regimes unless you are an expert.

INSOMNIA

Look for and treat underlying cause
Determine normal pattern for each patient
Then establish routine to suit patients pattern of sleep
and avoid stimulants, e.g. coffee
and, but only as a last resort use
   either Diazepam 2-30 mg at night
   or Chloral hydrate 0.5-1.0 g (well diluted with water) at night
   or Triclofos 0.5-1.0 g at night
   or Dichloralphenazone 0.65-1.3 g at night
NB: THERE ARE MULTIPLE DRUGS THAT INDUCE SLEEP, BUT IT IS
     BEST TO USE THE SIMPLEST AND SAFEST.
WHEN SLEEP PATTERN RE-ESTABLISHED STOP TABLETS.

MANIC DEPRESSION

Acute
To control mania
   Haloperidol 5 mg i.m. repeated as necessary
     or Chlorpromazine 25-100 mg 6 hourly
   May need ECT

When controlled
   Haloperidol 1.5-3.0 mg daily
     or Chlorpromazine 25-100 mg 6 hourly
   and Lithium 900 mg for 1 day
   then Lithium 1200 mg for 1 day
   then Lithium 600-3000 mg per day depending on
   serum level (0.5-1.2 mmol/l) and clinical response.

When response
Reduce dose of Lithium to two thirds of maximum needed
AIM for once daily dosage and review regularly
Monitor serum levels frequently (0.5-1.2 mmol/l)

Prophylaxis
Lithium – maintain serum level between 0.5-1.2 mmol/l
usual dosage range needed 600-1500 mg per day.

Depressive episode
Continue Lithium and Amitriptyline 50-150 mg daily

ORGANIC BRAIN SYNDROME

Acute
Haloperidol 0.5 mg 12 hourly increasing dose as necessary.

Chronic
Chlorpromazine 25-100 mg 8 hourly
   or Diazepam 2-5 mg 8 hourly
Parenteral administration sometimes helpful.
Adjust dose in either case to control symptoms.

SCHIZOPHRENIA

Acute

Hyperactive
Chlorpromazine 25-100 mg 8 hourly
Change to once daily dose when dosage level determined

Underactive
Flupenthixol 3-9 mg 12 hourly
   or Trifluoperazine 4-30 mg daily
   or Thiothixene 10-30 mg daily
May need Orphenadrine 50-100 mg 8 hourly in addition to control
side effects.

Chronic
Find lowest dose of drug which maintains patient symptom free.
Consider using Fluopenthixol deconoate which is a long acting
agent given by i.m. injection.
OBTAIN EXPERT HELP.

FURTHER READING

Sargent, W. & Slater, E. (1973) *An Introduction to Physical Methods
   of Treatment in Psychiatry,* New York. Arrowson-Jason
Silverstone, T & Turner, P. (1974) *Drug Treatment in Psychiatry*
   London: Routledge.

Rheumatology

ANKYLOSING SPONDYLITIS

Maintain mobility
with daily exercise (under supervision)
and an active job (if possible)

Mild
Phenylbutazone 100-200 mg 8 hourly with meals
  or Indomethacin 25-50 mg 8 hourly with meals
either drug is used INTERMITTENTLY for 1-2 months at a time
when pain severe. Once ankylosis has occurred pain is no longer a
problem.
>   *rarely* Corticosteroids – usually intra-articularly in affected
>   peripheral joints
>   *rarely* Radiotherapy – *NB:* 10 fold increase in incidence of
>   leukaemia
>   *rarely* Surgery, e.g. hip replacement

When pain is bad at night or there is marked early morning
stiffness:
Indomethacin 75-100 mg taken with food on retiring
  or Indomethacin 100 mg suppository on retiring

CARPAL TUNNEL SYNDROME

Find cause and treat as appropriate, e.g. Myxoedema
Frusemide 40 mg daily
and Splints, particularly at night to relieve pain
  and Hydrocortisone injections locally
  or Surgery, to relieve compression on nerve.

DERMATOMYOSITIS

Look for underlying neoplasm.
Prednisone 50-80 mg daily until muscle enzymes normal
  then reduce the dose slowly to maintenance level, monitoring
  activity with serial muscle enzyme estimations.
Methotrexate may occasionally help.
BEWARE aspiration pneumonia secondary to pharyngeal muscle
involvement.

DISSEMINATED LUPUS ERYTHEMATOSIS (D.L.E.)

Exclude drug causes, e.g. Procainamide, Hydrallazine, Isoniazid, Anticonvulsants or Methyldopa.

Mild
Synovitis or Skin Disease
 Hydroxychloroquine 200 mg 8-12 hourly
  or Chloroquine Phosphate 250 mg 12-24 hourly
 Use SMALLEST EFFECTIVE dose
 Use for NO LONGER THAN 1 YEAR
NB: REGULAR OPHTHALMOLOGICAL TESTING IS
  NECESSARY – AT LEAST EVERY 3 MONTHS
 Occasionally:
 Aspirin 300-600 mg 4-8 hourly
NB: POSSIBLE INCREASED HEPATOTOXICITY IN D.L.E.

More severe
Prednisone initially 60-80 mg daily
 then reduce dose to lowest possible that controls symptoms.
 and occasionally:
 Azathioprine 2.5 mg/kg/day

Renal disease
When all else fails: Transplantation

ERYTHEMA NODOSUM

Find cause and treat as appropriate (Sarcoid, Streptococcal infection, Tuberculosis etc.)
Rest
Aspirin 300-600 mg 4-8 hourly
 and/or occasionally:
Prednisone 15-20 mg daily for a short period

GIANT CELL ARTERITIS

Prednisone 60 mg per day, initially.
Then, reduce dose to maintenance dose which keeps ESR less than 20mm/hr.
Continue therapy for 2-3 years.
Then, attempt to withdraw Prednisone, using ESR to assess activity.
NB: OFTEN ASSOCIATED WITH POLYMYALGIA RHEUMATICA (q.v.)

GOUT

Acute attack
Start treatment as early as possible
Maintain high fluid intake

and either Phenylbutazone 200 mg 6 hourly with food x 4
> then 100 mg 6 hourly with food x 4
> then 100 mg 8 hourly with food until attack better

or Indomethacin 50 mg 8 hourly with food until attack better
or Colchicine 1 mg stat
> 0.5 mg hourly or 2 hourly until better or diarrhoea
> or *total of 10 mg given*
> Followed by 0.5 mg 8 hourly to prevent relapse

or A.C.T.H. 100 units stat
followed by Colchicine 0.5 mg 8 hourly to prevent relapse

Prevention
Reduce to ideal body weight
Reduce alcohol intake
Only start DRUG THERAPY
> if Frequent attacks
> or Serum Uric Acid level more than 550 μmol/l
> or Renal damage
> or Tophi

NB: THERAPY IS FOR LIFE
Colchicine 0.5 mg 8 hourly for 2-3 months to prevent attacks which
may be precipitated by other drugs.
and Allopurinol 100-200 mg 8 hourly
(Inhibits Xanthine oxidase)
and/or a uricosuric agent
> either Probenecid 0.5-2.0 g daily
> or Sulphinpyrazone 50-400 mg daily
> Both drugs work better if the urine is Alkaline
> (use Sodium Bicarbonate or Potassium Citrate)
> Neither drug works in RENAL FAILURE

In Tophaceous Gout surgery is occasionally necessary.
Drugs may take many months to become effective.
NB: ASPIRIN IN LOW DOSES (LESS THAN 4 g PER DAY) CAUSES
URATE RETENTION AND OFFSETS THE ACTION OF THESE
DRUGS.
THEREFORE IT SHOULD BE AVOIDED.

Chronic hyperuricaemia or secondary hyperuricaemia
Find cause and treat as appropriate, e.g. stop thiazide therapy.
if symptoms
or evidence of organ damage
or serum uric acid levels more than 550 μmol/l
> Allopurinol 100-200 mg 8 hourly

When improvement occurs, reduce dose to 100 mg 8 hourly.

HAEMOPHILIA

Acute haemarthrosis
bed rest
splint joint in position of function
replace anti-haemophiliac globulin (Factor VIII)
with either anti-haemophiliac globulin
   or Cryoprecipitate
   or Fresh frozen plasma
   enough to give 15-30 units of factor VIII per kilogram per day.
When factor VIII level restored
Aspirate Joint
Physiotherapy to maintain mobility and prevent muscle weakness.

Chronic haemarthrosis
physiotherapy to maintain mobility and strengthen muscles thereby
preventing deformity.
splinting if necessary, to prevent deformity and maintain position of
function.
avoid surgery.

INFECTIVE ARTHRITIS

Aspirate joint fluid for bacterial culture
Culture blood (positive in 25%)
Relieve pain using either Aspirin 300-900 mg 4-8 hourly
     or Soluble Aspirin 300-900 mg 4-8 hourly
  or Ibuprofen 400 mg 8 hourly
     or Fenoprofen 300-600 mg 6-8 hourly
  or Phenylbutazone 100-200 mg 8 hourly with food
     or Indomethacin 25-50 mg 8 hourly with food
  or Pethidine 50 mg 8 hourly
     or Morphine 10 mg 8 hourly
     or Diamorphine 5 mg 8 hourly
Reducing the dose when infection is better.
Rest joint in position of function with splints if necessary.
If on long term steroids may need to increase dosage.

Treat with Appropriate antibiotics (See Table 1, pp. 84 and 85)
Before bacteriological result available start treatment with:
   Benzyl Penicillin 2 mega units 6 hourly
  or Cephaloridine 500 mg 8-12 hourly
When laboratory results available, reassess therapy:
   patient better; continue therapy
   patient not better, or worse, change to antibiotic suggested by
   laboratory result.
When inflammation settled reduce analgesia and start
physiotherapy to mobilise joint and rehabilitate muscles.
Allow weight bearing when joint no longer swollen or tender.
NB: SURGICAL DRAINAGE MAY BE NECESSARY
   (Especially when disease advanced or thick pus in joint)

Table 1 Suggested antibiotics for infective arthritis

Organism	ADULTS 1st Choice	2nd Choice	Comments
Gonococcus	Benzyl Penicillin 10-20 mega units/day i.v. for 3 days. then Amoxycillin 0.5 g 8 hourly for 5 days		Expert help needed
Meningococcus	Benzyl Penicillin 1-3 mega units 6 hourly	Cephaloridine	
Brucella	Tetracycline 500 mg 6 hourly. +Streptomycin 1 g daily	Co-Trimoxazole	Treatment should be continued for 3 or 4 weeks.
Tuberculosis	INAH 300 mg + Rifampicin less than 50 kilograms 450 mg daily more than 50 kilograms 600 mg daily + Streptomycin less than 40 years – 1 g daily more than 40 years – 0.75 g daily or Ethambutol 15 mg/kg/day		All drugs being taken together ½ an hour before breakfast. After 4-8 weeks therapy continue with INAH and Rifampicin alone unless sensitivities suggest other therapy. Surgery may be needed. Therapy should be continued for at least 9 months.
Treponema pallidum	Procaine Penicillin 1 mega unit daily × 21.		usually *non* painful. Expert help needed.
Rubella	None	None	Usually responds to Aspirin alone.

Table 1 (contd.)

	1st Choice	2nd Choice	Comments
Mumps	None	None	Usually responds to Aspirin alone.
Actinomycosis	Benzyl Penicillin 1-3 mega units 6 hourly for 5 days.		Usually spread from soft tissue injury.

NEONATES

Organism	1st Choice	2nd Choice	Comments
Staphylococci	Cloxacillin + Gentamicin 2-3 mg/kg/12 hourly		GET EXPERT HELP
Gram negative or unknown	Cloxacillin 30 mg/kg/day + Gentamicin 2-3 mg/kg/12 hourly		GET EXPERT HELP

INFANTS

| Haemophillus influenzae | Ampicillin 40-100 mg/kg/6 hourly | | |

OSTEOARTHROSIS

Reassure, not a crippling disease
Reduce work of joints
  if obese reduce weight
Correct abnormal use (often induced by pain)
Avoid excess use
  – change job
  – change way of doing things
  – do not 'walk the pain off'
Use aid, e.g. walking stick, early.
Increase stability of joints with physiotherapy
Analgesia

Prophylactically half an hour before painful activity
either Aspirin 300-900 mg
   or Paracetamol 500 mg to 1 g
   or Dihydrocodeine 30 mg
   or Benorylate 750-2250 mg

Occasionally to relieve pain
either Aspirin 300-900 mg
   or Paracetamol 500 mg-1 g
   or Dihydrocodeine 30 mg
   or Benorylate 750-2250 mg 8-12 hourly
   or Indomethacin 75-100 mg orally with food (also useful on
     retiring for relief of night pain).
   or Indomethacin 100 mg suppositories (also useful on retiring for
     relief of night pain).

Regular dosage
either Aspirin 300-900 mg 8 hourly
    or Soluble Aspirin 300-900 mg 8 hourly
   or Ibuprofen 400 mg 6-8 hourly
    or Fenoprofen 300-600 mg 6-8 hourly
   or Indomethacin 25-50 mg with food 8 hourly
    or Phenylbutazone 100-200 mg with food 8 hourly

Local therapy
Occasionally local injection of Hydrocortisone into the affected joint
helps.
Splinting – to relieve pain.
Surgery: Osteotomy
  Joint replacement
  Rarely arthrodesis

OSTEOMYELITIS

Acute
Bed rest
Cloxacillin 1 g 6 hourly
and Benzyl Penicillin 2 mega units 6 hourly
Stop the inappropriate antibiotics when sensitivities known

Chronic
Erythromycin 0.5-1 g 6 hourly
and Sodium Fusidate 500 mg 8 hourly
    or Clindamycin 300 mg 6 hourly
Change therapy according to laboratory sensitivities
Continue therapy for 10 days
Surgery is often needed.

POLYARTERITIS NODOSA

Prednisone 60-80 mg per day, then reduce dose to lowest amount
possible to avoid symptoms.
Treat complications, e.g. hypertension as appropriate.

POLYMYALGIA RHEUMATICA

Prednisone 10-15 mg daily
Then reduce dose to maintenance dose, which keeps the ESR less
than 20 mm/hr.
Continue therapy for 2-3 ye rs, then attempt to withdraw using ESR
to assess activity.
May be associated with giant cell arteritis. (q.v.)

PSORIATIC ARTHRITIS

Treat joints separately from skin
First
either Aspirin 300-900 mg 4-8 hourly
    or Soluble Aspirin 300-900 mg 4-8 hourly
  or Ibuprofen 400 mg 8 hourly
    or Fenoprofen 300-600 mg 6-8 hourly
  or Indomethacin 25-50 mg 8 hourly
    or Phenylbutazone 100-200 mg 8 hourly
Then if fails
add Gold (Sodium Aurothiomalate)
    Initially 10 mg i.m. weekly, increasing by 10 mg weekly up to 50 mg
    weekly.
    Continue with 50 mg i.m. weekly to a total of 750 mg

D

Then, if benefit and no adverse reaction, continue same dose monthly.

NB: STOP IF ANY TOXIC SYMPTOMS.
TEST URINE AND CHECK PLATELETS AND WHITE CELLS BEFORE EACH INJECTION, OR CHANGE IN TREATMENT (AT LEAST MONTHLY)
STOP IF PROTEINURIA OR THROMBOCYTOPENIA OR LEUKOPENIA
IF INDUCES RASH – STOP TRY TO RE-ESTABLISH THERAPY LATER.

ANTIMALARIALS ARE CONTRAINDICATED BECAUSE THEY MAY EXACERBATE THE SKIN DISEASE

Then if both fail

Corticosteroids occasionally help – use lowest possible dose.
  or Rarely cytotoxic agents
(Methotrexate might help both skin and joint disease).

PYROPHOSPHATE ARTHROPATHY

Aspirate joint and identify crystals.
If large joint, e.g. knee
  intra-articular steroids
Otherwise only treat symptoms.
Either Aspirin 300-900 mg 8 hourly
    or Soluble Aspirin 300-900 mg 8 hourly
  or Ibuprofen 400 mg 6-8 hourly
    or Fenoprofen 300-600 mg 6-8 hourly
  or Indomethacin 25-50 mg 8 hourly
    or Phenylbutazone 100-200 mg 8 hourly

REITER'S SYNDROME

Joints
Bed rest
Light splinting to relieve pain
Physiotherapy to prevent wasting
Joint aspiration with or without Corticosteroid instillation
Aspirin 300-900 mg 8 hourly
  or Indomethacin 25-50 mg 8 hourly
  or Phenylbutazone 100-200 mg 8 hourly
  or rarely Prednisone in minimal dosage

Non-specific urethritis
Tetracycline 500 mg 6 hourly for 10 days
Both the PATIENT and CONSORT

Conjunctivitis if evidence of infection
either Sulphacetamide eye drops 10% 2 hourly
  or Chloramphenicol eye drops 0.5% 2 hourly
Until fully cleared.

Iritis
Atropine eye drops 1% – to keep pupil dilated
  and Hydrocortisone eye drops – to reduce inflammation
Get expert help

Skin – Keratoderma blennorrhagica
Keep clean
No specific therapy

RHEUMATOID ARTHRITIS

Early disease
Once diagnosis established, control pain with:
Aspirin 300-900 mg 4-8 hourly
    or Soluble Aspirin 300-900 mg 4-8 hourly
  or Ibuprofen 400 mg 8 hourly
    or Fenoprofen 300-600 mg 6-8 hourly
    or Indomethacin 25-50 mg 8 hourly
    or Phenylbutazone 100-200 mg 8 hourly
There are now many compounds being produced with benefit to
some patients, e.g. Naproxen, Allofenac and Fenoprofen. It is
worthwhile trying these if pain is not controlled using the drugs
suggested here.
Continue to keep active.
Consider surgery (see later)

Acute attack
Bed rest until disease controlled
NB: MAINTAIN GOOD POSTURE IN BED
Splints to affected joints – to relieve pain – to keep in position of
function
Exercises to prevent muscle wasting.
Drugs as outlined above to control pain

If fails, and:
Disease still active – high ESR, joints inflamed, erosion on X-ray
Assess initial drug regime as outlined above and increase if possible.
Then consider second line drugs:
  Gold (Sodium Aurothiomalate) initially 10 mg i.m. weekly, then
    increased by 10 mg per week up to 50 mg weekly.
  Continue 50 mg weekly, to a total dose of 750mg
  Then if benefit and no adverse reaction, continue with same dose
  monthly.
NB: STOP IF ANY TOXIC SYMPTOMS
    TEST URINE, CHECK PLATELETS AND WHITE CELLS BEFORE
    EACH INJECTION OR CHANGE IN TREATMENT (AT LEAST
    MONTHLY)
    STOP IF PROTEINURIA OR THROMBOCYTOPENIA OR
    LEUKOPENIA
    IF INDUCES RASH STOP AND TRY TO RE-ESTABLISH
    TREATMENT LATER

Middle disease
Low grade activity
Analgesia as outlined above
and Hydroxychloroquine 200 mg 8-12 hourly
    reducing to 200 mg 12-24 hourly for maintenance therapy.
    Stop after one year
  or Choloroquine Phosphate 250 mg 12-24 hourly.
NB: MAY TAKE 2-3 MONTHS TO BECOME EFFECTIVE
    REGULAR OPHTHALMOLOGICAL CHECKS ARE NEEDED AT
    LEAST EVERY 3 MONTHS.
    STOP AFTER 1 YEAR AND REASSESS.

Established chronic active disease (When Gold has failed)
Penicillamine 125 mg a day increasing by 125 mg every month until
a daily dose of 750 mg reached.
Once effect obtained reduce dose slowly and then maintain on half
the dose which produced maximum benefit.
NB: MAY TAKE 2-3 MONTHS TO BE EFFECTIVE
    TEST URINE, CHECK PLATELETS AND WHITE CELLS AT EACH
    VISIT OR CHANGE IN THERAPY (AT LEAST MONTHLY).
    STOP IF PROTEINURIA PRESENT

Disease still active – despite 1st and 2nd line drugs
Prednisone – not more than 7.5 mg per day
  BEST USED FOR SHORT PERIODS ONLY
  Give 5 mg at night for maximum benefit
  Consider alternate day use
NB: GIVES IMMEDIATE BENEFIT, BUT LONG TERM
    COMPLICATIONS
or local Hydrocortisone after joint aspiration
or ACTH 10-20 units daily (use lowest dose possible)
or Tetracosactrin 0.1-0.2 mg daily or alternate days (use lowest
    dose possible, with maximum of 1 mg per week).
Review therapy regularly and STOP as soon as possible.

Disease severe – and unresponsive to other therapy
Try:
  Azathioprine 1.5-2.0 mg/kg/day
  or Cyclophosphamide 1.5-2.0 mg/kg/day
NB: MAY ALSO ALLOW PREDNISONE DOSE TO BE REDUCED
    CHECK PLATELETS AND WHITE CELL COUNT AT FREQUENT
    INTERVALS
  or Synovectomy
    either surgical
    or medical – Radioactive Yttrium into joint

Late stage disease
Continue analgesic drugs as outlined above to control pain
Maintain splints to affected joints – to relieve pain and to keep in
  position of function.

Treat any deformity with splinting and consider surgery if splinting
fails.
Keep as mobile as possible.
Help to modify life style if necessary
   at home
   at work
   at play

Inactive disease with deformity
Serial splinting
and/or Surgery

Surgery
Should be considered both early and late in the disease.
Early: synovectomy, which if done before advanced joint destruction,
   relieves symptoms and improves function.
   Surgery is also useful in prevention and early correction of
   deformity.
Late disease
Surgery is of use in correcting established deformity that does not
   respond to splinting

SCLERODERMA

Maintain function as much as possible
Analgesia as necessary, e.g. Aspirin 300-900 mg 4-8 hourly
In early stages with progressive disease:
   Avoid Cold
   Treat respiratory infection early
   Treat hypertension early
   Try treating steatorrhoea with
      Tetracycline 250 mg 6 hourly
Rarely with rapidly progressive skin disease or synovitis
      Prednisone 60 mg/day might help
      If effective, reduce dose slowly to lowest possible
      If not effective, reduce dose gradually and then stop.
   Occasionally:
   Penicillamine 125 mg a day increasing by 125 mg every month
      until daily dose of 750 mg reached.
      Once effect obtained reduce dose slowly and then maintain at
      lowest dose which continues to control the disease (often about
      ½ maximum dose used).
      MAY TAKE 2-3 MONTHS TO BE EFFECTIVE
      TEST URINE, CHECK PLATELETS AND WHITE COUNT AT EACH
      VISIT OR CHANGE OF THERAPY (AT LEAST MONTHLY).

SJOGREN'S SYNDROME

Treat joints as for rheumatoid arthritis
SYSTEMIC STEROIDS ARE NOT INDICATED
Local treatment to eyes:
  Either Artificial Tears
    0.3% or 1% Methyl Cellulose
  or 1% Gelatin
  or Local Hydrocortisone
    0.5-2% 3-6 times a day
  or Surgery
    to obliterate lacrimal duct.

SOFT TISSUE SYNDROMES (Non Articular Rheumatism)

Avoid precipitating factors.
  Then Aspirin 300-900 mg 4-8 hourly
  and Hydrocortisone injection into the area of maximal tenderness
    and/or Rest with or without splints
    and/or Local heat
    and/or Methyl Salicylate Liniment
        with massage

STILL'S DISEASE

Joint symptoms
Bed rest – during acute active phase only
and Splinting – to prevent deformity
              – to correct deformity
and Physiotherapy – to maintain joint function
                  – to prevent wasting
and either Aspirin 40-100 mg/kg/day according to clinical
  response (aim at serum level of 30 mg/100 ml)
      or Soluble Aspirin 40-100 mg/kg/day
      or Ibuprofen 20 mg/kg/day
        NB: IF CHILD LESS THAN 30 kg NOT MORE THAN
        500 mg PER DAY
      or Indomethacin 1.0-2.5 mg/kg/day
If fails:
  GET EXPERT HELP and either Gold (Sodium Aurothiomalate)
    Less than 6 years old 10 mg weekly x 10-20
    >6 years old 20 mg weekly x 20
If improvement:- continue with maintenance injection every 2-4
weeks depending on the activity of the disease.
STOP IF ANY TOXIC SYMPTOMS
CHECK URINE, PLATELETS AND WHITE CELLS AT EACH VISIT (AT
LEAST MONTHLY) AND CHANGE OF DOSAGE
STOP IF PROTEINURIA OR CHANGES IN HAEMATOLOGY.

or Chloroquine 100-200 mg daily for 6-12 months
NB: OPHTHALMALOGICAL CHECKS MUST BE MADE AT LEAST
   EVERY 3 MONTHS
or Penicillamine:-

Weeks of therapy	less than 20 kg	More than 20kg
0 - 2	50 mg/day	100 mg/day
2 - 4	100 mg/day	200 mg/day
4 - 6	200 mg/day	300 mg/day
6 - 10	300 mg/day	450 mg/day
10 - 14	450 mg/day	600 mg/day

Use minimum dose that will control disease
MAY TAKE SEVERAL WEEKS OR MONTHS TO BE EFFECTIVE
CHECK URINE, PLATELETS AND WHITE CELLS AT EACH VISIT AND
CHANGE IN THERAPY (AT LEAST MONTHLY).
STOP IF PROTEINURIA, THROMBOCYTOPENIA OR LEUKOPENIA

Severe generalised disease or progressive joint disease
Prednisone in minimal dosage for shortest possible time.
NB: CAUSES GROWTH RETARDATION, EVEN IN ALTERNATE DAY
   DOSAGE.

FURTHER READING

Boyle, J.A. & Watson Buchanan, W. (1978) *Clinical Rheumatology* London: Blackwell Scientific
Copeman, W.S.C. (ed.) (1978) *Textbook of Rheumatic Disease* Edinburgh: Churchill Livingstone
Mason, M. & Currey, M.L.F. (1976) *Introduction to Clinical Rheumatology* Tunbridge Wells: Pitman Medical
Medical Education (International) Ltd. (1979) *Medicine* (Third series) Nos. 12 & 13
Pearson, C. & Carson Dick, W. (1975) Current management of rheumatoid arthritis. In *Clinics in the Rheumatic Disease,* August 1975 London: W.B. Saunders

Endocrinology and metabolism

ADRENAL DISEASE

Corticosteroid insufficiency (Hypotension. Low serum sodium. High serum potassium.)

PRIMARY

Acute (Addisonian Crisis)
0.9% Sodium Chloride i.v. ½-1 litre as quickly as possible. Then volume and rate of administration according to degree of dehydration and cardiovascular state.
and Hydrocortisone sodium succinate 100 mg i.v.
    then 50 mg i.m. 6 hourly.
and If total adrenal failure
add Aldosterone 1 mg i.v. or i.m.
    or Deoxycorticosterone acetate 5 mg in oil i.m.

Chronic:
Hydrocortisone 20 mg b.d.
    Reducing to 20 mg each morning and 10 mg at night after a few weeks.
And Fludrocortisone 0.1 mg daily

The doses need to be assessed individually using blood pressure, urea and electrolytes as indices of control. The measurement of plasma cortisol levels if available is also very helpful. The dosage should be adjusted so that the plasma level has a peak value of 700-970 mmol/l (25-35µg/100 ml) after the morning dose, a value of 160 mmol/l (6 µg/100 ml) just before the evening dose with a peak value of 320-480 mmol/l (12-17 µg/100 ml) after the evening dose.

In times of stress: more Hydrocortisone will be needed.
minor febrile illnesses
    double dose and continue until afebrile.
vomiting (unable to retain tablets)
    Hydrocortisone sodium succinate 100 mg i.v. or i.m. and then 50 mg i.m. 6 hourly until able to take tablets.
pregnancy
    maintain usual therapy.
labour
    Hydrocortisone 50 mg i.m. 6 hourly until delivered.
surgery

Hydrocortisone sodium succinate 100 mg i.v. or i.m. with the premedication, then:
50 mg i.v. or i.m. 6 hourly until able to resume oral therapy.

THERAPY IS NECESSARY FOR LIFE

SECONDARY

Acute (usually due to stopping steroid therapy or 'stress')
Hydrocortisone sodium succinate 100 mg i.v.
   then 50 mg i.m. 6 hourly until able to take oral therapy.
and 0.9% Sodium Chloride infusion, the quantity and rate of
   infusion being determined by the degree of dehydration and the
   cardiovascular state of the patient.
and Treatment of the precipitating cause if possible.

Chronic:
Hydrocortisone 20 mg each morning and 10 mg each night
NO Fludrocortisone is needed as Aldosterone still produced
Hydrocortisone therapy should be monitored as outlined on p. 94

In times of stress:
minor febrile illness
if due to infection treat with appropriate antibiotic.
if maintenance dose is less than 40 mg of Hydrocortisone per day,
   double dose until afebrile.
if maintenance dose greater than 40 mg of Hydrocortisone per day,
   probably no need to change the dose, but watch the blood pressure.

surgery
Maintenance dose less than 40 mg of Hydrocortisone per day.
   Hydrocortisone sodium succinate 100 mg i.v. or i.m. with the
   premedication
then 50 mg i.m. 6 hourly until able to take oral medication
Maintenance more than 40 mg of Hydrocortisone per day double
   dose until convalescent.

NB: THESE REGIMES SHOULD BE FOLLOWED IN ANY PATIENT
   WHO HAS HAD EITHER STEROID THERAPY OR ACTH WITHIN
   THE LAST YEAR OR IN THE PAST FOR A YEAR OR LONGER.

Steroid withdrawal
The rate of withdrawal depends on the peak dose and the length of
treatment. The higher or longer the slower the rate of withdrawal
should be.
During withdrawal, Note:
Relapse of the disease for which therapy is given
   and/or Evidence of hypoadrenalism (hypotension, low serum
   sodium and high potassium).
Unless only on treatment for a short time reduce dosage of
Prednisone each month by 2.5 mg per day until on 7.5 mg per day
(unless relapse).

Then after another month reduce by 1.5 mg per day (unless relapse).

Then reduce each month by 1 mg per day (unless relapse), until on 3 mg per day.

Then check residual adrenal function.

If not present or minimal continue same dose for 3 months and then repeat assessment.

If adrenal activity present:

Reduce by 1 mg per day every 2 months until off treatment (or relapse).

NB: ALTERNATE DAY THERAPY CAUSES LESS ADRENAL SUPPRESSION THAN DAILY DOSAGE, BUT DOES NOT ALWAYS CONTROL THE UNDERLYING DISEASE AS WELL. THERAPY GIVEN AT 8.00 AM CAUSES LESS ADRENAL SUPPRESSION THAN EVENING DOSES.

Throughout this section on withdrawal of corticosteroids the dosage has been that appropriate to Prednisone or Prednisolone and these are the drugs most commonly used in corticosteroid therapy. The following table gives the comparative dosage of other cortiscosteroids using their anti-inflammatory activity:

Prednisone 5 mg
Prednisolone 5 mg
Hydrocortisone 20 mg
Cortisone 25 mg
Triamcinolone 4 mg
Dexamethasone 0.8 mg
Betamethasone 0.6 mg

Cortisosteroid excess: Cushing's Syndrome (Hypertension, Moon face, high midnight cortisol level).
BEST INVESTIGATED AND TREATED IN SPECIALIZED UNIT.

PRIMARY
If severe Amino-Glutethimide 250 mg 8 hourly for a few weeks will temporarily reduce the cortisol level (by reducing adrenal synthesis) which may be useful before definitive treatment can be under taken.

Adenoma or Hyperplasia
Surgery with corticosteroid 'cover':
Hydrocortisone 100 mg 6 hourly i.m. on the day of operation
then hydrocortisone 75 mg 6 hourly i.m. for two days
then hydrocortisone 50 mg 6 hourly i.m. or orally for 3 days
then slowly reduce over a few weeks to 60 mg per day, then more slowly to 30 mg per day.
and Fludrocortisone 0.1 mg per day.
or Metyrapone 3 g/day
then, surgery

Carcinoma
Surgery if possible with cover as above
or Mitotane (op'DDD) 3 g daily initially, gradually increasing to
maximum dose tolerated. (Up to 15 g per day).
If serum cortisol level reduced at tolerated dose give
Dexamethasone. DO NOT reduce dose of Mitotane.
If serum cortisol level not reduced at maximum tolerated dose add
Aminoglutethimide 250 mg 8 hourly.
or Metyrapone 3 g/day
then Surgery

SECONDARY
a. Iatrogenic
Review need for treatment and reduce dose of corticosteroid if at all
possible.
b. Pituitary or Hypothalamic over-activity
(i) no obvious tumour
Surgery to pituitary with steroid 'cover' as described above.
or External irradiation (proton beam)
+ Metyrapone 3 g/day
or Radioactive implantation (Gold or Yttrium)
+ Metyrapone 3 g/day
or Bilateral adrenalectomy with corticosteroid 'cover' and life long
replacement as described above.
+ Pituitary irradiation to prevent Nelson's Syndrome. (excess
ACTH)
(ii) obvious tumour (usually invasive)
Surgery to pituitary with steroid 'cover' as described above.
and External irradiation
+ Metyrapone 3 g /day
If this fails to control Cushing's Syndrome and the pituitary tumour
is contained, bilateral adrenalectomy with conticosteroid 'cover' and
replacement as described above may be beneficial.
c. Ectopic ACTH Production (pigmentation, oedema, diabetes, low
serum potassium)
Remove primary tumour if possible
or Metyrapone 3 g per day
or Aminoglutethimide 250 mg 8 hourly
or Spironolactone 400 mg daily
with or without potassium supplements
or RARELY if prognosis otherwise very good, bilateral
adrenalectomy.

Aldosterone excess (hypertension and hypokalaemia)

Adenoma
Surgery

Bilateral hyperplasia
Spironolactone 50-100 mg 6 hourly reducing once hypertension is controlled to maintenance level, but therapy needs to be continued indefinitely.
   or RARELY bilateral adrenalectomy (under corticosteroid cover) see above

Phaeochromocytoma (paroxysmal hypertension and raised catecholamine levels)

Adenoma

   Acute attack
   1. Hypertension – Phentolamine 5 mg i.v. repeated as necessary
   2. Tachycardia – Propranolol 2.5 mg i.v.

   Definitive therapy
Surgery after adequate medical preparation which should precede angiography if this is contemplated.
Phenoxybenzamine 10 mg 6 hourly increasing to 200 mg daily as an alpha sympathetic blocker and
Propranolol 40-160 mg 6 hourly to control pulse rate as a beta sympathetic blocker.
NB: 1. DOSES ARE INCREASED UNTIL BLOOD PRESSURE IS CONTROLLED.
      2. THERAPY SHOULD BE ESTABLISHED AT LEAST TWO WEEKS BEFORE ANGIOGRAPHY AND SURGERY TO ALLOW REPLETION OF THE BLOOD VOLUME.
         LIAISON WITH THE ANAESTHETIST IS ESSENTIAL (CYCLOPROPANE AND TRICHLORETHYLENE ARE BEST AVOIDED DURING SURGERY).

Inoperable tumour or metastases
Alpha and beta sympathetic blockade as outlined above and Alpha-Methyl Tyrosine 2.5-3.5 g per day. (not commercially available)

BONE DISEASE

Hypercalcaemia
Rehydration (essential and always first)
and Frusemide 40-120 mg (not Thiazide)
then establish diagnosis.

Hyperparathyroid
See later, p. 107.

Non-hyperparathyroid
Prednisone 40 mg daily
Then adjust dose to control serum calcium level
if fails:

Get EXPERT help
and consider Sodium Phosphate 0.75 mmol/kg over 8-12 hours
or Mithramycin 25 μg/kg/day i.v.
(BOTH ARE DANGEROUS AND SHOULD ONLY BE USED WITH
EXPERT ADVICE)

Hypocalcaemia

Acute
Calcium Gluconate 10% 20 ml i.v.

Severe symptoms
Calcium Gluconate 20% 100 ml diluted with 1 litre
Dextrose 5% and infused over 12-24 hours.
Repeat as necessary

Osteomalacia

Nutritional deficiency
Tabs. Calcium Vitamin D BPC 2, 8 hourly

Renal osteodystrophy
Get Expert help.
1 α Hydroxycholecalciferol 1 μg daily

Malabsorption
Correct underlying condition (if possible)
then Tabs Calcium Vitamin D BPC 2, 8 hourly

Post gastrectomy
Tabs Calcium Vitamin D BPC 2, 8 hourly

Osteoporosis

Pain
Aspirin 300-600 mg 4-6 hourly
or Paracetamol 0.5-1.0 g 4-6 hourly
and Physiotherapy

Paget's disease

Pain
Paracetamol 0.5-1.0 g 4-6 hourly
or Dihydrocodeine 30-60 mg 6 hourly

Pain uncontrolled and disease active (Alkaline Phosphatase and
Urinary Hydroxyproline increased)
add Salmon Calcitonin 100 MRC units s/c x 3 per week
Stop after 12 weeks (since maximum pain relief by this time)
If fails:
Get EXPERT help.

DIABETES

'Juvenile' (Insulin dependant or Ketone prone) type

Diet
With enough calories to allow growth and maintain a weight appropriate to the patient. The calories should be distributed throughout the day in a manner which the patient can follow regularly so that Insulin dosage can be adjusted accurately.

Insulin
The dose of Insulin needs to be tailored to each patient.
NB: 1. Initially diabetic control is best obtained using either Isophane or Soluble Insulin and twice daily injections. The renal threshold should if possible be established for all patients so that the urine can be used to monitor therapy.
   2. Urine should be collected using a double voiding technique (pass urine and discard, pass urine as soon as possible and test), so that it reflects more closely the blood sugar at the time of collection. The patient should be taught to test their urine first thing in the morning, after breakfast, lunch and the evening meal and again before going to bed. The results of the tests should be recorded and are used to monitor therapy. Initial therapy should be 20 units of Insulin before breakfast and 10 units before the evening meal. Every 4 or 5 days the Insulin dosage should be adjusted according to the results of urine testing. Once control appears to have been obtained a switch can be made to long acting Insulin, e.g. Lente Insulin, usually on a unit for unit basis, but best control is obtained by continuing twice daily injections. Having established apparent control a blood sugar series throughout the day should be estimated to ensure optimum control.
   3. If more than 50 units of long acting Insulin are required it would be preferable to continue with twice daily injections to obtain better control.
   4. If less than 20 units of Insulin required per day, alternative means of therapy, particularly in the elderly, might be possible but not necessarily better.

Pregnancy

Antenatal
Rigid control is essential to keep fetal loss to a minimum
Keep RANDOM blood sugar less than 8.5 mmol/l
Admit at 32 weeks, then maintain random blood sugar at less than 5.5. mmol/l
This requires strict control of diet, and
   twice daily Soluble Insulin almost always with
   Isophane Insulin
NB: Renal threshold falls in 20 per cent of patients and therefore blood sugar measurements are essential.

Labour
Night before delivery: normal dose of Insulin
Morning of delivery: Breakfast as usual and start i.v. infusion of
Dextrose 10 per cent 10 g per hour and Insulin 1.5, 3 or 7 units per
hour
Measure blood sugar hourly and adjust Insulin infusion rate as
necessary.
Maintain blood sugar between 4 and 6 mmol/l.

Post delivery
Continue Insulin and Dextrose infusion until the next morning.
Then return to PRE PREGNANCY regime.
Later, adjust as necessary.

Surgery
Either half normal dose of Insulin on morning of surgery and infuse
10% glucose throughout operation.
  or Infuse Insulin at 1-5 units per hour and maintain fluid balance.
  or (if low dose) omit Insulin on day of surgery
      Check blood sugar regularly
      Restart Insulin next morning
NB: ONLY DANGER IS UNRECOGNISED HYPOGLYCAEMIA

Ketoacidosis/Coma
Fluid replacement (a central venous pressure measurement might
be helpful).
Start with 0.9% Sodium Chloride 1 litre in 30 minutes
then if:
serum sodium less than 155 mmol/l: continue with 0.9% Sodium
  chloride 1 litre per hour for 4 hours.
orserum sodium more than 155 mmol/l: continue with 0.45%
  Sodium chloride 1 litre per hour until serum sodium less than
  155 mmol/l then 0.9% Sodium chloride 1 litre per hour.
In either instance when blood glucose less than 14.0 mmol/l
change to 5% Dextrose 1 litre in 2 hours and continue until
rehydrated.
Add Potassium 13 mmol (1 g KCL = 13.4 mmol potassium) to each
litre but observe the following rules:
If serum potassium more than 6.0 mmol/l STOP potassium
  infusion.
If serum potassium more than 5.0 mmol/l reduce potassium
• infusion to 6.5 mmol/l.
If serum potassium less than 4.0 mmol/l increase potassium
  infusion to 26.0 mmol/l.
If serum potassium less than 3.0 mmol/l increase potassium
  infusion to 39.0 mmol/l.
Maximum rate of infusion should not exceed 98 mmol/hr.
Continue potassium replacement for several days after stopping
  intravenous therapy.

Insulin:

Initially 20 units of Soluble or Act-Rapid Insulin i.m. If hypotensive
10 units i.v. and 10 units i.m.

then 5 units i.m. per hour
or 2-6 units i.v. hourly using an infusion pump.

When blood glucose has fallen to 14.0 mmol/l change to sliding
scale s/c Insulin according to urine concentration measured every 4
hours,

e.g. urine concentration 2% – 28 units   1% – 16 units   ½% – 8 units

With an additional 4 units if the urine contains ketones.

NB: Also need:

TO EMPTY STOMACH IF PATIENT UNCONSCIOUS – because of
gastric dilatation and ileus and consequent risk of inhalation.

TO MAINTAIN AIRWAY IF PATIENT UNCONSCIOUS.

LOOK for precipitating cause, e.g. infection, heart attack or
stroke.

CATHETERISE IF NECESSARY to get urine samples.

CONSIDER HEPARIN if risk of thrombosis high, e.g. elderly
and/or deeply unconscious patient.

Non-ketotic hyperosmolar coma

Treat as for ketotic coma

except Start with 0.45% sodium chloride solution until serum
sodium less than 155 mmol/l

Heparinise unless contra-indicated to prevent disseminated
intravascular coagulation or deep venous thrombosis.

NB: It is wise to monitor central venous pressure especially in the
elderly.

Maturity onset

Obese:

Diet – low calories to ensure weight loss (until ideal weight
obtained).

If weight loss not obtained and diabetes not controlled add
Metformin 0.5-1.5 g daily

If still uncontrolled change to Insulin

NB: DRUGS SHOULD ONLY BE USED IN OBESE PATIENTS WHEN
ALL ATTEMPTS AT CALORIE RESTRICTION HAVE FAILED.

Slim:

Diet – balance to maintain ideal body weight

and a Sulphonylurea:

either Chlorpropamide 100-375 mg daily
or Tolbutamide 0.5-1 g 8 hourly
or Glibenclamide 2.5-20 mg daily

and If still uncontrolled: Consider adding

Metformin 0.5-1.5 g daily (not if evidence of renal or hepatic
disease).

Or change to Insulin

If still remains uncontrolled or weight not maintained change to
Insulin

Hypoglycaemia

In a diabetic

Conscious
Carbohydrate by mouth, e.g. Glucose tablets, sweets or sweetened tea.
Unconscious
either 20 ml of 50% Dextrose given i.v. and repeated as necessary
   or if at home Glucagon 1 mg i.m.
When regained consciousness supplement with oral carbohydrates.
NB: HYPOGLYCAEMIA DUE TO CHLORPROPAMIDE MAY LAST FOR SEVERAL DAYS.

In a non-diabetic
Find cause and treat as appropriate

Insulinoma:
Surgery or Diazoxide initially 5 mg/kg/day then adjusted to patients
   requirements.
      The addition of Chlorthiazide 0.5-2 g daily may be of benefit
   or *if Malignant:* Streptozotocin – as last resort 1.5-4 g by infusion
i.v.

Essential reactive hypoglycaemia:
Diet with reduced carbohydrate content (especially sucrose and glucose)

HYPOTHALAMIC/PITUITARY DISEASE

Anterior pituitary
Get EXPERT help early to help with diagnosis and treatment.

Anterior pituitary deficiency
Usually several or all hormones are affected so that combined
therapy may be necessary. The usual order of loss being
gonadotrophins, growth hormone, prolactin, ACTH and TSH.

Gonadotrophins (no rise in Luteinizing hormones or follicular
stimulating hormones after Clomiphene 3 mg/kg/day for 10 days or
Growth hormone releasing hormone)
   Male
   Human chorionic gonadotrophins 4000 units i.m. for 5 days per
   week. (2000 units into each buttock) Continued for 5-7 months.
      or Human menopausal urinary gonadotrophins (FSH and LH)
         2-4 ampoules i.m. three times a week.
      and human chorionic gonadotrophins 500 units i.m. twice a
      week
      Both being given for 6-12 months
      If no benefit or injections become undesirable, either

Testosterone enanthate 200-400 mg i.m. every 4 weeks
> or Testosterone cypionate 200-400 mg i.m. every 4 weeks
> or Fluoxymesterone 1-10 mg daily by mouth in divided doses.

Female
Oestriol 0.5-2.0 mg daily
> or Stilboestrol 1-3 mg daily
> or Ethinyloestradiol 0.1 mg daily

Infertility (Female)
LH and FSH may be given, but only in specialist centre.

Growth hormone
Children
Need fully investigating
Treat any organic cause found (rare and usually associated with other deficiencies).
Growth hormone injections, but only under the control of specialist centres.
NB: Growth Hormone is species specific and therefore is in very short supply.
Adult
Treat cause if found
No specific therapy is needed

Adreno-Cortico-Trophic-Hormone
Hydrocortisone 20 mg each morning and 10 mg at night
NO Mineralocorticoid is needed
The serum level should be monitored to give
A peak value of 700-900 mmol/l (25-35 μg/100 ml) after the morning dose.
A value of 160 mmol/l (6 μg/100 ml) just before the evening dose.
A peak value of 320-480 mmol/l (12-17 μg/100 ml) after the evening dose.
NB: In children especially those on growth hormone therapy, high serum cortisol levels should be avoided because cortisol will inhibit growth hormone and lead to stunting of growth.
Androgen given by mouth will slow the rate of utilisation of cortisone and will therefore lead to higher blood levels.
In times of stress
Dose will need to be increased (see p. 94)

Thyroid stimulating hormone
Aged less than 50
L. Thyroxine 100 μg daily
Then increasing as described below
Aged more than 50 or Ischaemic Heart Disease
L. Thyroxine 50 μg daily

In either case increase the dose by 50 μg daily every 4 weeks until clinically euthyroid. (usually 200-300 μg daily)

NB: In patients with ischaemic heart disease – angina may be made worse by treatment and therefore full replacement therapy may not be possible. The addition of Propranolol 10 mg 8 hourly with slow increments will allow the dose of L. Thyroxine to be increased without the patient developing angina.

Anterior pituitary excess

Gonadotrophin
Children (Precocious puberty)
Find cause: usually a hypothalamic or Pineal tumour
Irradiation
  or Medroxyprogesterone 200-300 mg i.m. every 2 weeks

Growth hormone (Acromegaly or Giantism)
Acromegaly
Assess degree of hypopituitarism before treatment as treatment may reveal deficiency of hormones and make the patients condition worse.
Visual field defects present
Surgery with corticosteroid cover as described on p. 96
  When patient convalescant assess need to continue corticosteroid therapy by stopping treatment for 24-48 hours and then measuring the plasma cortisol at 9.00 am
  If less than 160 mmol/l (6 μg/100 ml) they need therapy for life
If after surgery growth hormone remains high:
Irradiation
Visual field defects not present
External irradiation
    or implantation with Yttrium or Gold
    or Surgery as outlined above
    or Bromocriptine which is:
      given with food, initially
      1.25 mg nocte for 1 day
      then 2.5 mg nocte for 1 day
      then 2.5 mg 12 hourly for 2 days
      then 2.5 mg 8 hourly for 2 days
      then 2.5 mg 6 hourly for 2 days
      then 5.0 mg 6 hourly for 3 months
      then Reassess activity.
      May need increasing up to 60 mg per day
Giantism
No treatment needed
Adreno-Cortico-Trophic-Hormone (Cushing's Syndrome)
In severe cases a few weeks' treatment with
Aminoglutethamide 250 mg 8 hourly reduces the cortisol level temporarily and allows full assessment to be made.

In less severe cases with no obvious tumour:
  either Surgery to remove the adenoma with corticosteroid cover
        as described on p. 96
        When the patient is convalescent the corticosteroid
        should be stopped for 48 hours and the plasma cortisol
        level measured at 9.00 am.
        If it is less than 160 mmol/l (6 μg/100 ml)
        corticosteroids should be restarted and continued for life.
  or External irradiation (Proton beam)
  or Radioactive implant with Gold or Yttrium
  or Bilateral adrenalectomy with corticosteroid cover as described
     on p. 96 and life time therapy with corticosteroids including
     Fludrocortisone 0.1 mg daily.
In presence of an obvious tumour:
  Surgery with corticosteroid cover as described on p. 96
  and External irradiation
If control not obtained:
Bilateral adrenalectomy with the precautions as described on p. 96

Thyroid stimulating hormone (Very Rare)
Treat as for thyrotoxicosis

Prolactin (induces hypogonadism)
(Found in 20% of secondary amenorrhea)
Stop cause if possible, e.g. Phenothiazine
                           Resperine
                           Methyldopa
                           Metoclopramide
  or Bromocriptine (very effective) initially 1.25 mg nocte
     then increase every 2-3 days until effective
     Usual dose needed being 2.5-5.0 mg 8-12 hourly
NB: If the patient has a pituitary tumour and wishes to become
      pregnant, irradiate the tumour first because swelling of the
      gland occurs during pregnancy and can cause visual field defects.

Posterior pituitary

Oxytocin deficiency or excess
No known disease state

Vasopressin
Deficiency (Diabetes Insipidus)
NB: May be temporary therefore test for pituitary function every 3
      months. May also be modified by associated ACTH deficiency.
  either Desmopressin 10-20 μg intranasally at night and/or
         in the morning (acts for 12-24 hours).
  or Lysine vasopressin nasal spray. 20 units given as 2 sprays
     per nostril as often as necessary. (Acts for approx. 4 hours).
  or Pitressin Tannate in oil 5 to 10 units i.m. every one to three
     days
NB: Active drug settles in ampoule and may therefore not be taken

up into syringe. This is best avoided by placing ampoule in water which has just boiled and then shaking vigorously to resuspend powder.

NB: No longer available in the UK

  or Chlorpropramide 100-350 mg daily – delay of 3 days before effect noted.

  – patient needs to have regular carbohydrate intake to prevent hypoglycaemia.

  or Bendrofluazide 5-10 mg daily – only in mild cases.

PARATHYROID DISEASE

Deficiency (Hypoparathyroidism)

All causes
Dihydrotachysterol 1-2mg by mouth daily
  and Calcium gluconate 1-2 g daily
Until calcium (measured x 2 a week) nearly normal.
  then Dihydrotachysterol 0.05 mg daily – dose is then adjusted until a maintenance level is found, usually between 0.25 and 1.0 mg
NB: TREATMENT IS FOR LIFE

Excess (Hyperparathyroidism)

Primary
Surgery, once diagnosis is established

Post operatively
1. Osteitis Fibrosa absent
   High calcium diet, e.g. 2-3 pints of milk per day until serum calcium normal
2. Osteitis Fibrosa present
   High calcium diet using calcium tablets
     if hypocalcaemia:
   Dihydrotachysterol 8 mg daily for 2 days
     then Dihydrotachysterol 4 mg daily for 2 days
     then Dihydrotachysterol 2 mg daily until plasma calcium normal
     then Dihydrotachysterol 1 mg daily until bones healed and alkaline phosphatase normal
   and Aluminium Hydroxide mixture 30 ml 4 times a day with meals for 7-14 days.

Secondary
Find cause and treat as appropriate
  and Vitamin D

Tertiary
Surgery with post operative treatment as outlined above.

THYROID DISEASE

Goitre

Simple
Prophylaxis
   Iodine in the diet. If not naturally present should be added, e.g. in
   table salt.
Curative
   either L. Thyroxine 100-200 μg per day to suppress TSH and
   prevent further enlargement.
   or Surgery for cosmetic reasons.
      (Iodine is not effective).

Multinodular
No therapy
or Surgery for cosmetic reasons.

Solitary nodule
Remove unless 'hot' on scanning

Primary hypothyroidism

Initially
Aged less then 50
   L. Thyroxine 100 μg/daily
Aged 50 or more, or with ischaemic heart disease
   L. Thyroxine 50 μg daily for 4 weeks
Then increasing to 100 μg daily

Maintenance
When established on 100 μg of L. Thyroxine daily check TSH level.
If normal continue that dosage.
If high increase dose by 50 μg to 150 μg daily
Then 4 weeks later repeat TSH level and continue to increase
L. Thyroxine dosage until patient euthyroid and TSH level is in the
normal range.
Most patients need 250 μg daily or less.
CAUTION: In patients with ischaemic heart disease or angina, who
may be made worse and are unable to tolerate the full dosage, add
Propranolol 10 mg 8 hourly. Then increase Propranolol dosage
slowly until the pulse rate falls. Then increase L. Thyroxine by 50 μg
and reassess.

Myxoedema, coma or psychosis
Lio-Thyronine (T_3) up to 100 μg 12 hourly, initially i.v. and then by
mouth (when conscious), and Hydrocortisone 100 mg
NB: Shorter onset of action than L. Thyroxine and more likely to
   precipitate angina.

Cretin
L. Thyroxine 25 μg daily increasing by 25 μg every 2 weeks.
The optimum dose being just less than that which causes diarrhoea.

TREATMENT FOR ALL HYPOTHYROID PATIENTS MUST CONTINUE
FOR LIFE, AND THE PATIENT AND RELATIVES MUST BE TOLD
THIS.

Hyperthyroidism

Young
Propranolol 40 mg 8 hourly whilst confirmatory tests being
performed and definitive therapy started.
Then Carbimazole 15 mg 8 hourly
   or Propylthiouracil 100 mg 8 hourly
   or Potassium perchlorate 300 mg 8 hourly

Middle aged or elderly
Propranolol 10 mg 8 hourly, increasing over a few days to control
symptoms.
Treatment can be maintained whilst confirmatory tests being
performed and definitive therapy started.
Then Carbimazole 15 mg 8 hourly
   or Propylthiouracil 100 mg 8 hourly
   or Potassium perchlorate 300 mg 8 hourly
   or Radio active iodine.

In either group when euthyroid consider
   either maintenance therapy with:
Carbimazole 10-20 mg daily
   or Propylthiouracil 50-100 mg daily
   or Potassium perchlorate 100-200 mg daily
Adjusting dosage of any of the drugs to maintain the patient
euthyroid.
   or Maintain therapy with enough of their drug to suppress thyroid
   activity and in addition give L. Thyroxine 200 μg daily as
   replacement.
Either type of therapy should be continued for 1-2 years and then
tailed off to see if the disease has 'burnt out'.
If disease not burnt out consider Radio iodine or partial
thyroidectomy – after making euthyroid with drugs as described
above.

Partial thyroidectomy
10 days pre-operative treatment with Potassium Iodide 180 mg daily
makes the operation easier, but should not be used after Potassium
Perchlorate as sudden severe relapse can occur.

IN ALL CASES FOLLOW FOR LIFE TO DETECT EARLY
HYPOTHYROIDISM.

Eye signs:
Avoid hypothyroidism
Usually no treatment necessary
Occasionally 5% Guanethidine eyedrops
Rarely limited lateral tarsorrhaphy

Failing visual acuity:
Admit to endocrine unit
Prednisone 60 mg daily. If no effect change to
Dexamethasone 20 mg daily. If no effect
Decompress orbit.

Thyroid storm:
Prophylaxis, prepare patient fully before surgery.
Treatment, get expert help if readily available.
Correct fluid balance
   and Propranolol 5-15 mg slowly i.v. – titrated against the patients
   response.
   and Carbimazole 15 mg 8 hourly
   and Potassium Iodide 20 mg 8 hourly
When euthyroid continue therapy as outlined above.

FURTHER READING

Avery, G. (1975) *Drug Treatment* Edinburgh: Churchill Livingstone
Clinics in Endocrinology and Metabolism London: W.B. Saunders
Evered, D. (1976) *Diseases of the Thyroid* Tunbridge Wells: Pitman
Medical
Hall, R., Anderston, J., Smart, G. A. ad sser, M. (1974)
Fundamentals of Clinical Endocrinology Tunbridge Wells: Pitman
Medical
Jeffcoate, N. (1975) *Principles of Gynaecology* London: Butterworths
Oakley, W.G., Pyke, D.A. & Taylor, K.W. (1978) *Diabetes and Its
Management* London: Blackwell Scientific
Williams, R.M. (ed.) (1974) *Textbook of Endocrinology* London: W.B.
Saunders

Gynaecology and obstetrics

With A.M. Jequier

AMENORRHOEA

Primary
Find cause and treat as appropriate

Secondary
Exclude pregnancy or menopause
   then Clomiphene 50-200 mg daily for 5 days
   or Tamoxifen 10 mg 12 hourly from day 2-5 of cycle
MUST MONITOR FOR PREGNANCY THROUGHOUT THERAPY. STOP IF OCCURS.
If these fail get Expert help.

Hyperprolactinaemia
Exclude pituitary macroadenoma
   then Bromocriptine 2.5 mg at night
Increase dose slowly until prolactin level falls to normal.

DYSMENORRHOEA

Primary
either Analgesics:
   Paracetamol 0.5-1.0 g 4-6 hourly
      or Dihydrocodeine 30-60 mg 4-6 hourly
or Menstrual suppression

   either Partial
Dydrogesterone 5-10 mg daily for days 5-25 of cycle.
   or Complete
Oestrogen – Progesterone mixture (oral contraceptive)

or if fails:
Full surgical investigation and treatment.

Secondary
Needs full investigation.

Membraneous
Needs full investigation.

Mid cycle pain (Mittelschmerz)
Reassurance, and:
Paracetamol 0.5-1.0 g
    or rarely, Oestrogen – Progesterone mixture (oral contraceptive)
        for ovulation suppresssion.

ENDOMETRIOSIS

Large masses
Surgery

Small masses or inaccessible areas
either Norethisterone 15 mg per day
    or Medroxyprogesterone acetate 15 mg per day
    or Danazol 200-800 mg per day (Very expensive)
    Menstruation must be totally suppressed.

INFECTIONS

Candida albicans
either Nystatin pessaries (100000 units) 1, 12 hourly for 10 days
    or Clotrimazole 100 mg pessaries 1 nocte for 6 days
    or Miconazole Nitrate 2% nocte for 14 days
and examine consort
    then treat if indicated with
    general hygiene
    and Nystatin ointment

Clostridia
See Chapter on Infections. – Gas gangrene p. 6.
Hysterectomy may be indicated.

Gonorrhoea
See Chapter on Infection. p. 6

Non specific salpingitis
Exclude gonorrhoea and syphilis.
then Ampicillin 500 mg 6 hourly x 10 days
    or Amoxycillin 250 mg 8 hourly x 10 days
    or Cephalexin 500 mg 6 hourly x 10 days
    or Co-Trimoxazole 2, 12 hourly x 10 days
If fails Get Expert Help
    and exclude ectopic pregnancy.

Post menopausal – non-specific infection
Triple-sulpha vaginal tablets 1, 12 hourly x 10 days
    or Povidone Iodine pessaries 1, 12 hourly x 10 days
    or Noxythiolin gel

Syphilis
See chapter on infection. p. 14

Trichomonas Vaginalis
either Metronidazole 200 mg 8 hourly x 14 days for women
   and Metronidazole 200 mg 8 hourly x 7 days for men
   or Metronidazole 2 g stat for both
NB: Disulfiram effect
   or Nimorazole 2 g with a meal—for both partners

Tuberculosis
As for other tuberculous infections.
See Respiratory chapter for details p. 29.

MENOPAUSE

Marked symptoms
Explain cause then if essential:

Oestrogens
either local:
   Dienoestrol 0.01% to vagina and vulva 12 hourly for 2-4 weeks.
     or Dienoestrol 0.16% to vagina and vulva 12 hourly
     or Stilboestrol 0.5 mg in 5% lactic acid, pessaries 2 nocte
and/or: oral
   either Piperazine oestrone sulphate 1.5-4.5 mg daily
     or Oestrodiol valerate 1-2 mg daily for 3 weeks, then stop for
     one week
     Then repeat cycle.
   or Conjugated oestrogens 0.625-1.25 mg daily for three weeks,
   then stop for one week.
   Then repeat cycle.
     REDUCE DOSE in all cases once symptoms are controlled.
   or Combined oestrogen and Progesterone
     either oral contraceptive
     or Mestranol 12.5 μg for 5 days
     then   25 μg for 8 days
     then   50 μg for 2 days
     then   25 μg and Norethisterone 1 mg for 3 days
     then   30 μg and Norethisterone 1.5 mg for 6 days
     then   20 μg and Norethisterone 0.75 mg for 5 days
     Then repeat cycle.

Post menopausal bleeding
Obtain Expert Help
NEVER TREAT FOR MORE THAN SIX MONTHS WITHOUT FULLY
REASSESSING

MENSTRUAL PROBLEMS

Post coital bleeding
Find cause and treat as appropriate.

Intermenstrual bleeding
Find cause and treat as appropriate.

Menorrhagia
Find cause and treat as appropriate.

Dysfunctional uterine bleeding
Get Expert Help
and then either Norethisterone 10-15 mg per day from day 5-25 of cycle

       or Medroxyprogesterone 10-15 mg per day from day 14-21 of cycle
       If cycle shorter, start treatment earlier
       or Contraceptive Pill

Change date of period
Oral contraception taken continuously until date required.

ORAL CONTRACEPTIVE

If no history of breast carcinoma
  no excess risk of thrombo-embolism
  no active liver disease:
    Oestrogen – low dose (ethinyl oestradiol or Mestranol) and
    Progesterone, e.g. norethisterone or norgestrel
    from 5th to 25th day of cycle.
If breast feeding or risk of thrombo-embolism:
    Progestogen only (norethisterone acetate or norgestrel or
    ethynodiol diacetate daily).

PREMENSTRUAL TENSION

Reassurance, and:
    Bendrofluazide 5 mg daily for last 10 days of cycle
    or Spironolactone 25 mg 12 hourly for last 10 days of cycle.
    or Dydrogesterone 5-10 mg from day 12 to 26 of cycle.

THREATENED ABORTION

Rest
Avoid intercourse
  then if during 1st trimester
    Hydroxyprogesterone 250 mg i.m. weekly or twice weekly
    NOT Norethisterone acetate

Obstetrics

AVOID ALL DRUGS IF POSSIBLE

ANAEMIA

Iron deficiency
Ferrous Sulphate 200 mg 12 hourly

Megaloblastic
Folic Acid 5 mg 8 hourly

Prophylaxis
Only indicated if mother has poor diet
   then Ferrous Sulphate 200 mg daily
   and Folic Acid 5 mg daily

EPILEPSY

Phenytoin 200-600 mg once daily
adjust dose to maintain serum level between 10-20 $\mu g/ml$

HYPERTENSION

Essential
Methyldopa 250 mg 6-12 hourly and increase as necessary
   or Clonidine 0.05-0.1 mg 8 hourly and increase as necessary
   or Hydrallazine 25 mg 6 hourly and increase as necessary

Pre eclampsia
Rest
Chlormethiazole 0.5-1 g 6 hourly
   or Diazepam 2-5 mg 6-8 hourly
If fails:- Get expert help

Eclampsia
Chlormethiazole 0.8% infusion – at a rate to control fits
   or Diazepam 5-10 mg i.v. over 5 minutes
   repeated as necessary
Get expert help early

INFECTION

Trichomonas
Avoid Metronidazole
Use locally active agents only, e.g. Acetarsol pessaries 2 nocte for
2-3 weeks
   or Hydragraphen pessaries 2 nocte for 2-3 weeks
   or Clotrimazole pessaries 2 nocte x 3 days

Urinary infection
Obtain sample and treat as appropriate
Avoid Cotrimoxazole and Tetracycline – ? avoid sulphonamides

Other infections
Treat as appropriate

Herpes gestationis
Clioquinol 3% ointment to erosion
In puerpurium
Prednisone 10 mg 8 hourly, reducing dose as soon as possible.

INHIBITION OF LACTATION

Either tight binder with simple analgesia
      or Frusemide 40 mg daily for 3 days
      or Bromocriptine 2.5 mg daily for 2-3 days
            then Bromocriptine 2.5 mg 12 hourly for 14 days
      or rarely Quinestrol 4 mg within 6 hours of delivery
      Repeat 48 hours later
      or Stilboestrol 5 mg 8 hourly for 5 days

NAUSEA AND VOMITING

Explain cause
Ensure small frequent meals with adequate fluid intake
Then, IF ESSENTIAL,
    Promethazine theoclate 25 mg at night
    If fails: and still essential
    increase to 25 mg 8-12 hourly

THYROTOXICOSIS

Carbimazole initially 15 mg 8 hourly,
then adjust dose to lowest possible,
aim to be a little toxic if anything at time of delivery.
Avoid Propranolol near to labour as it slows the fetal heart.
Measure LATS – if high suggests baby might develop thyroid crisis.

VENOUS THROMBOSIS

Heparin 10000 units 6 hourly i.v.
    or Heparin 5000 units subcutaneously 12 hourly
If impractical to continue with Heparin throughout pregnancy
Change to Warfarin until thirty sixth week, then restart Heparin

FURTHER READING

Barnes, C.G. (1978) *Medical Disorders in Obstetrics Practice* Oxford: Blackwell Scientific
Medical Education (International) Ltd. (1978) *Medicine* (Third Series) 8-11
Jeffcoate, N. (1975) *Principles of Gynaecology* London: Butterworths

Urology

With R. P. Burden

In this chapter on renal disease it is important to remember that a complete diagnosis is essential. It may well be that the patient has acute renal failure, and that the regime outlined in the chapter can be used to control this, but nevertheless, it is essential to establish the cause before definitive therapy is instituted.

The kidneys, being the main route of excretion of many drugs, have a profound effect upon their blood levels, and the incidence of side effects. At the end of this chapter is a table giving a list of drugs whose dosage intervals should be changed in the presence of renal impairment. The table also includes information about the efficacy of peritoneal or haemodialysis in removing the drug from the body. A second table lists drugs about which there is little evidence of the effects caused by changing the dosage intervals. The side effects likely to be encountered along with other comments are also given.

CALCULI

Acute renal colic
Morphine 5-10 mg subcutaneously
    and Atropine 0.3-0.6 mg subcutaneously
(available as a mixture BPC)
    or Pethidine 50-100 mg subcutaneously

Chronic calculi

Obstruction or structural abnormality present
Treat associated urinary infection with appropriate antibiotic and then surgery.

No obstruction or structural abnormality
Treat associated urinary infection with appropriate antibiotic and then find metabolic cause (if any) and treat as appropriate.

Metabolic causes

Hypercalcaemia: (see p. 98)

Hypercalcuria
high fluid intake and low calcium diet (restrict dairy products)
    and if no response either Bendrofluazide 5-10 mg daily
        and/or Cellulose Phosphate 12-15 g/day by mouth

Cystinuria
high fluid intake (greater than 1 litre/8 hours, throughout the 24
  hours). and Mist. Pot. Cit. 10 ml (well diluted) 8 hourly to
  maintain urine alkaline. (pH > 7.5)
  or Sodium Bicarbonate 5-15 g daily to maintain urine alkaline (pH
  > 7.5)
rarely D Penicillamine – dose being adjusted to maintain cystine
output less than 300 mg/day (*NB:* severe side effects).
Urates
high fluid intake (greater than 1 litre/8 hours, throughout the 24
  hours).
  and Allopurinol 100-300 mg 8 hourly
  and Mist. Pot. Cit. 10 ml (well diluted) 8 hourly to maintain urine
  alkaline. (pH > 7.5)

GLOMERULONEPHRITIS

With rare exceptions (e.g. steroids in minimal change nephropathy
and lupus nephritis) management is symptomatic depending on the
clinical presentation.
  e.g. Acute renal failure as on p. 121
       Chronic renal failure as on p. 123
       Nephrotic Syndrome as on p. 121
       Hypertension as on p. 36
USUALLY SPECIALIST ADVICE IS NECESSARY AND SHOULD BE
SOUGHT EARLY

Minimal change nephropathy

Relapse
Prednisone 60 mg daily for 7 days
  then Prednisone 40 mg daily for 7 days
  then Prednisone 30 mg daily for 7 days
  then Prednisone 20 mg daily for 7 days
  then Prednisone 10 mg daily for 7 days
  then Prednisone 5 mg daily for 7 days
  then STOP

Frequent Relapses
Induce remission with steroids as outlined above
Then consider adding:
Cyclophosphamide 3 mg/kg/day for 8 weeks
(*NB:* Severe side effects)
  or Long term Prednisone 5-10 mg per day

Lupus nephritis

Acute stage
Methyl Prednisone 1 g daily i.v. for 2-4 days
  then Prednisone 60 mg/day
  reduce dose according to response

E

Chronic stage
Prednisone 5-10 mg/day
Adjust dose according to clinical response, renal function and levels of DNA binding and C_3 complement
and if necessary:
Azathioprine 2 mg/kg/day to allow reduction in Prednisone dosage

Rapidly progressive glomerulonephritis
Prednisone, anticoagulants, immunosuppression, plasmaphoeresis are of value in some patients. Therefore refer for specialist advice.

Other forms of chronic glomerulonephritis
Symptomatic therapy as necessary
No specific therapy of proven use.

HAEMATURIA

Find cause, e.g.
  Infection
  Obstruction
  Stones
  Tumours – bladder and kidney
  Glomerulonephritis
Requires urinary examination, intravenous urography and cystoscopy in most cases.
If negative consider:
  Renal biopsy
Then treat as appropriate.

PREGNANCY IN RENAL DISEASE

OBTAIN EXPERT HELP AS SOON AS BECOMES APPARENT

PROTEINURIA

Postural

Plasma creatinine, blood pressure and urinary deposit normal
Ignore and reassure

Plasma creatinine, blood pressure or urinary deposit abnormal
Investigate

Persistent
Investigate including IVP and possibly refer for renal biopsy to
establish cause, e.g.
  infection
  tuberculosis
  obstruction
  analgesic nephropathy
  glomerulonephritis
Then treat as appropriate.

Nephrotic syndrome
Investigate including renal biopsy to establish cause
Then treat.
Symptomatic – high protein, low salt diet (unless in renal failure)
  and restricted fluid intake
  and either Frusemide 40-600 mg daily
    or Bumetanide 1-15 mg daily
  and in resistant patients
  salt free albumin infusion
    or Mannitol 10% infusion
  and Frusemide 40-600 mg i.v. daily
    or Bumetanide 1-15 mg i.v. daily
NB: BEWARE RISING CREATININE (HYPOVOLAEMIA) AND
    ELECTROLYTE DISTURBANCES WITH LARGE DOSES OF
    DIURETICS – DAILY WEIGHING AND BIOCHEMISTRY IS
    NECESSARY

RENAL FAILURE

Acute
Determine cause

Pre-renal (Hypovolaemia)
  Prevention: ensure replacement of fluid loss, e.g. during surgery
  or after burns.

  Cure: replace fluid loss with blood, plasma expanders or saline as
  appropriate.
Ensure that *CLINICALLY* the central venous pressure is positive.

NB: BEWARE OF FLUID OVERLOAD IF MYOCARDIAL DAMAGE.

Post-renal
Maintain fluid and electrolyte balance
Determine site of obstruction
Then surgery

Renal
Determine diagnosis (renal biopsy)

Established

General points
Get expert help for diagnosis and/or management EARLY
Preserve veins – minimize venepunctures, i.v. infusions, cannulae
etc., especially on the non-dominant forearm to allow subsequent
construction of fistulae if chronic renal failure ensues.

Specific measure
Maintain fluid and electrolyte balance (*NB:* measure all input and
losses, including drains etc.)
Assess balance with daily weight, blood and urine chemistry as well
as clinical findings
Maintain nutrition with naso-gastric or i.v. feeding if necessary. (*NB:*
Protein and calorie requirement greater than might be assumed
especially if hypercatabolic)

Dialysis. Better to dialyse early rather than late, especially if
hypercatabolic.

> *Indications*
> 1.   symptoms of uraemia, e.g. confusion,
>   nausea, itching, pericarditis   ⎫ depending
> 2.   Plasma urea 40 mmol/l   ⎬ on rate
>   or creatinine 900 μmol/l   ⎭ of rise
>   or Potassium > 6.5 mmol/l–ion exchange
>   resin may help temporarily.
>   or Bicarbonate < 12 mmol/l
> 3.   Fluid problems; may need to provide
>   'space' for feeding.

Hyperkalaemia
Prophylaxis.
Exclude potassium containing or retaining drugs
Then in emergency – Calcium Gluconate 10% 10 ml i.v.
   and/or Glucose 20 g with Insulin 40 units i.v.
   and/or Ion exchange resin (calcium resonium)
         15 g 6-8 hourly by mouth or 30 g
         rectally (acts more quickly)
   and/or Dialysis

Infection
Prophylaxis:
Use aseptic techniques whenever possible
Cure: Use appropriate antibiotic early and in adequate doses.
BEWARE INCREASED TOXICITY OF MANY ANTIBIOTICS, EITHER
ALONE OR WITH OTHER DRUGS. (see Tables 2 and 3, pp. 126-129)

Diuretic phase
Maintain fluid and electrolyte balance carefully matching input with
output and monitoring with daily weights, and plasma and urinary
biochemistry.

Chronic renal failure
Identify cause, looking for treatable lesions,
  e.g. Obstructions
       Excess analgesic intake
       Steroid responsive disorders
Look for correctable factors, which may make existing renal failure
worse,
  e.g. Salt and water depletion
       Drugs e.g. Tetracycline
       Hypertension
       Infection
NB: 1. Early referral if haemodialysis/transplantation is to be
        considered.
      2. Preserve veins – minimize venepunctures, i.v. infusion,
         cannulae etc., especially on the non-dominant forearm to
         allow subsequent construction of fistulae.
      3. Beware drugs (see Tables 2, and 3, pp. 126-129)
      4. Beware minor intercurrent illness which may lead to
         dehydration and aggravation of renal failure.
      Then diet:
Protein restriction (60 g/day initially) to improve symptoms of
      uraemia rather than biochemical values. (only used in patients
      unsuitable for haemodialysis).
      Better to dialyse early than to prolong dieting.
Calories – maintain calorie intake even if protein restricted.
Potassium – hyperkalaemia usually late unless potassium
      supplements or potassium retaining drugs given (e.g. Triamterene,
      Amiloride and Spironolactone).
      Beware Potassium containing calcium compounds and 'sodium free
      salt'
Salt and water – requirements vary; adjust according to weight,
      blood pressure, venous pressure, presence of oedema, urinary
      volume and electrolyte excretion.

Raised serum phosphate
Reduce phosphate in diet
      then reduce phosphate absorption with aluminium hydroxide
      mixture 10-20 ml 6 hourly with meals
and/or maintain Calcium intake of 1 g from all sources (if protein
      restricted supplement with Calcium Gluconate).
ATTEMPT TO MAINTAIN PLASMA PHOSPHATE LEVEL AT UPPER
LIMIT OF NORMAL

Symptomatic bone disease
Consider Vitamin D, e.g. 1,25 Dihydroxycholecalciferol 1-2 μg/day
      (reversible hypercalcaemia may occur)
    or 1 α Hydroxycholecalciferol 1 μg/day initially
    then according to response
IN ALL CASES GET EXPERT HELP EARLY RATHER THAN LATE

URINARY INFECTION

INVESTIGATE (i.e. IVP and ? cystoscopy) ALL CHILDREN, ALL MEN AND WOMEN IF RECURRENT ATTACKS AND/OR UPPER URINARY TRACT SYMPTOMS.

Asymptomatic

Pregnant
Appropriate antibiotic, then low dose prophylactic antibiotic throughout pregnancy.
NOT COTRIMOXAZOLE   NOT TETRACYCLINE

Not pregnant
The value of screening for and of treating asymptomatic infections has not been established.

Symptomatic

Initial attack
MSU for culture before antibiotics
High fluid intake
2 hourly double micturition to ensure complete bladder emptying

> *Lower tract symptoms*
> Sulphafurazole 2 g initially
>   then 1 g 4-6 hourly for 7 days
>   or Sulphamethizole 200 mg 4-6 hourly for 7 days
> If no response, antibiotic as indicated by lab. results

> *Upper tract symptoms*
> Cotrimoxazole 2 tablets 12 hourly
>   or if fails to respond antibiotics as indicated by lab. results

Recurrent attacks
> High fluid intake
> 2 hourly double micturition to ensure complete bladder emptying

> *Bacterial infection confirmed*
> Sulphafurazole 2 g initially
>   then 1 g 4-6 hourly for 7 days
>   or Sulphamethizole 200 mg 4-6 hourly for 7 days
> If fails antibiotic as indicated by laboratory result
> Followed by: low dose prophylaxis, e.g. Co-trimoxazole 1 tablet
> nocte
>   or if possibility of pregnancy
>   Sulphamethizole 100 mg daily

Bacterial infection NOT confirmed ('urethral syndrome')
Consider:
None bacterial infection – Trichomonas, Candida
Hypersensitivity to deodorants, e.g. soap etc.
Urethral stricture
Anxiety
Cystoscopy

Chronic pyelonephritis
Treat hypertension, recurrent infections, chronic renal failure as appropriate and suspect excess analgesic intake.

DRUGS IN RENAL FAILURE

The information contained in these tables is intended as a rough guide and should be interpreted with caution. The status of renal function should be checked with the recommendations before and during therapy to ensure that the patient receives adequate treatment without toxicity. This is especially important with the drugs of low therapeutic index, for example Digoxin and the aminoglycoside antibiotics. The more toxic drugs should only be used where there is no safe alternative and blood concentration monitoring carried out throughout the treatment period.

The dosage guidelines may not apply directly to elderly patients, where changes in drug disposition and renal function may result in an accumulation of the drug. Uraemic patients should also be carefully monitored for any unexpected toxic reaction. If any untoward events do occur, then the possibility that these are drug induced should be considered.

Table 2 A list of drugs which show increased toxicity in renal failure in which there is no indication of the effect of changing dosage interval. The comment column deals with problems which may occur, prepared by Mrs S. French, Information Pharmacist.

DOSES UNCHANGED IN RENAL IMPAIRMENT

DRUG	COMMENT
Amitriptyline	Sedation. Acute urinary retention possible
Benzhexol	May induce urinary retention in patients with prostatism.
Chloramphenicol	Bone marrow toxicity adds to uraemic marrow suppression.
	Some avoid especially if therapy longer than 10 days.
Chloroquine	Reduce dose if treatment prolonged.
Chlorpheniramine	Possible excessive sedation.
Codeine	Possible excessive sedation.
Corticosteroids	May increase azotaemia by enhancing catabolism
Diazoxide	Decrease dose size if given very frequently.
Doxycycline	Not useful in UTI's in moderate/severe renal failure.
Frusemide	Ototoxicity especially with aminoglycosides, and at high doses.
Heparin	Adds to bleeding tendency
Imipramine	Possible sedation, acute urinary retention
Indomethacin	May add to uraemic gastrointestinal symptoms.
Morphine	May cause excessive sedation
Naloxone	May cause excessive sedation
Nortriptyline	Sedation, acute urinary retention.
Pentazocine	Possible sedation
Pethidine	Possible sedation
Phenytoin	Monitor serum levels
Propranolol	May reduce renal blood flow
Pyrimethamine	Low renal clearance
Rifampicin	May cause acute renal failure

Table 3 A list of drugs which might be used in renal failure and recommended changes in dosage interval with varying degrees of renal impairment. The possible adverse effect are given in the comment column. Where there is information of the dialysability of the drugs it is also given. A blank indicating that no strong evidence is available. (Prepared by Mrs S. French Information Pharmacist.)

| DRUG | DOSAGE INTERVAL (hours) | | | | Significant Removal by Dialysis | | COMMENTS |
| | Normal | Renal Failure Serum Creatinine µmol/l | | | Haemo – | Perit – | |
		120-250	250-800	>800			
ACETAZOLAMIDE	6	6	12	Avoid			Ineffective with renal failure.
ALLOPURINOL	8	8	12	12-24			Nephrotoxicity, Rashes
AMANTADINE	12	12	reduce	dose			Neurotoxicity
AMILORIDE	12-24	24	24	Avoid			Hyperkalaemia
AMOXYCILLIN	8	8	12	16	YES		Fits with high serum levels
AMPHOTERICIN B	24	24	24	24-36	NO	NO	Nephrotoxicity
AMPICILLIN	6	6	9	12	YES		Fits with high serum levels
ASPIRIN	4	4	4-6	8-12	YES	YES	Nephrotoxicity GIT Symptoms
AZATHIOPRINE	24	24	24-36	24-48	YES	YES	Hyperuricaemia
BENZYL PENICILLIN	8	8	8	12	NO	NO	Fits with high serum levels
BETHANIDINE	1-2/wk	1-2/week	?	?			Monitor blood pressure
BLEOMYCIN	8	8	1/week	1/week			Hyperuricaemia
CARBENICILLIN	4	4	6-12	12-16	YES	NO	Fits with high serum levels
CEPHALOSPORINS	6	6	Avoid	Avoid	YES	YES	Nephrotoxicity with Aminoglycosides and loop diuretics

DRUG	DOSAGE INTERVAL (hours) Normal	Renal Failure Serum Creatinine μmol/l			Significant Removal by Dialysis		COMMENTS
CHLORDIAZEPOXIDE	8	8	8-12	12-24	NO	NO	Sedation. Urinary Retention
CHLORPROMAZINE	8	8	8-12	12-16	NO	NO	Sedation. Urinary Retention
CHLORPROPAMIDE	24	24-36	Avoid	Avoid		NO	Prolonged Hypoglycaemia
CLOFIBRATE	6	6-12	12-18	24			Myopathy
CLONIDINE	8	8	?	?			Monitor blood pressure
COLCHICINE	12	12	12	18			GIT symptoms
CO-TRIMOXAZOLE	12	12	24	Avoid	YES		Crystalluria. Nephrotoxicity
CYCLOPHOSPHAMIDE	12	12	12-18	12-24	YES		Hyperuricaemia
DIGOXIN	24	24-36	36-48	48-72	NO	NO	Arrhythmias
DIPHENHYDRAMINE	6	6	6-9	9-12			Sedation. Urinary Retention
EMEPRONIUM	6	8	Reduce	Dose			Acute urinary retention
ETHACRYNIC ACID	6	6	6	Avoid			Ototoxicity
ETHAMBUTOL	24	24	24-36	48	YES	YES	Ocular toxicity. Peripheral neuropathy
GENTAMICIN	8	8-12	12-36	48-72	YES	NO	Ototoxicity worse with Loop diuretics e.g. Frusimide
GOLD	24		Avoid	Avoid		NO	Proteinuria reduces renal blood flow
GUANETHIDINE	8	24	24-36	36-48	NO		Genetic variability
HYDRALLAZINE	8	8	8	8-16	YES	YES	
KANAMYCIN	8	24	24-72	72-96	NO	YES	Ototoxicity Nephrotoxicity
LINCOMYCIN	6	6	6	8-12	YES	NO	
LITHIUM	8	8-12	Avoid	Avoid	YES	YES	Nephrotoxicity CNS toxicity
METRONIDAZOLE	8	8	Reduce dose			YES	? Neurotoxicity
MEPROBAMATE	6	6	9-12	12-18	YES	YES	Sedation

Drug							Comments
METFORMIN	8-12	12	Avoid	Avoid			Lactic acidosis
METHADONE	6-8	8-12	12-16	16-24			Sedation
METHENAMINE MANDELATE	6	6	Avoid	Avoid			Ineffective
METHICILLIN	4	4	4	8-12	NO	NO	Fits with high serum levels
METHOTREXATE	24	24-36	36	48	YES	YES	Bone marrow depression, Hyperuricaemia
METHYLDOPA	6	6	9-12	12-24	YES	YES	Hepatitis
NALIDIXIC ACID	6	6	Avoid	Avoid	YES		
NEOMYCIN	6	6	12	18-24	YES	NO	Ototoxicity Nephrotoxicity
NITROFURANTOIN	8	8	Avoid	Avoid	YES		Peripheral neuropathy, Pulmonary toxicity
PENICILLAMINE	6	6	9-12	12-24	YES	YES	Nephrotic syndrome
PHENOBARBITONE	8	8	8	8-16	YES	YES	Sedation
PHENYLBUTAZONE	8	8	Avoid	Avoid			
POLYMYXIN B	12	24	36-60	60-96	YES	YES	Nephrotoxicity Neurotoxicity
PRIMIDONE	12	12	12-18	18-24	YES	YES	Sedation
PROBENECID	12	12	Avoid	Avoid			Ineffective
PROCAINAMIDE	3	3	4.5-6.0	6-9	YES		Active metabolite persists
PROMETHAZINE	12	12	12-18	18-24			Sedation
PROPYLTHIOURACIL	8	8	12-16	16-24			Cardiotoxicity
SALBUTAMOL	6-8	6-8	Reduce Dose	Avoid			Tachycardia
SPIRONOLACTONE	6	6	6	Avoid			Hyperkalaemia
STREPTOMYCIN	12	24	24-72	72-96	YES	YES	Ototoxicity
SULPHAMETHIAZOLE	6	6	Reduce	Avoid			Crystalluria
SULPHINPYRAZONE	6-8	8	Avoid	Avoid			Ineffective
SULTHIAMINE	8	?	?	?			Neurotoxicity
TETRACYCLINES	Avoid	Avoid	Avoid	Avoid	NO	NO	Nephrotoxicity
THIAZIDES	12	12	12	Avoid	NO		Hyperuricaemia ineffective
TOLBUTAMIDE	8	8-12	8-12	8-12			
TRIMETHADIONE	8	8	8-12	12-18			Neurotoxicity

FURTHER READING

Bennett, W.M., Singer, I. & Coggins, C.J. (1974) *A guide to drug therapy in renal failure.* J. Am. Med. Assoc, **230**, 1544.
Brenner, B.M. & Rector, F.C. (1976) *The Kidney* London: W.B. Saunders.
de Wardener, M.E. (1973) *The Kidney: An Outline of Normal and Abnormal Structure and Function* Edinburgh: Churchill Livingstone.

Haematology and oncology

J. Fletcher and M.B. McIllmurray

Unlike other chapters in this book a brief explanation of the
principles of treatment will be given before dealing with the general
problems and then specific regimes. Only the more common and
treatable cancers are discussed. Tumours of childhood are not included.

Principles of therapy

Cytotoxic drugs act on replicating cells both normal and abnormal
and they fall into two main groups. The first group, e.g. vinca
alkaloids, methotrexate, 6 Mercaptopurine, 6 Thioguanine and
cytosine arabinoside act during specific parts of the replication cycle
and are called phase specific. These drugs kill cells that happen to
be in the sensitive phase of the cycle and therefore their effects are
not dose-dependent once an initial threshold value is reached
provided they are given over a short period of time. The second
group, e.g. Cyclophosphamide, Mustine, Doxorubicin act during all
phases of the replication cycle and are called cycle specific. The
toxicity of these drugs is dose-dependent.

In general the proportion of cells in cycle (the growth fraction)
determines the sensitivity of both normal and tumour tissues to
cytotoxic therapy. If the growth fraction is small and growth is slow
then continuous treatment may be appropriate. If growth is rapid
with a high growth fraction then it is more effective to give drugs
intermittently in maximally tolerated doses with an interval of 3-4
weeks which allows normal tissues, particularly the bone marrow,
to recover. There is a further advantage in giving a combination of
drugs which act in different ways and have different side effects.
However combinations of cycle specific drugs may be additionally
toxic to the bone marrow and the dosage may need to be reduced
accordingly.

One of the major side effects of treatment is alopecia. This can be
helped by providing the patient with a wig.

IN ALL CASES GET EXPERT HELP.

General problems of chemotherapy

Route of administration

Because of the risk of local tissue damage if given extravascularly
most drugs are given into the side arm of a rapidly running i.v.
infusion of either
0.9% Sodium Chloride or 5.0% Dextrose

BLOOD COUNT MANDATORY BEFORE EACH COURSE OF
THERAPY

Modify dose
If white cell count less than 3000/cmm
If platelet count less than 100000/cmm
If renal or hepatic disease.

Nausea and vomiting
Metoclopramide 20 mg i.v. before treatment
   or Prochlorperazine 10 mg orally as necessary
   or Prochlorperazine 25 mg suppositories as necessary

Hyperuricaemia (Tissue breakdown)
Allopurinol 200 mg 8 hourly starting 24 hours before therapy
   then Allopurinol 100 mg 8 hourly when mass of tissue reduced

Bleeding
With rapidly falling platelet count
   or Purpura:
Fresh platelet infusion

Infection
Neutrophil count less than 800/cmm
   and unexplained pyrexia:
Take samples for culture
   Then Getamicin i.v. according to Mawer Nomogram (p. 323)
   and Cloxacillin 1 g i.v. 4 hourly
Then check Gentamicin serum level after 3-4 doses
If no response:

   Culture positive: Change therapy as appropriate

   Culture negative: add Clindamycin 150 mg 6 hourly by mouth
   Continue for 5 days then stop and reassess

Effectiveness
In this section we have only included treatment regimes which have
been shown to have some effect, although survival is not always
improved. Where possible patients should be included in the many
treatment trials that are currently being conducted.

ANAEMIA

Iron deficiency
Find cause and treat if possible.
Then Ferrous Sulphate 200 mg 12 hourly
If total oral intolerance

Iron Dextran 100 mg i.m. weekly and repeated until stores replete
or Iron Sorbitol Citrate 100 mg i.m. weekly and repeated until
stores replete

Megaloblastic anaemia
Find cause and treat as appropriate

Pernicious anaemia
Hydroxocobalamin 1000 μg i.m. daily for one week
   then Hydroxocobalamin 1000 μg i.m. every 3 months FOR LIFE

Folic acid deficiency
Initially Folic Acid 5-15 mg daily
   then Folic Acid 5 mg daily

Haemolytic anaemia
Find cause and treat as appropriate

Auto-immune
Prednisone 15 mg orally 6 hourly
then slowly reduce dose to 5-10 mg 12 hourly
depending on haemoglobin.
If fails:
Consider splenectomy.

Hereditary spherocytosis
Consider splenectomy

Aplastic anaemia
Find cause and treat if possible.
NB: TOXINS
   then Oxymethalone 50-100 mg 8 hourly
   May take 3-9 months to cause effect.

ACUTE LYMPHOBLASTIC LEUKAEMIA

At presentation
Vincristine (oncovin) 1.5 mg/m^2* i.v. weekly for 5 doses
   and Prednisone 40 mg/m^2 daily – tailing off after 4 weeks.

CNS prophylaxis
Start 10 weeks after remission induction.
Cranial irradiation 2300 rads
and Methotrexate 10 mg/m^2 intrathecally, weekly x 4
   or Cytosine arabinoside 50 mg/m^2 intrathecally at 2 week
   intervals x 4 doses

* Do not exceed 2 mg/dose. If aged 60+ reduce dose by 0.05 mg/year. Omit
when less than 1 mg (i.e. aged 80+)

Maintenance

Vincristine (Oncovin) 1.5 mg/m²* i.v. weekly for 5 doses
  and Prednisone 40 mg/m² daily – tailing off after 4 weeks
    then 6 Mercaptopurine 70 mg/m² orally daily for 3 weeks
    then Methotrexate 15 mg/m² orally daily for 3-5 days
Repeat 6 Mercaptopurine and Methotrexate regime x 2 (total of 3 cycles)
    then Repeat Vincristine and Prednisone as outlined above.
Then repeat whole cycle and continue with repeats for 3 years.

ACUTE MYELOID LEUKAEMIA

Toxicity to bone marrow is inevitable. Patient should be treated in a specialised unit. Pyrexia – see general comments on infection above.

At presentation

Daunorubicin 55 mg/m² i.v. day 1
  and Cytosine arabinoside 70 mg/m² i.v. days 1-5 inclusive
    Then repeat, starting on day 11
  and then continue repeated courses until remission is induced (elimination of blast cells from peripheral blood and bone marrow) or total Daunorubicin dose of 550 mg/m².

When remission induced

Repeat drugs as above, but at 28 day intervals (until total Daunorubicin dosage 550 mg/m².)
  or Thioguanine 70 mg/m² orally days 1-3
    then no treatment on day 4
    then Cyclophosphamide 100 mg/m² orally single dose days 5-7
Then repeat every 28 days until relapse.

Relapse

Repeat treatment as at presentation.
When Daunorubicin maximum dose is reached substitute Thioguanine 70 mg/m²

BLADDER CANCER

Local disease

Surgery with pre-operative radiotherapy in those with deeply infiltrating tumour.

Advanced disease

5 Fluorouracil 500 mg/m² i.v. day 1
Adriamycin 50 mg/m² i.v. day 1
Repeated at 21 day intervals.

*See footnote on p. 133.

BREAST CANCER

Local disease
Enter into clinical trial
or
Simple mastectomy and axillary node clearance
  and Local radiotherapy post operatively.

Nodes showing no tumour
No further treatment

Nodes showing tumour present
Chemotherapy for 1 year. See below.

Advanced disease
Treatment includes radiotherapy, surgery, hormone and
chemotherapy.

Premenopausal women
Ovarian ablation (surgical or radiotherapy)

NB: Ovarian ablation is more likely to be effective if:
Regular periods
Long disease free interval
Generalised disease (especially bone)
Presence of oestrogen receptors in tumour cells.

Poor initial response Chemotherapy. See below.

Good initial response Watch
    if RELAPSE
Tamoxifen 10-20 mg 12 hourly
    if RELAPSE
Chemotherapy. See below.

Perimenopausal women (0-5 years after last period)
Norethisterone 10-15 mg 6 hourly
  or Tamoxifen 10-20 mg 12 hourly

    if RELAPSE
Chemotherapy. See below.

Postmenopausal women
either for soft tissue or lung involvement
    Ethinyloestradiol 0.5-1 mg 8 hourly
    or Tamoxifen 10-20 mg 12 hourly
    or Nandrolone 50 mg i.m. weekly
or for hepatic metastases and lymphangitic infiltration of the lung
    Prednisone 10 mg 6 hourly

Poor response or relapse Chemotherapy. See below

Relapse after initial good response Hypophysectomy or
adrenalectomy

Chemotherapy schedule
Cyclophosphamide 100 mg/m² orally days 1-14 inclusive
    and Methotrexate 40 mg/m² i.v. days 1 and 8
    and 5 Fluorouracil 600 mg/m² i.v. days 1 and 8
± (Prednisolone 40 mg/m² orally days 1-14 inclusive)

or 5 Fluorouracil 500 mg/m² i.v. days 1 and 8
    and Adriamycin 50 mg/m² i.v. day 1
    and Cycloposphamide 500 mg/m² i.v. day 1
Repeated at 21 day intervals.
Continue for 1 year (if useful tumour RESPONSE).

CHORION CARCINOMA

Treatment should be in specialised centre.

Methotrexate 20-25 mg by mouth days 1-7 inclusive
Courses repeated at 14-21 day intervals
At least 3 further courses are given after the urinary human
chorionic gonadotrophin level has fallen to less than 50 iu/24 hrs.

CHRONIC GRANULOCYTIC LEUKAEMIA

At presentation
Busulphan 4-6 mg daily until WBC less than 20000/cmm
    and platelets less than 500000/cmm
The dose is adjusted to control the rate of fall in cell count.
This can be predicted by plotting the counts on semi-log paper.

Maintenance
Busulphan 0.5-2 mg daily
Adjust dose to maintain white cell and platelet count satisfactory

Acute transformation
Hydroxyurea 250 mg daily
Adjust dose to maintain white cell and platelet count satisfactory.

Blastic transformation
When lymphoblastic
    Treat as for acute lymphoblastic leukaemia (see p. 133)

CHRONIC LYMPHATIC LEUKAEMIA

At presentation
Treat if anaemia and/or enlarged uncomfortable glands and/or
splenomegaly.

Chlorambucil 4 mg orally daily
  Reduce dose and slowly stop when white cell count controlled and
  the haemaglobin restored.
and Prednisone 10 mg orally 6 hourly
  Slowly reduce and stop once disease responding.

Maintenance
Repeated short course of:
  Chlorambucil 2-4 mg/day lasting for a few weeks
Occasionally:
  Prednisone 5-10 mg daily will control disease.

Auto-immune haemolytic anaemia
Prednisone 10 mg orally 6 hourly
Reduce dose to maintenance level when anaemia controlled.

COLO-RECTAL CANCER

Local
Surgery

Advanced
5-fluorouracil 500 mg/m^2 at weekly intervals

DISSEMINATED INTRAVASCULAR COAGULATION

Find cause and treat as appropriate.
  then Heparin 10000 units 6 hourly i.v.
  and Blood and/or platelets as necessary

HENOCH-SHONLEIN PURPURA

Exclude Drug Causes

If streptococcal
Phenoxymethyl Penicillin 250 mg 6 hourly

If joints painful
Rest
Consider Prednisone 25-30 mg daily
  When joints controlled
  Reduce dose.

HEPATOMA

Adriamycin 60 mg/m^2 i.v. day 1
Repeated at 21 day intervals.

HEREDITARY HAEMORRHAGIC TELANGECTASIA

If bleeding a problem
Ferrous Sulphate 200 mg 12 hourly
Ethinyloestradiol 0.25 mg daily for 4 weeks
    then Ethinyloestradiol 0.5 mg daily

In males
    add Methyl testosterone 5 mg daily

LUNG CANCER

Local
Surgery

Advanced
Small cell anaplastic carcinoma and adenocarcinoma are more responsive than either epidermoid or large cell anaplastic carcinoma.

		days
Cyclophosphamide 500 mg/m^2	i.v.	1
and Methotrexate 50 mg/m^2	i.v.	1 and 4
and Lomustine (CCNU) 50 mg/m^2	orally	1

Cycle repeated at 21 day interval and Lomustine omitted from alternate courses.

LYMPHOMAS

Hodgkins disease
    Type of treatment is determined by extent of disease.
    Clinical staging is mandatory.
    Stage I – Single lymph node region
    Stage II – Two or more lymph node regions on the same side
            of the diaphragm or localised involvement of extra
            lymphatic organ.
    Stage III – Several lymph node regions on both sides of
            diaphragm.
    Stage IV – Dissemination with involvement of extra lymphatic
            organs.
    NB: The spleen is counted as a lymph node.
Staging is subdivided into those without (A) and those with (B) symptoms, such as night sweats, fever or a greater than 10% weight loss.
Staging procedures include chest X-ray, lymphangiograms, bone biopsy, liver scan and laparotomy (with splenectomy).

    Stages I, II and IIIa
    Radiotherapy

Stages IIIB and IV
Chemotherapy with MVPP

			days
Mustine hydrochloride	(M)	6 mg/m^2 i.v.	1 and 8
and Vinblastine	(V)	6 mg/m^2 i.v.	1 and 8
and Procarbazine	(P)	100 mg/m^2 orally	1 – 14 inclusive
and Prednisolone	(P)	25 mg/m^2 orally	1 – 14 inclusive

Repeat course at intervals of 42 days (between the first day of consecutive courses).
Continue to repeat courses x 3 after clinical remission (no signs, normal investigations including lymphangiogram).
IF WHITE CELL COUNT LESS THAN 4000/cmm AND/OR PLATELET COUNT LESS THAN 100000/cm:
Reduce dose of Mustine and/or Vinblastine
Then repeat course keeping same interval.

Relapse or failure to respond
Either: BVB

			days
BCNU (Bischloronitrosourea)(B)		50 mg/m^2 i.v.	1
(Carmustine)			
and Vinblastine	(V)	6 mg/m^2 i.v.	1 and 8
and Bleomycin	(B)	15 mg/m^2 i.m.	1 and 8

NB: BCNU is diluted in 200 ml 0.9% Soduim chloride before injection
Repeat cycle every 28 days
Or BACOP

				days
Bleomycin	(B)	5 mg/m^2	i.v.	15 – 22
and Adriamycin	(A)	25 mg/m^2	i.v.	1 and 8
(Doxorubicin)				
and Cyclophosphamide	(C)	650 mg/m^2	i.v.	1 and 8
and Vincristine	(O)	1.4 mg/m^2*	i.v.	1 and 8
(Oncovin)				
and Prednisone	(P)	60 mg/m^2	orally	15 – 28

Repeat cycle every 28 days.

Non-Hodgkin lymphoma
The value of staging in determining treatment is less certain than for Hodgkins Disease, because Non-Hodgkin lymphoma follows a less predictable clinical course.

* Do not exceed 2 mg/dose. If aged 60+ reduce dose by 0.05 mg/year. Omit when less than 1 mg (i.e. aged 80+)

Stages I and II:
Radiotherapy
Stages III and IV:
Are divided according to the histology into:

(1) Good Prognosis Group (i.e. follicular lymphomas, diffuse well differentiated lymphocytic lymphomas, including chronic lymphatic leukaemia).
Only those with progressive disease, or with symptoms or complications are treated.

Lymphocytic lymphomas
Chlorambucil 4 mg daily orally, continuously
  and Prednisolone 40 mg daily orally, continuously
The dose of each being titrated against the clinical response, Prednisolone being withdrawn before Chlorambucil.

Follicular lymphomas
Treatment as outlined above.
Or COP

				days
Cyclophosphamide	(C)	800 mg/m²	i.v.	1
and Vincristine	(O)	1.4 mg/m²*	i.v.	1
(Oncovin)				
and Prednisolone	(P)	50 mg/m²	orally	1 – 5

Repeat course, starting next course on day 22

(2) Bad Prognosis Group (i.e. all other diffuse lymphomas regardless of cell type).
CHOP

				days
Cyclophosphamide	(C)	800 mg/m²	i.v.	1
and Adriamycin	(H)	50 mg/m²	i.v.	1
(Doxorubicin)				
and Vincristine	(O)	1.4 mg/m²*	i.v.	1
(Oncovin)				
and Prednisolone	(P)	50 mg/m²	orally	1 – 5 inclusive

At least 6 courses at intervals of 21 days
Radiotherapy may be required to deal with bulk disease.
or MVPP (as described under Hodgkins Disease)

MACROGLOBULINAEMIA

Chlorambucil 4 mg daily
Continue until macroglobulin level reduced

*Do not exceed 2 mg/dose. If aged 60+ reduce dose by 0.05 mg/year Omit when less than 1 mg (i.e. aged 80+)

Then reduce to 2 mg daily or STOP
  and Prednisone 10 mg orally 6 hourly
Tail off after a few weeks when haemoglobin rises, if white cell and
platelet counts maintained.

MULTIPLE MYELOMA

At presentation
Melphalan 10 mg orally days 1-7 inclusive
and Prednisolone 40 mg orally days 1-7 inclusive
  Then repeat courses starting on day 29
  and continue for 1 year.
Then either:
Stop and watch for recurrence
or:
Repeat course every 3 months.

If no remission (At least 50% reduction in Para-Protein), or relapse
Melphalan 6 mg/m^2 orally days 1-3
and Prednisolone 40 mg/m^2 orally days 1-3
and Cyclophosphamide 250 mg/m^2 orally days 1-3
and Lomustine (CCNU) 50 mg/m^2 orally day 4 only
Repeat course starting on day 29
and continue repeats for 1 year.
Then stop and reassess.

Hypercalcaemia
Maintain hydration
and Prednisolone 60 mg daily
and see section on Hypercalcaemia, p. 98.

Bone pain due to deposits
Radiotherapy

Hyperviscosity
Plasma-phoresis

MYELOID METAPLASIA (Myelosclerosis)

Folic Acid 5 mg daily may help anaemia

OVARIAN CANCER

No combination regime has been shown to be better than an
alkylating agent used alone, though few have been evaluated.
  Melphalan 0.2 mg/kg orally days 1 to 5 inclusive
  Repeated at 3-5 week intervals
or Chlorambucil 0.2 mg/kg orally daily
or Cyclophosphamide 50-150 mg/day orally daily

NB: Remissions are less frequent with undifferentiated tumours and are of shorter duration.
A high dose intermittent regime is no better than low dose continuous treatment.

POLYCYTHEMIA RUBRA VERA

Haematocrit greater than 55%
   or symptoms
Venesection 1 pint (500 ml) weekly
   then Radio Phosphorous (^{32}P) 5-7 millicuries i.v.
   or Busulphan 4-6 mg orally daily
when haematocrit controlled
Reduce dose and stop.

PROSTATIC CANCER

   Stilboestrol 1 mg 8 hourly orally daily
or Phosphorylated Methyl Stilboestrol (Fosfestrol) 250-500 mg i.v.
for rapid relief of bone pain
or subscapular orchidectomy

SOFT TISSUE SARCOMAS

For all tumour types:

			days
Cyclophosphamide	500 mg/m^2	i.v.	1
and Adriamycin (Doxorubicin)	50 mg/m^2	i.v.	1
and Vincristine (Oncovin)	1 mg/m^2*	i.v.	1
and Dacarbazine	250 mg/m^2	i.v.	1 – 5 inclusive

   At intervals of 28 days.
NB: Soft tissue sarcomas are much less responsive in adults than in children.
Chemotherapy given pre-operatively may make surgery easier by reducing the tumour bulk.

TESTICULAR TERATOMA

Clinical staging mandatory
TREAT IN SPECIALISED CENTRE
Orchidectomy followed by radiotherapy
and chemotherapy
with

			days
Vincristine(Oncovin)	1 mg/m^2*	i.v.	1
and Methotrexate	300 mg/m^2	i.v.	1
and 5 hours later			
Folinic Acid Rescue	9 mg/m^2	i.m.	repeat x 4 5-6 hourly
and Bleomycin	15 mg/m^2	infusion 2 – 4 inclusive	

THROMBOCYTOPENIA

Find cause and treat as appropriate.

Idiopathic
Prednisone 10 mg/m^2 6 hourly
Reduce to maintenance dose according to platelet count.

If fails: or dose needed too high:
Consider splenectomy.

THROMBOCYTHAEMIA (Platelet count more than 10^6/cmm)

Radiophosphorous (^{32}P) 5-7 millicuries i.v.
  or Busulphan 4-6 mg daily
Reduce dose and stop when platelet count controlled

Thrombotic lesions
Aspirin 600 mg orally 12 hourly
  and/or Dipyridamole 100 mg 8 hourly

FURTHER READING

Cancer Treatment Reveiw (1975) 2, 159-175
De Gruchy, G.C. (1978) *Clinical Haematology in Medical Practice*
London: Blackwell Scientific
Holland, J.F. & Frei, E. (1974) *Cancer Medicine* Philadelphia: Lea & Febiger
Priestman, T.J. (1977) *Cancer Chemotherapy—An Introduction*
Barnet: Montedism Pharmaceuticals

*Do not exceed 2 mg dose; if aged 60+ reduce dose by 0.05 mg/year; Omit when less than 1 mg (i.e. aged 80+)

Ear, nose and throat

In writing this chapter I have attempted to deal with common conditions which will be seen by a general physician. The only treatments I discuss are medical and in many instances it will be necessary to obtain surgical help.

ACUTE EPIGLOTTITIS (Emergency in Children)

Ampicillin 1 g i.m. 6 hourly for 48 hours or until swallowing normal then Amoxycillin 500 mg 8 hourly
NB: DO NOT ATTEMPT EXAMINATION UNTIL FACILITIES FOR
   TRACHEOSTOMY AVAILABLE.

ACUTE SINUSITIS

Symptomatic
either Xylometazoline 0.1% nasal spray
   or Oxymetazoline 0.05% nasal spray
NB: MAOI INTERACTION
   and Inhalations, e.g. Pine

Viral
No specific treatment

Bacterial
Phenoxymethyl Penicillin 500 mg 6 hourly by mouth for 7 days
   or Amoxycillin 250 mg 8 hourly for 7 days
   or Erythromycin 500 mg 6 hourly by mouth for 7 days.

ALLERGIC RHINITIS

Define cause if possible and then either avoid exposure or desensitize
   If fails:
   Sodium Cromoglycate nasal spray 1, 6 hourly
   If fails:
   Diphenhydramine 25-50 mg by mouth 6-12 hourly
      or Triprolidine 2.5-5.0 mg by mouth 8 hourly
      or Chlorpheniramine 4 mg 6 hourly
   and Phenylpropanolamine 25 mg 4 hourly by mouth
      or Pseudoephedrine 60 mg 8 hourly by mouth
NB: MAOI INTERACTION
   If fails:
   Beclomethasone diproprionate nasal spray 1 spray/nostril 6 hourly
   (may take several days to be effective)

or Prednisone 10 mg 8 hourly for 4 days
then Beclomethasone diproprionate nasal spray 1 spray/nostril 6
hourly

CHRONIC SINUSITIS

Establish bacteriological cause and treat as appropriate.
If does not respond:
Obtain expert help.

CROUP

Symptomatic
Reassure child and parents
Sedation for child may help, e.g. Promethazine Elixir 5-25 mg
Humidify atmosphere

Viral – common
No effective treatment

Bacterial
Amoxycillin 250 mg 8 hourly by mouth for 7 days
   or Ampicillin 500 mg 6 hourly i.m.

EPISTAXIS

Pressure over Littles area
and/or Modified Trotter's Method
   Sit up
   Squeeze nose for 5 minutes (by the clock)
   Spit saliva and blood into bowl

If fails:
Obtain expert help

LARYNGITIS

Symptomatic
Inhalations, e.g. Pine

Viral (usual)
No specific treatment

Bacterial (rare)
Amoxycillin 250 mg 8 hourly by mouth for 7 days
or Co-Trimoxazole 2 tablets 12 hourly for 7 days

If fails:
Get expert help – may be carcinoma

MASTOIDITIS

Acute
Obtain expert help early.
Obtain material for culture if possible
Then antibiotics as appropriate
  If no material for culture:
  Ampicillin 1 g 6 hourly i.v. or i.m.
  If no response after a short period:
  Surgery.

Chronic
Get expert help.

MOTION SICKNESS

Hyoscine 0.6 mg by mouth 1 hour before starting
  or Hyoscine 0.2 mg i.m. at any time
  or Promethazine theoclate 25 mg orally 1 hour before starting

NASAL BLOCKAGE

Find cause and treat as appropriate.

Symptomatic
either Phenylpropanolamine 25 mg 4 hourly by mouth
  or Pseudoephedrine 60 mg 8 hourly by mouth
NB: MAOI INTERACTION
or Xylometazoline 0.1% nasal spray for a short period only
  or Oxymetazoline 0.05% nasal spray for a short period only
  NB: MAOI INTERACTION

NASAL DISCHARGE

Find cause and treat as appropriate.

OTITIS EXTERNA

EXCLUDE DERMATOLOGICAL AND GENERAL CAUSES, E.G. DIABETES

Acute oedematous (Swimmers Ear)
Clean canal with Acetic Acid 1%
then insert wick with solution/ointment of Corticosteroid
plus Framycetin
  or Neomycin
  or Polymyxin
and continue application of solution/ointment 8 hourly for 7 days
and Promethazine 25 mg orally nocte (to relieve irritation)
and if marked oedema
Prednisone 10 mg 8 hourly for 3-4 days

Infected
Take material for culture
Clean canal with Acetic Acid 1%
then Aluminium Acetate Solution 8 hourly for 3 days
then instil appropriate antibiotic/corticosteroid solution
and Promethazine 25 mg nocte by mouth
Continue treatment for at least 1 week

Recurrent infection
After control as described above continue antibiotic/corticosteroid
ointment for prolonged period.

Fungal
Clean canal
Then wipe with either Diamethazole solution
   or Tolnaftate solution
Then either paint with Gentian Violet 1.0%
   or Clotrimazole 1% cream
   or puff in Nystatin powder
   or Clioquinol powder
Repeat treatment weekly
Keep canal as dry as possible

'Malignant'
Control diabetes mellitus (usually associated)
Obtain material for culture
Clean canal with Acetic Acid 1%
Carry out any debridement necessary
Pack with Gentamicin ointment
   then douche daily with Gentamicin solution
   and start on systemic antibiotics as appropriate
When infection controlled:
Daily alcohol drops 95% as prophylaxis.

OTITIS MEDIA

Acute
Stop pain with
   either Aspirin 300-900 mg orally 6 hourly
   or Paracetamol 0.5-1 g 6 hourly orally
   or Dihydrocodeine 30 mg orally 6 hourly
   or occasionally:
   Pethidine 25-50 mg i.m.
and
   In adult:
   Benzyl Penicillin 1 mega unit 6 hourly i.m.
      or Phenoxymethyl Penicillin 500 mg 6 hourly by mouth
      or Erythromycin 500 mg 6 hourly by mouth

In child under 5:
Amoxycillin 250 mg 8 hourly
    or Erythromycin 10 mg/kg 6 hourly
and to clear Eustacian tube
    either Phenylpropranolamine 12.5-25 mg 4 hourly orally 3-4 days
        or Pseudoephedrine 30-60 mg 8 hourly orally 3-4 days
        NB: MAOI INTERACTION

    and/or Xylometazole 0.1% nasal spray for 3-4 days
    or Oxymetazoline 0.05% nasal spray for 3-4 days
        NB: MAOI INTERACTION
If not cleared in one week continue antibiotics for 10 days
If not cleared at end of 10 days:
or Deafness persists:
or Complications suspected:
GET EXPERT HELP as surgery often necessary

Chronic
Obtain material for culture
Clean canal with Acetic Acid 1%
then irrigate canal and middle ear (via perforation which is
invariably present) with appropriate antibiotic solution.
and systemic antibiotics if organism not pseudomonas or proteus.
Look for and treat any causes of Eustachian tube obstruction.
    OBTAIN EXPERT ADVICE as surgery often necessary.

Serous
OBTAIN EXPERT ADVICE: surgery often necessary.

'Glue ear' in children
    either Diphenhydramine 6.25-50 mg depending on age by mouth
        6-8 hourly
    or Triprolidine 1-3 mg depending on age orally 8 hourly
    or Chlorpheniramine 1-2 mg depending on age 8-12 hourly
and Phenylpropanolamine 12.5-25 mg depending on age 4
hourly
    or Pseudoephedrine 15-30 mg depending on age 6 hourly
NB: MAOI INTERACTION
If persists: for more than 1 month
Get expert help

PHARYNGITIS

Acute

Viral
No effective treatment

Bacterial
Adults – Penicillin V 500 mg 6 hourly by mouth for 7 days
  or Erythromycin 500 mg 6 hourly by mouth for 7 days
Children – Amoxycillin 250 mg 8 hourly by mouth for 7 days

NB: 'Penicillin Rash' common with glandular fever

Chronic

Exclude
Blood dyscrasias
Glandular Fever
Specific infection

Then symptomatic treatment
e.g. Domiphen gargle

If fails
Get expert help

TONSILLITIS

Symptomatic
Saline gargle

Viral
No effective treatment

Bacterial
Phenoxymethyl Penicillin 500 mg 6 hourly by mouth for 7 days
  or Erythromycin 500 mg 6 hourly by mouth for 7 days

Recurrent streptococcal
Phenoxymethyl Penicillin 125 mg twice a day to prevent Rheumatic
fever.

VASOMOTOR RHINITIS

Look for and treat any infection as appropriate
  and Phenylpropanolamine 25 mg 4 hourly by mouth
  or Pseudoephedrine 60 mg 8 hourly by mouth
  NB: MAOI INTERACTION
  With or without

Diphenhydramine 25-50 mg by mouth 6-12 hourly
  or Triprolidine 2.5-5.0 mg by mouth 8 hourly
  or Chlorpheniramine 4 mg by mouth 6 hourly
  or Beclomethasone diproprionate nasal spray 1 spray/nostril
  6 hourly (may take several days to become effective)
and at night if necessary
  Xylometazoline 0.1% nasal spray for short period only
    or Oxymetazoline 0.05% nasal spray for short period only
NB: MAOI INTERACTION

VERTIGO

Find cause and treat as appropriate.

Symptomatic
Prochlorperazine 5-10 mg 8 hourly
  or Cyclizine 50 mg 8 hourly
  or Cinnarizine 15-30 mg 8 hourly
  or Acetazolamide 250 mg daily for 2 days
No therapy for one day and then repeat
  or Thiazide diuretic
  or Diazepam 2-5 mg 8 hourly
  or Chlordiazepoxide 10 mg 8 hourly
  or Amitriptyline 25 mg 8 hourly.

Menière's syndrome
Betahistine 8 mg 8 hourly
  or any of the drugs listed above, either alone or in combination.

WAX IN EAR

Dioctyl Sodium Sulphosuccinate 5%
Fill ear and plug with cotton wool
Repeat next night, then syringe out softened wax.

Eyes

In this chapter I deal with the common conditions of the eye which can be treated by medication. There are obviously many other conditions that require expert surgical help but I have not attempted to cover these.

ARTERITIS

(Medical emergency)
Prednisone 20 mg 8 hourly
then reduce dose to lowest possible to control evidence of arteritis, e.g. ESR
Maintain ESR less than 20 mm/hr

BLEPHARITIS

Obtain material for culture
Remove scales with
   Sodium Bicarbonate lotion
then antibiotic/steroid cream to lid margins
   e.g. Neomycin or Erythromycin
   Use only for short courses.
and treat dandruff.

CONJUNCTIVITIS

Acute
Obtain material for culture
Irrigate the eye with Saline
Many cases resolve with no further treatment.
If does not start to resolve in 1-2 days:
   either Chloramphenicol eye drops hourly
   or Neomycin/Polymyxin eye drops hourly
   or Antibiotic according to cultural results
In ALL CASES ointment with a similar antibiotic should be instilled at night.
If not better after 3-4 days:
GET EXPERT HELP.

Chronic
Establish cause and treat as appropriate
and Zinc Sulphate 0.25% solution
GET EXPERT HELP.

F

Gonococcal
Establish diagnosis
Then:
Benzyl Penicillin 15000 units/kg i.m. 6 hourly for 7 days
and after Saline irrigation
Chloramphenicol eye drops every 15 minutes until response
 or Tetracycline eye drops every 15 minutes until response
 or Penicillin eye drops every 15 minutes until response

CORNEAL OEDEMA

Find cause:
 e.g. Glaucoma
     Corneal dystrophy
     Herpes simplex
     Post traumatic
and treat as appropriate
symptomatic treatment:
 Acute
Glycerol eye drops
 Chronic
 Sodium Chloride 2-8% eye drops
  or Albumin eye drops
  or Cellulose gum
 and soft contact lenses which facilitate action of drops

CORNEAL ULCER

Obtain material for culture
Then start local antibiotics
 either Sulphacetamide eye drops hourly
 or Neomycin/Polymyxin eye drops hourly
 or Tetracycline eye drops hourly
 or Framycetin 0.5% eye drops hourly
 or Chloramphenicol eye drops hourly
 or Gentamicin 0.3% eye drops hourly
May need systemic antibiotics
May need subconjunctival antibiotics

DILATATION OF THE PUPIL (For Retinoscopy)

Tropicamide 0.5% eye drops 1-2 drops repeated in ½ hour if
necessary
 or Phenylephrine 2.5-10% eye drops 1 drop as necessary
NB: MAY PRECIPITATE NARROW ANGLE GLAUCOMA

To reverse effect:
Pilocarpine 1.0% 1-2 drops
 or Physostigmine 0.25% 1 drop

DRY EYE

Find cause and treat as appropriate
  and Methyl Cellulose eye drops hourly
  and soft contact lenses
Occasionally surgical closure of punctum may be needed

EXOPHTHALMOS

Find cause and treat as appropriate.

Thyrotoxic
Treat thyroid disease see p. 109.

Associated lid retraction
Guanethidine 5% eye drops 12 hourly

Associated with visual failure or ophthalmoplegia
GET EXPERT HELP AT ONCE

GLAUCOMA

Narrow angle
GET EXPERT HELP

Pilocarpine 2-4% every 15 minutes until pressure controlled
  then Pilocarpine 2-4% 6-12 hourly
and Glycerol 50% 1 mg/kg in fruit juice orally
  or Mannitol 20% 5 ml/kg i.v. over 1 hour
and Acetazolamide 500 mg i.v.
and Acetazolamide 500 mg orally
then when pressure under control:
  Surgery

Open angle
GET EXPERT HELP
Pilocarpine 1% 6 hourly at least
  When resistance develops increase dosage or frequency
  Maximum dose 4% 6 hourly
  If possible use Pilocarpine Ocusert
If not hypertension or narrow chamber angle
add Adrenaline 1-2% 8-24 hourly
and Guanethidine 5% 12 hourly
If loss of control:
  either Acetazolamide 250 mg 6 hourly i.v. or i.m.
    or Acetazolamide 500 mg orally
  or change Pilocarpine for either
  Echothiopate 0.125-0.25% 12 hourly
    or Demecarium bromide 0.25% 12 hourly
If all medical treatment fails:
  Surgery

HERPES SIMPLEX

Idoxuridine 0.1% eye drops
  1 drop hourly during day
  and 1 drop 2 hourly or 0.5% ointment at night
  (until does not stain)
    then Idoxuridine 0.1% eye drops
    1 drop 2 hourly during day,
    and 1 drop 4 hourly or 0.5% ointment at night for 3-5 days
  or Vidarabine 3% eye ointment 5 times a day
    then when re-epithelialised 12 hourly for 7 days
AVOID STEROIDS WHEN CORNEAL EPITHELIUM BREECHED

HERPES ZOSTER

GET EXPERT HELP from Ophthalmologist EARLY
Hydrocortisone ointment 1%
and Idoxuridine eye ointment
  or Vidarabine eye ointment.

ISCHAEMIC PAPILLITIS

Find cause and treat as appropriate
e.g. Giant Cell Arteritis (Medical emergency)
  Prednisone 20 mg 8 hourly
  Reducing dose when ESR falls to maintain
  it less than 20 mm/hr

OPTIC NEURITIS

Find cause and treat as appropriate
e.g. Multiple Sclerosis see p. 65.

PAPILLOEDEMA

Find cause and treat as appropriate.

RETINAL THROMBOSIS

Arterial
If diagnosed within 15 minutes
  CO_2 rebreathing
  Tolazine injection retrobulbally
EXPERT HELP NEEDED
Then:
  Look for association factors and treat as appropriate,
  e.g. oral contraceptives and hypertension.

Venous
No specific treatment
Look for associated factors and treat as appropriate,
e.g. oral contraceptives and hypertension.

STYE (hordeolum)

Symptomatic treatment only.

TRACHOMA

Tetracycline 250 mg 6 hourly by mouth for 3-6 weeks
   or Sulphadimidine 0.5 g 6 hourly by mouth for 3-6 weeks
and Sulphacetamide eye drops 10% 6 hourly

UVEITIS

Find cause and treat as appropriate
   Whilst establishing diagnosis dilate pupil with:
   either Atropine 1% eye drops
      or Hyoscine 0.2-0.5% eye drops
      or Phenylephrine 10% eye drops
and either: Dexamethasone 0.1% eye drops 4 hourly
      or Prednisolone 0.5% eye drops 4 hourly
   with appropriate ointment at night

Severe
Get expert help
Sub conjunctival injections
and Prednisone 0.5% eye drops hourly

Bilateral
Get expert help
   add Prednisone 20 mg 8 hourly
then slowly reduce dose

Chronic refractory iritis
Prednisone in lowest dose possible to control inflammation.

FURTHER READING

Duke-Elder, S. (1976) *System of Opthalmology,* Vol. 7. London:
Kimpton

Skin

B.R. Allen

Topical steroids
In many places in this chapter steroid ointments of varying sorts have been suggested. As there are a multitude of these we have only indicated the strength of the steroid ointment appropriate for the condition being discussed and at the end of the chapter is a table indicating into which group the various steroid ointments and creams available fall. This means a wider variation of possible choices of therapy in many of the conditions.

Bases
The base of a topical preparation is not necessarily completely inert and occasionally adverse reactions occur to such ingredients as lanolin and preservatives.
The rate at which an active constituent is released will vary according to the base. As a rule creams are more potent than ointments and gels, and lotions are more potent than creams for an equal concentration of a drug.
Patient acceptability must also be considered. An ointment may be unacceptable in a hot climate but the base of choice for a patient with a dry skin living in a temperate climate. Gels and lotions containing alcohols, are generally unsuitable for eczema and conditions where the skin surface is not intact.

ACNE

Adult
Remove cause (e.g. oil) or exacerbating factors (e.g. drugs)
Then remove surface grease with
    either soap and water
      or 2% Cetrimide
and unblock glands (blackheads) with
    either a rough flannel
      or Comedo Expressor
    NOT FINGERS
and if fails
    Tetracycline 250 mg orally 6 hourly for 4-6 weeks
    NOT IF PREGNANT
if fails
    Tretinoin (Retinoic acid) ointment 0.025% 12 hourly
    or Benzoyl peroxide 5 or 10% cream 12 hourly
    or Benzoyl peroxide 10% with sulphur 5% cream 12 hourly
if fails
    Get expert help

Infantile
Exclude sexual precosity
Reassure – resolves by 2 years

ACRODERMATITIS ENTEROPATHICA

Infants
Zinc sulphate elixir 100 mg daily after food

Over 5 years
Zinc sulphate 220 mg daily after food.

ACTINIC RETICULOID

Acute
Nurse in total darkness (15 watt filament bedside lamp only)
and strong or very strong steroids (see p. 176)
When inflammation settled:
Sun screening ointment, e.g. Titanium Dioxide 5%
Red Ferric Oxide 0.5%
Cetomacrogol Cream to 100%
before allowing light exposure

Chronic
Avoid light exposure
Remove fluorescent lights
and use sun screen ointment 3 hourly—even if not exposed
either Mexenone ointment
or Padimate A ointment or lotion
or Titanium Dioxide ointment as outlined above.
and Medium strength steroid at night (see p. 176).
and if relapses frequent:
Prednisone orally – in minimal dosage.

ACTINOMYCOSIS

Phenoxymethyl Penicillin 500 mg 6 hourly for 6 weeks
or if patient Penicillin sensitive:
Tetracycline 250 mg 6 hourly for 6 weeks
or Erythromycin 250 mg 6 hourly for 6 weeks
If fibrous tissue present:
Surgery – early rather than late.

ALOPECIA

Areata, totalis and universalis (Usually spontaneously remits)
Allay anxiety and wait

Cicatricial
Exclude underlying skin disease
No effective treatment

Congenital
No effective treatment

Diffuse
Telogen Efluvium – self limiting – Reassure
Endocrine – find cause and treat as appropriate
Drug induced – review therapy and stop if indicated
Pre-senile – no effective treatment

Traumatic
Traction – change hair style
Friction – treat itchy skin as appropriate
Habit – 'crew cut' for 2-3 months
DO NOT TIE HANDS

ANAPHYLAXIS

Lie patient down
Maintain airway
then Hydrocortisone 100 mg i.v. repeat as necessary
and Chlorpheniramine 10-20 mg i.m.
   or Promethazine 25-50 mg i.m.
Remove cause
Replace blood volume with 0.9% Sodium Chloride i.v.

ANHIDROSIS

No effective treatment
Beware Hyperpyrexia

ANTHRAX

See Infectious Disease Chapter p.2

APHTHOUS ULCERS

Exclude underlying cause
then Hydrocortisone pellets 2.5 mg allowed to disolve on lesion 6
hourly
or Tetracycline 250 mg in 15 ml of water
   hold in mouth for 5 minutes
   then spit out. Repeat 6 hourly.

or *Betamethasone Mouth wash 15 ml
   hold in mouth for 5 minutes
   then spit out. Repeat 6 hourly.

BALANITIS

Exclude venereal disease
Keep clean
and soak in Potassium Permanganate 1:1000 5 minutes daily
and Povodine Iodine ointment 10%
   or Clinoquinol ointment 3%
Examine consort
and treat as appropriate.

BOILS

Limited
Determine sensitivity of organism
Then bath in
   either Cetrimide 15% and Chlorhexidine gluconate 1.5% 30
   ml/bath
      or Hexachlorophane 10% 30 ml/bath
and antibiotic ointment
If pain and inflammation severe
   either Flucloxacillin 500 mg orally 6 hourly
      or appropriate antibiotic
If abscess formation
Drain

Recurrent
Treat as above
and determine carrier status – including family
then treat with either
   Clinoquinol 3% ointment
      or Neomycin ointment
   to nose and perineum as appropriate

CALCINOSIS

Treat underlying condition (if any)
   and Surgery

*(Betamethasone tablets 5 mg. Compound Tragacanth Powder 6 g.
Double strength chloroform water 75 ml. Water to 100 ml.)

CANCRUM ORIS

Get expert help.
Treat malnutrition and or infection.

CANDIDIASIS

Cutaneous
Keep clean
and Nystatin ointment 6 hourly
    or Clotrimazole 1% cream or solution 6 hourly
    or Miconazole 2% cream 6 hourly
If inflammation severe
    combine above with Hydrocortisone ½-1% ointment hourly

Oral
Babies
Usually harmless and self limiting
Nystatin suspension 100000 units/ml 3 hourly

Young Adults
Find cause
Then Aqueous Gentian Violet ½-2%

Edentulous
Adjust dentures
then apply ¼ inch Nystatin ointment to top of upper Denture each morning.

CELLULITIS

Treat underlying disease
and Phenoxymethyl Penicillin 500 mg 6 hourly for 2 weeks
    or if patient Penicillin sensitive
    Erythromycin 500 mg orally 6 hourly for 2 weeks

CHEILITIS (sore lips)

Look for underlying cause
and stop habit of licking
and Soft Paraffin ad. lib. during day
and mild steroid ointment (see p. 176) at night

CHILBLAINS

Warm clothing

CRADLE CAP

Olive Oil daily
Remove with shampoo (not soap) twice weekly
If resistant
    2% Sulphur and 2% Salicylic Acid in Oily Cream
If inflammed
    treat as infantile seborrhoeic eczema

CRUSTS

Treat cause as appropriate
To remove
    Eusol solution
        or Aqueous Chlorhexidine Gluconate 0.05%
    Then lift off
If resistant
    Apply Lead plaster 50% and Yellow soft paraffin
    50% thickly on lint
        – leave for 12 hours
        then peel off

CYSTS

Surgery

DERMATITIS ARTEFACTA

Occlusive dressing
and if indicated Psychiatric help.

DERMATITIS HERPETIFORMIS

Gluten free diet
and Dapsone 25-100 mg daily
    or Sulphapyridine 0.5-2 g daily

ECZEMA

Acute (inflammation and serous exudate)
    Rest
    Daily bath
        NO SOAP
    2 lbs Sodium Chloride/20 gallons water if very bad.
    and wet dressing with
    Lead lotion 6 hourly

If infected
either ½ strength Eusol
   or Potassium Permanganate 1:8000 for wet dressing
Change to subacute regime when exudate stopped.

Sub acute (little exudate)
   Weak or moderate steroid ointment (see p. 176)

If infected add
Topical antibiotic
      or Clioquinol 3%

If severe or extensive
Cover

Chronic (little inflammation)
Strong steroid ointment (see p. 176)
      or Crude coal tar 1-6% in Lassars Paste
      or Occlusive bandage with zinc and coal tar for
      a week at a time.

Acute primary irritant
Remove cause
then treat as above

Atopic
Use weakest possible steroid ointment (see p. 176)
Avoid soap – use Emulsifying ointment
Treat infection early with topical antibiotic/steroid ointment

Asteototic
Avoid all degreasing agents
Avoid soap – use Emulsifying ointment
Mild steroid ointment (see p. 176)

Contact
Remove cause
Then as above
NEVER use tar

Chronic primary irritant
Remove cause
Avoid soap – use Emulsifying ointment
Then as chronic above
NEVER use tar

Discoid
Crude Coal Tar 1-6% in Lassars Paste
   or Occlusive dressing with zinc and coal tar for
   a week at a time
   or Strong steroid ointment (see p. 176)

Hand
As for chronic primary irritant
If hyperkeratotic
Salicyclic Acid 5% in soft paraffin frequently during the day

Seborrhoeic
Adult
Mild
2% sulphur and 2% Salicylic Acid in Oily Cream daily
on scalp 12 hourly before shampooing
    or 1% sulphur in 1% Hydrocortisone cream
    or 1% Hydrocortisone plus Clioquinol 3%
Severe
either Chlortetracycline ointment 3%
    or Moderate steroid/antibiotic (see p. 176)

Infant
Reassure parents
and 1% Hydrocortisone plus Clioquinol 3% ointment
or Hydrocortisone plus Nystatin ointment

If exfoliative GET EXPERT HELP
    and Betamethasone 0.1% plus Clioquinol 3% ointment
        or Fluocinolone 0.025% plus Clioquinol 3% ointment
    For short periods only

When resolving Zinc and Castor Oil ointment

IN ALL CASES once disease is under control reduce, and if possible stop steroid application.

ERYTHEMA MULTIFORME

Mild
No treatment needed

Severe
Prednisone 30-60 mg daily
When controlled reduce dose

Oral lesion
Tetracycline mouth wash 6 hourly
(250 mg in 15 ml of water held in mouth for 5 minutes)

ERYTHEMA NODOSUM

Find cause and treat as appropriate
    and Aspirin 300-600 mg 8 hourly
        or Indomethacin 25-50 mg 8 hourly
Rarely Prednisone 60 mg daily – reducing dose once resolution has started.

GRANULOMA ANNULARE

Leave alone.

HERPES SIMPLEX

Primary infection

Lips or mouth
Symptomatic treatment only

Ocular
Idoxuridine eye drops 0.1% hourly during the day and 2 hourly at night

Whitlow

Prophylaxis:
Wear gloves
Wash hands in Providone Iodine solution

Treatment:
Analgesia for pain
    If early:
    Wet dressing with 40% Idoxuridine in Dimethyl
    Sulphoxide

Kaposi
Get expert help

Recurrent infection

Cold sore
Povidone Iodine locally
or rarely at first symptom:
    5% Idoxuridine in Dimethyl Sulphoxide 2 hourly

Ocular
Idoxuridine eye drops starting with earliest symptoms

HERPES ZOSTER

See shingles in Infectious Disease Chapter p. 13

IMPETIGO

See Infectious Disease Chapter p. 7.

INSECT BITE

Eradicate cause
then calamine lotion to lesion
then if still irritant
   Crotamiton ointment

INSECT STING

Ensure sting removed
   if not remove by SCRAPING

Severe local reaction
   Splint limb
   Apply wet dressing

Anaphylaxis
See separate entry p. 158

INTERTRIGO

Separate skin surfaces
Then aqueous eosin 2% paint 6-8 hourly
When dry
   1% Hydrocortisone with 3% Clioquinol ointment
When cleared
   keep dry with Boric Acid 5% in talc.

ITCHING

see PRURITUS p. 169

KERATODERMA BLENHORRHAGICA

Inflamed – moderately strong corticosteroid plus antiseptic ointment
(see p. 176)

Hyperkeratotic lesion
Salicyclic Acid 5-10% in soft paraffin.

LEPROSY

Lepromatous
Dapsone 25 mg twice weekly, gradually increasing over 3-4 months
to 400 mg twice weekly.
   and Rifampicin 600 mg daily for 2-3 weeks (renders non-infective)
and to suppress lepra reaction:
Clofazimine 100 mg three times a week, increasing slowly to
maximum of 400 mg daily if necessary for at least 6 months
Continue Dapsone for life.

Tuberculoid
Dapsone 25 mg twice weekly
Continue for 2 years, or until all activity absent for 1 year –
whichever is the longer.

LICHEN PLANUS

Intense irritation
   Potent topical steroid ointment (see p. 176)
   (Occlusion may be necessary)
Widespread eruption
   Prednisone 20 mg daily
   reducing as soon as relief obtained
Otherwise
   No treatment necessary

LUPUS ERYTHEMATOSUS – DISCOID

Avoid direct sunlight
and Mexenone ointment prophylactically
   or Padimate A. ointment prophylactically
Occasionally Beclomethasone 0.5% ointment
Occasionally, during the summer, Chloroquine 250 mg 12 hourly
   or Hydroxychloroquine 200 mg 12 hourly
NB: OPHTHALMIC TESTING AT LEAST EVERY 3 MONTHS
MANDATORY

MOLLUSCUM CONTAGIOSUM

(Self Limiting)
Tretinoin (Retinoic Acid) to lesion
   or Pricking with wooden point dipped in liquid Phenol 6%
   or Painting with Podophyllin 25% in Tinct Benz Co.
   or Minor surgery

MYCOSIS FUNGOIDES

Get expert help.

NAEVI

Capillary
Ignore

Cavernous
Resolve spontaneously
Treat infections as appropriate

Cellular
Ignore

Epidermal
Surgery

Spider
Look for underlying cause
   then ignore

ONCOCERCIASIS

Get Expert help.
   Diethylcarbamazine 1 mg/kg for 2 days
      then 2 mg/kg for 2 days
      then 3 mg/kg for 2 days
      then 4 mg/kg for 15 days
   and Chlorpheniramine 4 mg 6-8 hourly for first 5 days (to prevent
   adverse reaction)
   BEWARE WORSENING OF EYE INVOLVEMENT

ONYCHOLYSIS

Find cause and treat as appropriate
(Remember trauma)

PARONYCHIA

Acute
Stop the pain with either Aspirin 300-900 mg 4-6 hourly
   or Paracetamol 0.5-1.0 g 4-6 hourly
   or Dihydrocodeine 30-60 mg 4-6 hourly
   and antibiotics as appropriate
May need surgery

Chronic
Reduce exposure to water
   and soft paraffin to nail fold ad lib during the day
   and 0.5% Hydrocortisone with Clinoquinol 3% and Nystatin
100 000 units at night
Continue treatment for 3 to 4 months

PEDICULOSIS

Capitis
Malathion 0.5% solution

Corporis
Autoclave all clothes and bedding

Pubic
Malathion 0.5% solution

PEMPHIGOID

Prednisone 50-100 mg daily
When under control reduce dose cautiously at weekly intervals to minimal possible dose
Occasionally
  Azathioprine 2 mg/kg/day will allow the Prednisone dose to be reduced.

PEMPHIGUS

Foliaceus
Moderate to strong steroid ointment (see p. 176)
Occasionally Prednisone 5-20 mg daily may be necessary

Vulgaris
Prednisone 20-30 mg 6 hourly
  When controlled
  Reduce dose to minimum necessary
and Azathioprine 2 mg/kg/day to allow Prednisone dose to be at minimum
and cover lesions
and bath in isotonic solution with 2 lbs of Sodium chloride in 20 gallons of water (900 g in 100 litres)

Secondary infection:
Treat as appropriate

Oral lesion:
Tetracycline 250 mg in 15 ml of water
Used as a mouth wash.

PITYRIASIS

Capitis
Sulphur 2% + Salicylic Acid 2% in oily cream BP 12-24 hours before shampooing

Rosea
(self limiting)

Severe irritation
    Mild/moderate corticosteroid cream (see p. 176)

PORPHYRIA

Congenital
Avoid all light exposure
Splenectomy may help

Acquired hepatic (Cutanea Tarda)
Avoid all alcohol
Look for cirrhosis or hepatoma
Venesection of 1 unit (500 ml) every 2 weeks until mild Iron
deficiency

Erythropoietic
Avoid all light exposure
ß carotene may help.

Variegate
Avoid barbiturates and sulphonamides
Avoid trauma and direct sunlight.

PRURITUS

Ani
Exclude metabolic or bowel disease
Exclude local skin disease
Wash on alternate days
Avoid soap – using emulsifying ointment
Then if fails:
    1% Hydrocortisone with Clioquinol 3% ointment
    or 1% Hydrocortisone with Clioquinol 3% and Nystatin 100000
    units
    Occasionally 0.1% Betamethasone plus Clioquinol 3%
Rarely need:
    Radiotherapy 70 rads at 100KV weekly x 3
    (often only temporary relief)

Generalised
Look for underlying cause and treat as appropriate.

Symptomatic
    Menthol $\frac{1}{4}$-1% in aqueous cream
        or Phenol $\frac{1}{4}$% in calamine
        or Crotamiton 10%

Senile
Exclude 'internal' cause
Reduce frequency of washing
Avoid soap – using emulsifying agents
Occasionally:
  Topical steroids
Rarely:
  Prednisone 10 mg daily

Vulvae
Exclude gynaecological disease and glycosuria
Then as for pruritis ani

Obstructive jaundice
Cholestyramine 4-6 g 6-8 hourly

PSORIASIS

AVOID OVER TREATING
AVOID STEROIDS if possible because of untoward effects

Guttate
Coal tar 2% and Salicylic Acid 2% in emulsifying ointment 12
  hourly
  or Salicylic Acid 5% in soft paraffin 12 hourly
  or Liquor picis carbonis 10% in emulsifying ointment 12 hourly
If following sore throat:
  Phenoxymethyl Penicillin 500 mg 6 hourly for 5 days
If persists:
  Ultra violet radiation

Nummular
? need to treat
Daily baths with liquor picis carbonis in water
and to lesions immediately after drying
Coal tar 2% and Salicylic acid 2% in emulsifying ointment
  or Salicyclic Acid 5% in soft paraffin
  or Liquor picis carbonis 10% in emulsifying ointment
If no benefit after 4-6 weeks:
  Ultra violet radiation in increasing suberythema doses 3 times
  weekly for 3 weeks.
If no improvement:
  Use Dithranol in Lassars paste in place of ointment above
  Start with Dithranol 0.25%
    and increase by 0.25% per week until effective
    or soreness develops.

Acute eruptive
When still spreading
  As for guttate

Scalp lesions

Mild
Daily lotion of equal parts of liquor picis carbonis, spirit and water

Severe
Add 3% sulphur and 3% Salicylic acid in oily cream 12 hourly
before shampooing.

Resistant
Daily pyrogallic acid compound ointment (messy)

Erythrodermic
Get expert help

Pustular

Palms and soles:
Crude coal tar 4-6% in Lassars paste
   or Dithranol as described under nummular p. 170

Generalised:
Get expert help

Nails
No specific treatment

Flexural
Moderate or strong topical steroids permitted (see p. 176)

PYODERMA GANGRENOSUM

Treat underlying cause
Then steroid and antibiotic ointment
Occasionally:
    Prednisone 10-15 mg 6 hourly to stop spread.

RADIODERMATITIS

Acute
Keep washing to minimum for 3-4 weeks after radiotherapy

 with blisters:

 Clioquinol 3% ointment

Chronic
Protect from further damage

RINGWORM

Human – tinea pedis, tinea corporis, tinea cruris

Acute exudative
Castellani's Paint 6-8 hourly for 3-4 days

Sub acute and chronic
Benzoic Acid compound ointment daily for 3-4 weeks

Resistant
Griseofulvin 250 mg 12 hourly for 4 weeks

Nails

  Fingers
  Griseofulvin 250 mg 12 hourly for 3-6 months

  Toes:
  Griseofulvin 250 mg 12 hourly for 6-12 months

Animal – tinea capitis (in children) tinea barbae, tinea corporis

In all cases

Children
Griseofulvin 125 mg 12 hourly

Adults
Griseofulvin 250 mg 12 hourly

In both cases continue until all signs of infection eradicated

Local lesion
Treat as for human infections as described above

ROSACEA

Stop all topical steroids
Then Tetracycline 250 mg 12 hourly
  or Metronidazole 200 mg 12 hourly
Continue until skin clear, or 2 months, which ever is longer

SCABIES

Adult
Paint whole body from neck to sole of feet with
Benzyl Benzoate emulsion B.P.
Repeat next day
Treat close contacts similarly

Children
Use gamma Benzene Hexachloride 1% solution & apply as above.

In both cases
On second day launder underwear and bed linen only

SUNBURN

Prophylaxis
Titanium Dioxide 5% plus
Red Ferric Oxide 0.5% plus
Cetomacrogol Cream to 100% applied as necessary

Mild
Calamine lotion

Moderate
Mild Topical Steroid (see p. 176)

Severe
Get expert help
Treat as for burns

TUBERCULOSIS

Treat as for systemic infection
see Respiratory chapter p. 29

TUMOURS

Get expert help.

ULCERS

Arterial
Adequate analgesia
Then get expert help

Venous

General
Elevate leg
Support with bandage whenever upright

Local
Clean with Eusol solution 6 hourly
When clean use Eusol in 50% emulsion with liquid paraffin 12 hourly
Reduce frequency of dressings as heals
Protect surrounding skin with
Lassars paste softened in 10% olive oil

If infected
with Pseudomonas use Polymixin B ointment
with Streptococci use Phenoxymethyl Penicillin 500 mg 6 hourly for 5 days

Pressure

Prophylaxis
Regular turning of patients at risk
Distribute pressure more evenly with sheepskins, water beds or ripple beds.
BEWARE of deep sedation
Avoid coarse linen, in particular 'draw sheets'.

Early lesions (Erythema, no necrosis)
    As for prophylaxis
        and Protection with 1% Ichthyol in Zinc paste spread thickly on calico.

Shallow necrosis
Avoid all pressure
Remove slough with wet dressings of Eusol applied 6 hourly

When granulating
Bland dressing with either paraffin gauze BPC
    or 'M & M tulle'

Deep necrosis
As for shallow necrosis
    and Surgery may be necessary to obliterate deep cavities

URTICARIA

Look for cause, e.g., drugs
Avoid friction and extremes of temperature

Symptomatic
Chlorpheniramine 4 mg 8-12 hourly
    or Diphenhydramine 25 mg 8-12 hourly
Start with lowest dose and increase on alternate days until symptoms controlled
Avoid steroids

VITILIGO

White skinned people
To prevent sunburn of depigmented areas:
Mexenone ointment
or Padimate A ointment
or Titanium Dioxide 5%, Red Ferric Oxide 0.5%, Cetomacrogol
Cream to 100%

Black skinned people
Prevent sunburn as above
and either attempt to repigment with
either Methoxypsoralen 10-20 mg orally
then 2 hours later controlled exposure to sunlight
initially 5 minutes and slowly increasing to at least ½ an hour.
CARE OR BURNING MAY OCCUR
or occasionally:
Betamethasone ointment
or to make depigmentation uniform:
use Monobenzone 5% in emulsifying ointment

WARTS

Perianal and perivulval
Podophyllin in tinc. Benz. Co 25-50% apply every 2 weeks (avoid in
Pregnancy)

Most sites
Salicylic Acid 20-50% in suitable base daily for 2 weeks
leave one week
then repeat until clear

Plantar
As above

Hands
Liquid Nitrogen
or Carbon Dioxide Snow

Table 4 Topical Corticosteroids

Non-Proprietary Name (General)	*Proprietary Name* (Trade)
MILD POTENCY	
Hydrocortisone base or acetate 0.1% – 2.5%	
	Cobadex 0.5% 1%
	Cortril 0.5% 1% 2.5%
	Dome-Cort 0.125%
	Efcortelan 0.5% 1% 2.5%
	Hydrocortistab 1%
	Hydrocortisyl 1%
	Hydrocortone 1%
MODERATE POTENCY	
Methylprednisolone 0.25%	Medrone
Clobetasone Butyrate 0.05%	Eumovate
Fluocinolone Acetonide 0.01%	Synandone
Fluocortolone Hexanoate/Pivalate 0.1%	Ultradil
Flurandrenolone 0.0125%	Haelan
Hydrocortisone 1% with urea	Alphaderm
	Calmurid HC
POTENT	
Beclomethasone Dipropionate 0.025%	Propaderm
Betamethasone Valerate 0.1%	Betnovate
Desonide 0.05%	Tridesilon
Diflucortolone Valerate 0.1%	Nerisone
	Temetex
Fluclorolone Acetonide 0.025%	Topilar
Flucinolone Acetonide 0.025%	Synalar
Fluprednylidene Acetate 0.1%	Decoderm
Hydrocortisone Butyrate 0.1%	Locoid
Flucortolone 0.25% + F. Hexanoate 0.25%	Ultralanum Plain
Flurandrenolone 0.05%	Haelan X
Triamcinolone Acetonide 0.1%	Adcortyl
	Ledercort
VERY POTENT	
Clobetasol Propionate 0.05%	Dermovate
Fluocinonide 0.05%	Metosyn
Halcinonide 0.1%	Halciderm
ESPECIALLY POTENT	
Beclomethasone Dipropionate 0.5%	Propaderm Forte
Diflucortolone Valerate 0.3%	Nerisone Forte
Fluocinolone Acetonide 0.2%	Synalar Forte
Flurandrenolone 4 μg per cm^2	Haelan Tape

Most of the corticosteroids above are also available in combinations with antibiotics and antiseptics.

Stronger corticosteroids may be diluted to reduce their potency but care must be taken to ensure that the diluent is compatible with the base of the corticosteroid preparation.

Corticosteroid/Antibiotic or Antiseptic mixtures must not be diluted.

The potency of topical preparations varies with the base. As a rule creams are more potent than ointments.

FURTHER READING

Barker, D.J. & Millard, L.J. (1979) *The Essentials of Skin Disease Management* Oxford: Blackwell Scientific.
British Medical Association. Today's Treatment No. 1.
Rook, A., Wilkinson, D.S. & Ebling, F.J.G. (1972) *Textbook of Dermatology* Oxford: Blackwell Scientific.
Wilkinson, D.S. (1977) *The Nursing and Management of Skin Diseases* London: Faber & Faber

Poisoning

In this chapter the management of various types of poisoning is presented. In most cases all that is necessary is the general management as described below. In only a few instances are specific measures helpful. Under the various headings these specific measures are indicated but these are only employed if there is evidence that the poison is harming the patient. In the majority of instances it is better just to maintain vital function and allow the patient to eliminate the poison.

If in doubt Get EXPERT help
  either locally
  or from one of the Poison Centres
  Telephone numbers of which are:
  BELFAST 0232-40503
  CARDIFF 0222-33101
  DUBLIN 45588
  EDINBURGH 031-229-2477
  LONDON 01-407-7600
  LEEDS 0532-32799
  MANCHESTER 061-740-2254
  NEWCASTLE 0632-25131

GENERAL MANAGEMENT

Clear airway and turn on side.

Conscious
Wash out with warm water* if within 4 hours of taking tablets
(With Aspirin never too late)
then any specific therapy

Unconscious
Insert endotracheal tube
then wash out with warm water* (never too late with Aspirin)
then insert i.v. line
and maintain airway
then any specific therapy

*for material used with cyanide, iron, glutethamide, opiates, sodium hypochlorite, oxalic acid, and phenol and phosphorous, please see appropriate section.

If respiratory failure
Oxygen by face mask
Try effect of Naloxone 400 micrograms intravenously and repeat if effective
If no benefit – Ventilate (early rather than late)
If respiratory depressant, see relevant section

If shock
Oxygen by face mask
Elevate legs
If no benefit in ½ hour – either Sodium Chloride 0.9% 500 ml i.v.
   and/or Dextran '40' 500 ml i.v.
     or occasionally:
     Metraminol 5 mg i.m, repeated if necessary after 20 minutes.

If acidaemia

Respiratory
Ventilate

Non-respiratory
Sodium Bicarbonate 8.4% 100 ml i.v. slowly
Repeated x 1 if necessary
If fails – Hydrocortisone 100 mg i.v. 6 hourly

If hypothermia
Keep warm and cover with 'space blanket'

In all cases
General nursing care
Regular turning
Regular physiotherapy to limbs and to chest
Rehydrate (if necessary)
and maintain water and electrolyte balance.

ANTICOAGULANTS

General care: as outlined above

Special care:

Coumarins
Vitamin K_1 2.5 mg slowly i.v. repeated as necessary according to coagulation tests.
occasionally need:
Coagulation factors
   either fresh frozen plasma
   or factor concentrates

Heparin
Protamine sulphate (1 mg ≡ 80 units of Heparin)
Aim to neutralize half of Heparin dose
Inject slowly i.v. to a maximum of 50 mg
Repeat after 10 minutes if necessary.

ANTIHISTAMINES

General care: as outlined above

Special care

If CNS stimulation
Diazepam 5-20 mg i.m. or i.v. as necessary.

ARSENIC

General care: as outlined above.

Special care
Dimercaprol 4 mg/kg i.m. 4 hourly x 12
then Dimercaprol 2 mg/kg i.m. 12 hourly for 8 days
(Painful and irritant, therefore use different sites for injection).
May require Morphine for abdominal pain.

ATROPINE

General care: as outlined above.

Special care

Central effects
Physostigmine 1-2 mg sub/c, i.m. or i.v. repeated in 1-2 hours if
necessary
(also blocks peripheral effects)
and either Diazepam 2-10 mg.i.m. or i.v.
   or Paraldehyde 5 ml i.m. repeated as necessary

Peripheral effects
Physostigmine 1-2 mg i.m. or i.v. or sub/c, repeated in 1-2 hours if
necessary
(also blocks central effects)
   or Neostigmine 0.25 mg sub/c
and Carbachol 0.5 mg sub/c repeated as necessary

BARBITURATES

General care: as outlined above

Special care
(Phenobarbitone or Barbitone)
If unconscious or deepening coma
To shorten period of coma
either
Renal function thought to be normal
Catheterise
then forced alkaline diuresis:
1. 500 ml 1.4% Sodium Bicarbonate i.v. over ½ hour with Frusemide* 40 mg
then 2. 500 ml 5% Dextrose i.v. over ½ hour + Potassium Chloride as necessary.
then 3. 500 ml 0.9% Sodium Chloride i.v. over ½ hour + Potassium Chloride as necessary.
then 4. 500 ml 20% Mannitol i.v. over ½ hour.
Then repeat 1-4 with an hour for each infusion.

*The dose of Frusemide should be adjusted to ensure marked diuresis.

Maintain electrolyte and water balance.
or
Renal function thought to be abnormal
Dialyse

BENZODIAZEPINES

General care: as outlined above.

Special care
None helpful

CARBAMATES e.g. Meprobamate

General care: as outlined above.

Special care (rarely needed – as metabolised/excreted within 24 hours)
Occasionally Osmotic alkaline diuresis as described for Barbiturates above.
or Haemodialysis NOT peritoneal dialysis.

CARBON MONOXIDE

General care: as outlined above.

Special care: Oxygen 100% by face mask
or Hyperbaric oxygen – if available

If cerebral oedema
Dexamethasone 10 mg i.m. or i.v. stat
then Dexamethasone 2-4 mg i.m. or orally 6 hourly
   or 500 ml of Mannitol 20% i.v. over 15 minutes
then 500 ml of Dextrose 5% i.v. 4 hourly

CHLORAL

General care: as outlined above

Special care
Very occasionally with severe poisoning.
Osmotic alkaline diuresis as described for barbiturates on p. 181.

CONTRACEPTIVE PILLS

General care: as outlined above.

Special care
None specific necessary.

CYANIDE

Special care
START AT ONCE
amyl nitrite by inhalation for 30 seconds every minute.
AS SOON AS POSSIBLE
Cobalt edetate 600 mg i.v.
   then via the same needle
Dextrose 50% 50 ml i.v.
If not recovered in one minute
Cobalt edetate 300 mg i.v.
   then via the same needle
Dextrose 50% 50 ml i.v.

If fails, or not available:
Sodium nitrite 3% 10 ml i.v. over 3 minutes
   then via the same needle
25 ml of Sodium Thiosulphate 50% i.v.
Repeat with ½ doses if no response
   and Ventilate with Oxygen if necessary.
NB: DO NOT STOP UNTIL ALL CARDIAC ACTIVITY HAS CEASED.

General care: as outlined above.
WASHOUT as soon as possible with Sodium Thiosulphate 25%
leaving 300 ml of Sodium Thiosulphate 25% in stomach.

DIGITALIS

General care: as outlined above.

Special care
Monitor cardiac rhythm
Potassium Chloride 1 g orally every 20 minutes
   or Potassium Chloride 1 g in 200 ml of 5% Dextrose i.v. every 30
   minutes.
   (depending on serum level)

Bradycardia
Atropine 0.6 mg i.m. repeated as necessary
May need pacemaker

Ventricular ectopics
Lignocaine 100 mg stat i.v.
   then Lignocaine infusion 1-3 mg/min i.v.
   or Phenytoin 50-250 mg i.v. slowly
   then Phenytoin 200-400 mg orally daily

ETHYL ALCOHOL

General care: as outlined above

Special care
Severe poisoning:
   Peritoneal dialysis
   or Haemodialysis

GLUTETHIMIDE

General care: as outlined above.
BUT when washing out (never too late) use a mixture of equal parts
of Water and Castor Oil, then leave
50 ml of Castor Oil in stomach.

Special care
Acidosis: 100 ml Sodium Bicarbonate 8.4% i.v. slowly
   Repeated as necessary.
Cerebral oedema: Treat on slightest suspicion, with
   either Dexamethasone 10 mg i.m. stat
      then Dexamethasone 2-4 mg orally or i.m. 6 hourly
   or 500 ml Mannitol 20% i.v. over 20 minutes
      then 500 ml Dextrose 5% i.v. for 4 hours.
NB: LEVEL OF CONSCIOUSNESS FLUCTUATES WIDELY

G

IRON

General care: as outlined above.
BUT always wash out using either Sodium Bicarbonate 1 g in 100 ml of water
   or Desferrioxamine 2 g in 1 litre warm water
then leave 10 g of Desferrioxamine in 50 ml of water in the stomach.

Special care
Desferrioxamine 2 g in 10 ml of water i.m.
then repeat 12 hourly
   and Desferrioxamine infusion 15 mg/kg/hr to a maximum of 80 mg/kg/24 hrs

KEROSENE AND PETROLEUM DISTILLATES

General care
DO NOT WASHOUT
250 ml of liquid Paraffin by mouth

Special care

Pneumonitis
Hydrocortisone 100 mg i.m. 6 hourly
   and Benzyl Penicillin 1 mega unit 6 hourly

LEAD

General care: as outlined above.

Special care

Chelation
Dimercaprol 4 mg/kg i.m.
then 4 hours later Dimercaprol 3 mg/kg i.m.
and Sodium Calcium EDTA 8 mg/kg i.v. or i.m. (Separate site)
Repeat Dimercaprol and Sodium Calcium EDTA 4 hourly for 1-3 days
(Given in separate sites)

Colic
10 mls of Calcium Gluconate 10% i.v.
   or Pethidine 25-100 mg i.m.
   or Morphine 15-30 mg i.m.

Encephalopathy
Give chelating agents (see above) i.m.
   and Dexamethasone 10 mg i.m. stat
then Dexamethasone 2-6 mg orally or i.m. 6 hourly
   or 500 ml Mannitol 20% i.v. slowly

Convulsions
Diazepam 5-20 mg i.m. or i.v. slowly
Repeated as necessary.

Convalescent
D-Penicillamine 20-40 mg/kg/day orally until serum lead levels
within normal range.

LITHIUM

General care: as outlined above.

Special care
either Osmotic Alkaline diuresis, as described for Barbiturates on
p.181
    or Prolonged peritoneal dialysis
(Monitor Plasma Level)

LYSERGIC ACID

General care: as outlined above

Special care
Chlorpromazine 100 mg i.m.
Repeat in 20 minutes if needed

MERCURY (rare as not well absorbed)

General care: as outlined above.

Special care
Dimercaprol 4 mg/kg i.m. 4 hourly x 12
then Dimercaprol 3 mg/kg i.m. 12 hourly for 8 days.
(painful and irritant therefore use different sites for injections).

METHAQUALONE (e.g. Mandrax)

General care: as outlined above.

Special care
None helpful.
AVOID FORCED DIURESIS as can induce pulmonary oedema.

METHYL ALCOHOL

General care: as outlined above.

Special care: Get EXPERT help early.

Acidosis
100 ml of Sodium Bicarbonate 8.4% i.v. repeated as necessary

Metabolism
Block with 50% Ethyl Alcohol 1 ml/kg orally
then 50% Ethyl Alcohol 0.5 ml/kg orally 2 hourly for 5 days or until
no Methyl Alcohol in blood

Impaired vision or failure of response
Haemodialysis
    or if not available Peritoneal dialysis
Protect eyes from strong light.

MONOAMINEOXIDASE INHIBITORS

General care: as outlined above.
BUT AVOID METRAMINOL – treat severe hypotension with
Dextran '40' 500 ml i.v.
    and Hydrocortisone 100 mg i.v. 6 hourly
    or Plasma

Special care

Sedate if necessary
with Chlorpromazine 25-100 mg i.m.

Convulsions
Diazepam 5-20 mg i.m. or i.v. as necessary

Hypertension
Pentolinium 3 mg s.c. repeated as necessary
(elevate head of bed)

If severe: Pentolinium 5-10 mg i.v. slowly
    or Phenoxybenzamine 10-20 mg i.v. slowly

Hyperthermia
Damp sponging
Chlorpromazine 25-100 mg i.m.
    and/or Hydrocortisone 100 mg i.m.

MORPHINE AND OPIUM ALKALOIDS including Dihydrocodeine
and Dextropropoxyphene

General care: as outlined above.

Special care
either Naloxone 400 μg i.v. every 2-3 minutes until recovery
   then if relapse repeat Naloxone 400 μg i.v.
(Worth trying whenever possibility of Opiate overdose)
or Nalorphine 10 mg i.v. every 15 minutes until recovery
   then if relapse repeat Nalorphine 15 mg i.v.
NB- MAY DEVELOP WITHDRAWAL SYMPTOMS

OXALIC ACID

General care: as outlined above.
BUT washout with Dilute Calcium Hydroxide (Lime Water)
and leave 100 ml in stomach.

Special care
10 ml of Calcium Gluconate 10% i.v.
May be needed in large quantities.
Monitor with ECG
Maintain tetany free
Maintain urine flow high
or Haemodialysis – early rather than late.

PARACETAMOL

General care: as outlined above.

Special care
If less than 4 hours since taking overdose:
L-Methionine 2.5 g orally (may only have DL Methionine therefore give 5.0g)
then osmotic alkaline diuresis as described for barbiturates. p. 181
If between 4-10 hours:
L-Methionine 2.5 g orally (may only have DL Methionine therefore give 5.0 g)
and take sample for plasma level.
Plot result on log scale against time.
Put in line 200 μg/ml (1320 mmol/l) at 4 hours to 70 μg/ml (462 mmol/l) at 10 hours (see Fig. 1 p. 188)

If more than 50 μg/ml below line
   Significant damage – rare
If on line or less than 50 μg/ml below line
   Significant damage – unlikely
   Repeat level in 2 hours.
   Check prothrombin time at 6 hours.
   If both normal
      Significant damage – rare

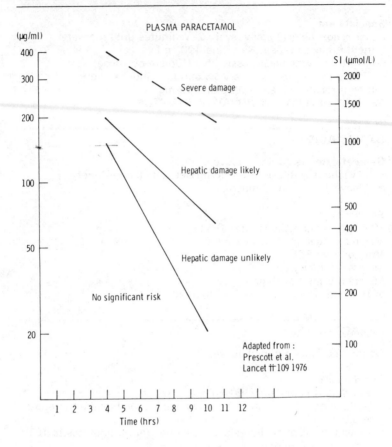

PLASMA PARACETAMOL

(μg/ml)

SI (μmol/L)

Severe damage

Hepatic damage likely

Hepatic damage unlikely

No significant risk

Adapted from:
Prescott et al.
Lancet ᵢᵢ 109 1976

Time (hrs)

If level above line (initially or secondarily)
   and still within 10 hours
     either N-acetylcysteine 150 mg/kg i.v. over 15 minutes
       then 50 mg/kg in 500 ml Dextrose 5% in 4 hours
       then 100 mg/kg in 500 ml Dextrose 5% in 16 hours
     or Cysteamine 2 g i.v. over 10 minutes
       then Cysteamine 800 mg i.v. over 4 hours
       then Cysteamine 400 mg i.v. over 8 hours x 2
     or Methionine 2.5 g orally 4 hourly x 4
Maintain fluid and electrolyte balance.
If more than 10 hours:
No special care helpful
Check liver function tests and treat as appropriate

PARAQUAT

General care: as outlined above,
but leave 500 ml of 7% Bentonite suspension in the stomach

Special care
GET EXPERT HELP QUICKLY
Avoid oxygen as long as possible
Magnesium Sulphate 10 g orally with 250 ml of water
    Then 200-500 ml of 7% Bentonite suspension orally
    Followed by Magnesium Sulphate 10 g orally
    Repeat every 2 hours for 24 hours,
    then every 4 hours for 24 hours.
Maintain fluid and electrolyte balance.
Haemodialysis or haemoperfusion, using a charcoal column may be of help.

PHENACETIN

General care: as outlined above

Special care

Methaemaglobinaemia
25 ml Methylene Blue 1% slowly i.v.
Repeated as necessary
OTHERWISE TREAT AS FOR PARACETAMOL.

PHENOL

General care: as outlined above,
BUT washout with a mixture of equal parts Water and Castor Oil.

Special care
None helpful

PHENOTHIAZINES

General care: as outlined above.
Ignore hypotension unless urine flow falls.

Special care
Cardiac arrhythmias
    Treat as described in chapter on cardiovascular system p. 30-34
Convulsions
    Diazepam 5-20 mg i.m. or i.v. as necessary.
Severe extra pyramidal reactions
    either Benztropine 1-2 mg i.v. slowly
        or Procyclidine 10 mg i.v. slowly
    Repeated x 1 if necessary.

PHENYTOIN

General care: as outlined above.

Special care
None helpful

PHOSPHORUS

General care: as outlined above,
BUT washout with 0.1% copper sulphate in water
  or 1:5000 Potassium Permangenate – do not leave in stomach.

Special care

Hepatic damage
Vitamin K_1 20 mg i.v. repeated according to prothrombin time
If severe refer to specialised centre.

Renal failure
Treat with dialysis if necessary

Burns
Wash with 1% copper sulphate in water.

PRIMIDONE

General care: as outlined above.

Special care
Severe poisoning:
  Osmotic alkaline diuresis as described for Salicylates below

SALICYLATES

General care: as outlined above,
  WASHOUT whenever tablets taken and take sample for blood level

Special care: If symptoms or signs
  Alkaline diuresis:
    1. 500 ml of Dextrose 5% i.v. over $\frac{1}{4}$ hour + Frusemide *40
       mg to increase diuresis
then 2. 500 ml of Sodium Bicarbonate 1.4% i.v. over $\frac{1}{4}$ hour with
       Potassium Chloride as necessary
then 3. 500 ml of Sodium Chloride 0.9% i.v. over $\frac{1}{4}$ hour with
       Potassium Chloride as necessary
then 4. 500 ml of Dextrose 5% i.v. over $\frac{1}{4}$ hour with Potassium
       Chloride as necessary
  1-4 can also be given together via one i.v. line over 1 hour
Maintain urine pH > 7.0

*Adjust Frusemide dosage to maintain high urine flow

If salicylate level > 50 mg/100 ml
  Repeat 1-4 x 3
  then repeat 1-4 but infusing each over ½ hour or altogether over
  2 hours
  Reassess with plasma level after 1 hour
If salicylate level 35-50 mg/100 ml
  Repeat 1-4 but infusing each over ½ hour or altogether over 2
  hours
  Reassess plasma level after 1 hour
    If rising or static continue
    If falling – stop
If salicylate level less than 35 mg/100 ml
  Stop infusion

NB: Maintain fluid and electrolyte balance throughout

In children
Infuse at the rate of 30 ml/kg/hr and watch potassium level
carefully.

In all cases
Maintain urine pH > 7.0
  encourage fluids by mouth and add effervescent potassium
  chloride to drinks.
Monitor salicylate level 4 hourly
  and adjust therapy according to results.
May develop severe hypoglycaemia.
If forced alkaline diuresis not possible:
  either peritoneal dialysis
  or haemodialysis
NB: If plasma pH falls or severe poisoning
    Consider haemodialysis early.

SODIUM HYPOCHLORITE

General care: as outlined above,
BUT washout with 2.5% Sodium Thiosulphate (Hypo)
  or Milk of Magnesia in water
  or Milk

Special care
None helpful

SYMPATHOMIMETIC AGENTS

General care: as outlined above.

Special care

Amphetamines
Acid diuresis:
      1. 500 ml Dextrose 5% ½ hourly with 1.5 g of Ammonium
         Chloride
then 2. 500 ml Dextrose 5% ½ hourly
then 3. 500 ml Sodium Chloride 0.9% ½ hourly
then repeat 1-3 with 1 hour for each infusion.

Cardiac
Control rate with Propranolol, initially 1-10 mg slowly i.v. under
ECG control.
then 10-40 mg orally 8 hourly.
May need α blocker, e.g. Phentolamine 5-10 mg i.v.
Repeated as necessary.

TRICYCLIC ANTIDEPRESSANTS

General care: as outlined above,
AVOID i.v. infusion unless mandatory.

Special care

Cardiac arrhythmias

  No haemodynamic effect
  Ignore

  Haemodynamic effect
  Initially Pyridostigmine 1 mg i.v. slowly with an ECG monitor
  If fails: repeat after ½ hour
  then if controlled: Pyridostigmine 1 mg i.m. 4 hourly
  If not controlled: use drugs as described in CVS chapter p. 30-34

Convulsions
Diazepam 5-20 mg i.v. as necessary
NB: PATIENT OFTEN HAS FIXED DILATED PUPILS

FURTHER READING

Matthews, H. & Lawson, A.A.H. (1974) *The Treatment of Common
Acute Poisoning* Edinburgh: Churchill Livingstone

Care of the Dying

In this chapter I deal with the use of medicines in the treatment of common symptoms encountered in patients who have terminal illnesses. Even when no curative treatment can be offered a great deal can be done to relieve symptoms. It should be realised that there is more to treating these patients than just treating the symptoms with medicine. The whole patient is important. Spiritual, mental and other needs require attention and there are as many possible treatments as there are patients.
One must also always remember that symptoms may not be due to the underlying disease and that full diagnosis is important so that the correct therapy can be prescribed.

ANOREXIA

Either Alcohol before meals
or Prednisone 5 mg 8 hourly

ANXIETY

Diazepam 2-5 mg 8 hourly
or Promazine 25 mg 8 hourly
or Chlorpromazine 10-25 mg 8 hourly

BONE PAIN

Add to basic analgesic regime:
    either Aspirin 300-900 mg 4 hourly
    or Phenylbutazone 200-300 mg 8 hourly with food
      reducing after 1 day to 100 mg 8 hourly if possible.
    or Indomethacin 25-75 mg 8 hourly with food
    or Ibuprofen 200-400 mg 6 hourly
    or Local radiotherapy

CONFUSION

Review all therapy
Stop as much treatment as possible
If fails Chlorpromazine 10-25 mg orally 6 hourly
    or Chlorpromazine 25-100 mg i.m.

Or in elderly
Thioridazine 10-25 mg orally 4-6 hourly.

CONSTIPATION

Common with narcotic analgesics
    Danthron with Poloxamer 188 (Dorbanex) 10-20 ml daily
    or Senna as Senokot 2 tablets nocte
    or Dioctyl forte 1-2 tablets 8 hourly
    or Magnesium sulphate 5-15 g in 250 ml of water before
    breakfast
    or Ispaghula Husk 3-5 g 12-24 hourly

COUGH

Treat local lesion if possible
and either Diphenhydramine expectorant 5-10 ml as necessary
    or Methadone 2 mg 4 hourly
    or Codeine Phosphate linctus 5 ml 6-8 hourly
    or Pholcodine 5-15 ml 6-8 hourly
and to liquify sputum:
    Bromhexine 8 mg 8 hourly

DEPRESSION

Control physical and mental problems, e.g. worries at home etc.
and Amitriptyline 25-100 mg nocte
(start with small dose as confusion may be precipitated).

DIARRHOEA

Rule out spurious diarrhoea with impaction
Then either Codeine Phosphate 30 mg when bowels open
    or Diphenoxylate with Atropine 2 tablets 6 hourly
or if due to pancreatic insufficiency:
    Pancreatin with meals

DRY MOUTH

Frequent drinks
or Ice to suck
Review therapy
    ? too much Phenothiazine

DYSPNOEA

Bronchospasm
Salbutamol 2-4 mg 8 hourly
or Aminophylline suppositories 1-2 as necessary
or Prednisone 10-15 mg 8 hourly
    reducing to smallest dose effective

Chest infections
Antibiotics as appropriate.

Effusions, etc.
(see Chapter on Respiratory System p. 23)

Symptomatic treatment
Morphine or Diamorphine as outlined under 'pain'
and an anxiolytic, e.g. Diazepam 2-5 mg 8 hourly

Excessive secretions
Hyoscine 0.4-0.6 mg i.m.
with if necessary Morphine or Diamorphine as outlined under 'pain'.

HICCOUGH

either Metoclopramide 10 mg orally or i.m., as often as necessary
    or Chlorpromazine 25 mg orally or i.m., as often as necessary
either drug in regular dosage may prevent relapse.

INSOMNIA

Diazepam 5-30 mg nocte
    or Dichloralphenazone 650-1300 mg at night
    or Chlorpromazine 25-50 mg at night

Or in elderly
Chlormethiazole 0.5-1 g at night

INTESTINAL OBSTRUCTION

Partial
Control pain and vomiting as outlined below.
and Dioctyl forte 1-2 tablets 8 hourly

Painful colic
Diphenoxylate with Atropine 2 tablets 6 hourly
Consider surgery

Complete
Control pain and vomiting as outlined below.

Painful colic
Diphenoxylate with Atropine 2 tablets 6 hourly
Consider surgery

ITCH

Local soothing lotions, e.g. Calamine
  or local antipruritic cream, e.g. crotamiton
or Chlorpheniramine 4 mg 8 hourly
or Prednisone 5-10 mg 8 hourly
or, if due to biliary stasis
  Cholestyramine 4 g 6 hourly – taken in fruit juice etc.

NAUSEA AND VOMITING

either Prochlorperazine 5-10 mg orally or i.m. 4 hourly
  or Prochlorperazine 25 mg suppositories 8 hourly
or Promazine 25 mg orally or i.m. 4 hourly
or Chlorpromazine 25 mg orally or i.m. 4 hourly
  or Chlorpromazine 100 mg suppositories 8 hourly
or Cyclizine 50 mg orally or i.m. 12 hourly
or Metoclopramide 10 mg orally or i.m. 8-12 hourly
or Thiethylperazine 10 mg orally 8-12 hourly
  or Thiethylperazine 10 mg suppositories 12 hourly

PAIN RELIEF

Give all drugs REGULARLY
Adjust FREQUENCY to prevent 'breakthrough' pain
Adjust DOSE to STOP ALL PAIN
(the right dose is that which relieves the pain)
Review AT LEAST WEEKLY

Moderate
either Aspirin 300-600 mg orally 4 hourly
  or Paracetamol 0.5-1 g orally 4 hourly
or if fails Dihydrocodeine 30-60 mg orally 4 hourly
or if fails Dipipanone + Cyclizine 1-2 orally 4 hourly
  or Dextromoramide 5 mg orally or by suppository 6 hourly

Severe
Morphine 7.5-100 mg orally 4 hourly
(Start with low dose then increase)
  or Diamorphine 5-75 mg orally 4 hourly
  (start with low dose then increase)
if fails Morphine at the same dose i.m. 4 hourly, increasing dose as
necessary.
  or Diamorphine at the same dose i.m. 4 hourly, increasing dose
  as necessary.
and in either case Prochlorperazine 5-10 mg orally 4 hourly
  or Chlorpromazine 12.5-25 mg orally 4 hourly
  (more sedative)

Severe pain with vomiting
either Morphine 7.5-100 mg suppositories or i.m. 4 hourly
(start with low dose and increase as necessary)
    or Diamorphine 5-75 mg i.m. 4 hourly
    (start with low dose and increase as necessary)
with Prochlorperazine 5-10 mg i.m. 4 hourly
        or Chlorpromazine 12.5-25 mg i.m. 4 hourly
        (more sedative)
    or Oxycodone pectinate suppositories 1-2 8 hourly

And/or mixtures
e.g. 'Brompton Cocktail – Morphine or Diamorphine
    with or without cocaine
    with or without a phenothiazine
    with or without alcohol
Best to adjust dose of drugs individually rather than use a fixed
combination, which stops therapeutic thought.

In all cases
Start with lowest dose and increase as necessary.
There is no place for p.r.n. medication.
Tailor the therapy to the patient and change frequently if necessary.
If oral route impractical, consider rectal route or injections.
A combination of strong analgesics with one of the weaker ones is
often helpful.
Ignore theoretical risks of addiction.

URINARY FREQUENCY

Rule out chronic obstruction with overflow
Treat infection with appropriate antibiotics
and Emepronium bromide 100 mg 8 hourly
    or Emepronium bromide 200 mg at night.

Section 2

Non-proprietary drug list

INTRODUCTION

In compiling this drug list I have used the non-proprietary name of the drugs, the use of which is described in the first section. Below each of these names I give a brief description of the type of drug, e.g. antibiotic, and below that a list of the proprietary names from both the United Kingdom and other countries. In preparing this list I have in most instances only included those preparations which contain a single substance and have not included mixtures. This follows the convention used in Martindale, which is the source of most of these drug lists.

Alongside each drug I give the major side effects and possible drug interactions. The first column deals with the side effects. I have not attempted to list the side effects in any order of frequency but have tried to group them together to conserve space. Thus nausea, vomiting, anorexia, diarrhoea or constipation are grouped as gastrointestinal disturbance, unless the side effect is more specific. I have only included side effects which appear in two of three publications, i.e. Martindale or Mylers *Side Effects of Drugs* Volume 8 or the Data Sheet Compendium 1978. In most instances the effects are noted in all three publications.

The second column deals with drug interactions. I have attempted in this column to group the effects so that, for instance, those interactions which enhance the action of the drug are listed together. As source material for these interactions I have again used Martindale, and in addition *Drug Interactions* by Phillip D. Hansten. I have tried to only include those interactions for which there is some evidence of clinical significance, but if there appears to be a doubt I have included the interaction because it seems better from the patient's point of view to consider the possibility of a noted adverse reaction being due to an interaction and being found wrong, rather than to ignore this possibility altogether.

In both these lists I have used CAPITAL LETTERS to bring out the important words and to make reading and rapid reference more easy.

I have also included at the end of this section details of calculations for the dosage of Gentamicin (The Mawer Nomogram) so that the correct dose can be given to patients who have renal impairment.

Drug	Major Side Effects	Interactions
ACETARSOL Trichomonacide Amoebicide SVC Stovarsol	LOCAL REACTION	None significant reported
ACETAZOLAMIDE Diuretic Carbonic anhydrase inhibitor Ocular hypotensive agent Diamox Defiltran Diazol Didoc Diuramide Glaucomide Glaupax Hydrazol	GIT DISTURBANCE FACIAL PARAESTHESIAE HYPOKALAEMIA HYPERURICAEMIA BONE MARROW DEPRESSION – rare Makes URINE ALKALINE RENAL COLIC	INCREASES effects of AMPHETAMINES REDUCES effects of HYPOGLYCAEMIC DRUGS CHANGES EXCRETION of many drugs due to ALKALINISATION of URINE
ACETIC ACID 1% Disinfectant	Local Discomfort	None significant reported

Drug	Major Side Effects	Interactions

ACTH
Corticotrophin
Acthar
Cortico-Gel
Corticotrophin ZN
Acortan
Acton
Alfatrofin
Isactid
Reacthin
Duracton
	HYPERPIGMENTATION
	CUSHING'S SYNDROME
	CATARACTS
	HYPERSENSITIVITY with injections
	SALT and WATER RETENTION
	HYPERTENSION
	HYPERGLYCAEMIA inducing diabetes or
	  making control difficult.
	IMMUNOSUPPRESSION leading to failure of
	  inflammatory response and reactivation of
	  some infection, e.g. tuberculosis
	OSTEOPOROSIS especially with long term
	  therapy.
	INCREASED CATABOLISM leading to wasting
	PEPTIC ULCERATION incidence increased
	EUPHORIA and DEPRESSION
	HYPOTENSION, 'shock' or an exacerbation of
	  disease IF STOPPED SUDDENLY.
	GROWTH RETARDATION in children
	MUSCLE WEAKNESS and ATROPHY
	SKIN ATROPHY and ECCHYMOSES
		ENHANCES HYPERGLYCAEMIC effect of THIAZIDES
		REDUCES effects of HYPOGLYCAEMIC agents
		REDUCES effects of SALICYLATES
		REDUCES effects of ANTICOAGULANTS
		RIFAMPICIN REDUCES effects due to enzyme
		  induction
		PHENYTOIN REDUCES effects due to enzyme
		  induction
		BARBITURATES REDUCE effects due to enzyme
		  induction

ADRENALINE (EPINEPHRINE)
Sympathomimetic
	TACHYCARDIA – dose related
	VENTRICULAR FIBRILLATION
	HYPERTENSION
	VASOCONSTRICTION
	HYPERGLYCAEMIA
		ENHANCES effects of other SYMPATHOMIMETIC
		  drugs
		MAOI induce HYPERTENSION
		RESERPINE ENHANCES effects
		GUANETHIDINE and RELATED DRUGS ENHANCE
		  effects

Drug	Major Side Effects	Interactions
ADRENALINE EYE DROPS Sympathomimetic Agent Eppy Isopto Epinal Lyophrin Simplene	HYPERSENSITIVITY MELANOSIS of CORNEA and CONJUNCTIVA DRY NOSE DILATATION of CONJUNCTIVAL VESSELS	MAOI induce HYPERTENSION
ALCOHOL Cerebral depressant	GIT DISTURBANCE CNS DEPRESSANT LIVER DAMAGE in PROLONGED EXCESS USE	ENHANCES effects of WARFARIN ENHANCES effects of HYPOGLYCAEMIC DRUGS ENHANCES effects of VASODILATORS SULPHONYLUREAS induce DISULFIRAM LIKE REACTION METRONIDAZOLE induces DISULFIRAM LIKE REACTION REDUCES effects of PHENYTOIN DISULFIRAM induces, NAUSEA, VOMITING AND HYPOTENSION TRICYCLIC ANTIDEPRESSANTS ENHANCE CNS depression BARBITURATES ENHANCE CNS DEPRESSION SEDATIVES ENHANCE CNS DEPRESSION MEPROBAMATE ENHANCES CNS DEPRESSION PHENOTHIAZINE ENHANCES CNS DEPRESSION NITROGLYCERINE ENHANCES HYPOTENSIVE effects SALICYLATES ENHANCE GASTROINTESTINAL BLEEDING METHOTREXATE has an ADDITIVE HEPATOTOXIC EFFECT MAOI CAUSE a HYPERTENSIVE CRISIS (with alcoholic drinks)

Drug	Major Side Effects	Interactions

ALDOSTERONE
Natural corticosteroid
(Mineralocorticoid)
Aldocorten
	SIDE EFFECTS SIMILAR TO THOSE OF PREDNISONE
	OCCUR IN LONG TERM USE AT HIGH DOSAGE, but DO
	NOT OCCUR IN NORMAL USE
		ENHANCES HYPERGLYCAEMIC effect of THIAZIDES
		REDUCES effects of HYPOGLYCAEMIC agents
		REDUCES effects of SALICYLATES
		REDUCES effects of ANTICOAGULANTS
		RIFAMPICIN REDUCES effects due to enzyme
		   induction
		BARBITURATES REDUCE effects due to enzyme
		   induction
		PHENYTOIN REDUCES effects due to enzyme
		   induction

ALLOPURINOL Xanthine oxidase inhibitor Zyloric Zyloprim Bloxanth Epidropal Foligan Urosin	GIT disturbance RASHES	ENHANCES effects of WARFARIN ENHANCES effects of AZATHIOPRINE ENHANCES effects of MERCAPTOPURINE INCREASED incidence of RASH with AMPICILLIN
ALPHA METHYL TYROSINE Competitive inhibitor of tyrosine hydroxylase	None significant reported	None significant reported
ALUMINIUM ACETOTARTRATE Astringent Acid Mantle Alsol Domeboro	None significant reported	None significant reported

Drug	Major Side Effects	Interactions
ALUMINIUM HYDROXIDE Antacid Alucap — Gelox Aludrox — Metem Adagel — Minajel Adrox — Mistalco Alox — Amphojel Alusorb — Chemgel Amphotabs — Palliacol Cremorin — Stomiline	CONSTIPATION	REDUCES effects of ASPIRIN REDUCES effects of TETRACYCLINES REDUCES effects of PHENOTHIAZINES REDUCES effects of ISONIAZID REDUCES effects of DIGOXIN REDUCES effects of IRON (All due to reduced absorption)
AMANTADINE Anti Parkinsonian Agent Anti Viral Agent Symmetrel Contenton PK – Merz Mantadix Virofal	LIVEDO RETICULARIS GIT disturbance CNS disturbance – Confusional states URINARY RETENTION OEDEMA and congestive cardiac failure HYPOTENSION	ENHANCES effects of ANTICHOLINERGICS
AMILORIDE Potassium conserving diuretic Midamor Modamide	HYPERKALAEMIA especially if POTASSIUM SUPPLEMENTS also given or in the presence of RENAL FAILURE	INHIBITS KALIURESIS of diuretics such as FRUSEMIDE and THIAZIDES
AMINOGLUTETHIMIDE Blocker of corticosteroid synthesis	GIT disturbance CNS Symptoms RESPIRATORY DEPRESSION LEUCOPENIA ADRENAL INSUFFICIENCY	None significant reported

Drug	Major Side Effects	Interactions
AMINOPHYLLINE Bronchodilator Cardophylin Ethophylline Phylodrox Andophyllin Phyllocontin Carine Reddoxydrin Carena Aminodur Euphylline Lixaminol Natrophyllin Miniix Peterphyllin Somophyllin Neophyllin Aminophyl Teofyllamin Coraphyllin	GIT DISTURBANCE CNS DISTURBANCE HYPOTENSION if given rapidly i.v. PROCTITIS with repeated suppositories PAIN with i.m. injections EASY to get an OVERDOSE IN CHILDREN	Incompatible with i.v. infusions of CHLORPROMAZINE INSULIN TETRACYCLINE PROMETHAZINE INCOMPATIBLE with STRONG ACIDS when injected Therefore should never be mixed in a syringe with another drug. SYMPATHOMIMETICS ENHANCE toxic EFFECTS

AMITRIPTYLINE
Tricyclic Antidepressant
Amizol
Domical
Lentizol
Saroten
Tryptizol
Annalytin
Deprex
Elatrol
Levate
Mareline
Novotriptyn
Elvail
Endep
Larozyl
Triptanol
	HYPOTENSION – ORTHOSTATIC
	CARDIAC ARRHYTHMIAS
	GIT DISTURBANCE
	DRY MOUTH
	URINARY RETENTION
	EPILEPTIC FITS in susceptible patients
	LOSS OF VISUAL ACCOMMODATION
	CHOLESTATIC JAUNDICE
	AGRANULOCYTOSIS – rare
	WEIGHT GAIN
		ENHANCES ANTICHOLINERGIC effects of
		  ANTIHISTAMINES
		ENHANCES ANTICHOLINERGIC effects of
		  PHENOTHIAZINES
		ENHANCES ANTICHOLINERGIC effects of
		  GLUTETHIMIDE
		ENHANCES ANTICHOLINERGIC effects of
		  ANTI PARKINSONIAN DRUGS
		BARBITURATES in normal dosage REDUCE effects
		BARBITURATES in overdosage ENHANCE effects
		CHLORDIAZEPOXIDE ENHANCES effects
		ENHANCES MARKEDLY the effects of
		  SYMPATHOMIMETIC drugs
		ENHANCES CNS DEPRESSANT effects of ALCOHOL
		MAY ENHANCE effects of WARFARIN
		REDUCES effects of BETHANIDINE
		REDUCES effects of DEBRISOQUINE
		REDUCES effects of GUANETHIDINE
		REDUCES effects of METHYLDOPA
		SEVERE REACTIONS with MAOI particularly if
		  over-dosage
		ENHANCED effect with THYROID HORMONE

Drug	Major Side Effects	Interactions
AMMONIUM CHLORIDE Acidifying Agent Ammonchlor SSW Chlorammonic	GIT DISTURBANCE HEADACHE HYPERVENTILATION	INDUCES CRYSTALLURIA with PARA-AMINOSALICYLIC ACID ENHANCES effects of SALICYLATES SPIRONOLACTONE ENHANCES effects
AMODIAQUINE Anti-Malarial Basoquin Flavoquine	*Normal dosage* GIT DISTURBANCE INSOMNIA *High dosage and Prolonged Therapy* CORNEAL DEPOSITS – reversible RETINAL REACTION – irreversible PERIPHERAL NEUROPATHY – rare LEUCOPENIA RASHES *NB:* REGULAR OPHTHALMOLOGICAL CHECKS ARE MANDATORY	None significant reported
AMOXYCILLIN Antibiotic Amoxil Clamoxyl Imacillin Larotid Polymox Pasetocin Sawacillin	GIT disturbance SKIN RASH Both are less common than with Ampicillin	PROBENECID ENHANCES blood levels by blocking Renal excretion. CROSS SENSITIVITY with other PENICILLINS
AMPHOTERICIN B Antifungal Fungilin Fungizone Ampho-Moronal	GIT disturbance CVS and CNS disturbance RENAL DAMAGE – usually reversible BONE MARROW DEPRESSION PAIN at SITE of INJECTION HYPOKALAEMIA THROMBOPHLEBITIS	ENHANCES DIGOXIN TOXICITY

Drug	Major Side Effects	Interactions
AMPICILLIN Antibiotic A-cillin Amfipen Austrapen Bristin Penbritin Pentrex Petercillin Polycillin Pentrexyl Synthecillin Vidopen Alpen Amperil D-Amp D-Cillin Omnipen Pen A Pensyn Principen QIDamp Ro-ampsen SK-Ampicillin Supen	Tctacillin Amblosin Binotal Deripen Pen-Bristol Penbrock Suractin Amcill Amcill-S Amipenex Domicillin Synpenin Ampen Ampexin Ampilean Ampilum Ampilux Ampipenin Doktacillin Panbritine Penicline Totapen	GIT disturbance SKIN RASH ESPECIALLY WITH lymphoproliferative disorders and GLANDULAR FEVER URTICARIA	PROBENECID REDUCES RENAL EXCRETION
AMYL NITRITE Vasodilator Anti-Cyanide		VASODILATATION HEADACHE TACHYCARDIA	ALCOHOL ENHANCES effects.
ANTI GAS GANGRENE ANTITOXIN Mixed or Monovalent Anti toxin available		ANAPHYLACTIC reaction	None significant reported

Drug	Major Side Effects	Interactions
ANTI HAEMOPHILIC GLOBULIN	AS FOR ALL BLOOD PRODUCTS	None specific reported
Blood Fraction	LESS THAN with less 'PURE' FRACTIONS	
Hemofil Factorate		
Kryobulin Humafac		
Profilate Koate		
ASPIRIN	GIT DISTURBANCE	ENHANCES effects of WARFARIN
(Salicylates)	ALLERGY with ASTHMA and ANGIONEUROTIC	ENHANCES effects of SULPHONYLUREAS
Antipyretic analgesic	OEDEMA – rare	INHIBITS effects of URICOSURIC AGENTS
Anti inflammatory	OCCULT GIT BLOOD LOSS	ENHANCES effects of METHOTREXATE
Aspergum	PROLONGED BLEEDING TIME	
Breoprin Dispril		
Caprin Instantine		
Claradin Premaspin		
Entorosalyl A.S.A.		
Levius Measurin		
Nuseals Aspirin Aquaprin		
Solprin Aspasol		
Acetophen Aspegic		
Acetyl-Sol Aspirisucre		
Ancasol Claragine		
Asodrine Ivepirine		
Cetasol Juvepirine		
Entrophen Seclopyrine		
Monasalyl Aspisol		
Neopirine 25 Bi-prin		
Nova-Phase Clariprin		
Novasen Codral		
Supasa Elsprin		
Triophen 10 Novosprin		
Acetylin Prodol		
Colfarit Provoprin 500		
Godamed Solcetas		
Albyl-Setlers Solusal		
Apernyl Babiprin		
Bamyl Ecotrin		
Rhonal		

Drug	Major Side Effects	Interactions
ATROPINE Anticholinergic Atropinol Atropisol	GLAUCOMA TACHYCARDIA CONSTIPATION BLURRING of VISION RASHES DRY MOUTH ACUTE URINARY RETENTION – if prostate enlarged FIXED DILATED PUPIL HALLUCINATIONS *NB*: AVOID IN CLOSED ANGLE GLAUCOMA	TRICYCLIC ANTIDEPRESSANTS have ADDITIVE effects REDUCES ABSORPTION of LEVODOPA REDUCES ABSORPTION of MANY DRUGS
ATROPINE EYE DROPS Cycloplegic & Mydriatic Atropt Minims Ophthalmic drops Isopto Atropine Opulets atropine Spersatrophine Atropisol Atroptol	GLAUCOMA TACHYCARDIA CONSTIPATION BLURRING of VISION RASHES DRY MOUTH ACUTE RETENTION (May occur with systemic absorption especially in children)	None significant reported with eye drops
AZATHIOPRINE Immunosuppressant Anti neoplastic Imuran Imurek Imural	GIT DISTURBANCE BONE MARROW DEPRESSION – reversible MACROCYTIC ANAEMIA PANCREATITIS – rare	ALLOPURINOL ENHANCES effects; therefore, reduce dose of AZATHIOPRINE to 25%
BACLOFEN Anti-spastic Agent Lioresal	GIT DISTURBANCE especially NAUSEA CNS DISTURBANCE Epilepsy MUSCLE WEAKNESS	None significant reported

Drug	Major Side Effects	Interactions
BECLOMETHASONE DIPROPIONATE Corticosteroid Inhalation Topical Corticosteroid Becotide Beconase Aldecin Viarox	ORAL CANDIDIASIS – usually responds rapidly to treatment. No other significant side effects yet reported.	None significant reported.
BENDROFLUAZIDE Diuretic – moderately potent Aprinox Berkozide Centyl Neo Naclex Aprinox M Bristuric Naturetin Naturine Pluryl Salures	GIT DISTURBANCE ALLERGIES RASHES HYPERGLYCAEMIA – making DIABETIC control difficult HYPERURICAEMIA – may precipitate acute GOUT HYPOKALAEMIA	ENHANCES DIGOXIN toxicity ENHANCES effects of ANTI HYPERTENSIVE agents REDUCES effects of HYPOGLYCAEMIA agents ADDITIONAL HYPOKALAEMIC effect with CORTICOSTEROIDS CHLORPROPAMIDE ENHANCES HYPONATRAEMIC effect
BENTONITE Adsorbent	None significant reported	None significant reported
BENZATHINE PENICILLIN Long acting Penicillin Penidural long acting Ben P Dulcepen – G Duapen LPG Megacillin Extencilline Bicillin Permapen Bicillin LA Tardocillin Penilente LA	GIT disturbance RASH which is COMMON ANAPHYLACTIC COLLAPSE and HYPOTENSION which is RARE	PROBENECID REDUCES renal EXCRETION

Drug	Major Side Effects	Interactions
BENZHEXOL (Trihexyphenidyl) Anticholinergic Artane Anti-Spas Aparkane Novohexidyl Trihexy Trixyl Pargitan Peragit Antitrem Tremin	DRY MOUTH CONSTIPATION BLURRED VISION DIFFICULTY with MICTURITION CNS DISTURBANCE TACHYCARDIA	AMANTADINE ENHANCES effects TRICYCLIC ANTIDEPRESSANTS ENHANCE effect ADDITIVE VAGAL BLOCKADE with QUINIDINE
BENZOIC ACID ointment Co. Local fungicide Whitfields ointment	None significant reported	None significant reported
BENZOYL PEROXIDE Keratolytic ointment Vanair Benzagel Desquam-x Persadox Oxy-5 Acne Panoxyl Benoxyl	CONTACT DERMATITIS – rare	None significant reported
BENZTROPINE Anticholinergic Cogentin Cogentinol	DRY MOUTH FIXED DILATED PUPILS TACHYCARDIA ACUTE URINARY RETENTION – if prostate enlarged HALLUCINATIONS	ENHANCES effects of other ANTICHOLINERGIC drugs

NB: AVOID IN CLOSED ANGLE GLAUCOMA

Drug	Major Side Effects	Interactions
BENZYL BENZOATE Insecticide Acaricide Ascarbiol Scabanca	LOCAL BURNING and ERUPTION – in sensitive people CNS STIMULATION – if ingested	None significant reported
BENZYL PENICILLIN Antibiotic Crystapen Therapen Abbocillin Wescopen Dymocillin Penevan Firepen Peniset Forpen Pensol Hylenta Hyasorb Ka-Pen Kesso-Pen Megacillin Specilline G NeoPens Novopen P-50 Pentids Pencitabs Pharmacillin Penioral	RASH – common ANAPHYLACTIC COLLAPSE and HYPOTENSION – rare	PROBENECID REDUCES RENAL EXCRETION
BETAHISTINE Histamine Analogue Serc Meginalisk Meniace Merislon	GIT DISTURBANCE HEADACHE	None significant reported

Drug	Major Side Effects	Interactions

BETAMETHASONE
Synthetic corticosteroid
Anti-inflammatory
 	
Betnelan
Betnesol
Betasolon
Bextasol
Celestan
Celestene
Celeston A
Celestone
Desacort-Beta
Minisone
Rinderon
Bentelan
Betapred
Betnovate
Betneval
Celestoderm
Betnovat
Celestroderm-V
Ecoval 70
Valisone
	COMMON ESPECIALLY IN LONGER TERM USE
	SALT and WATER retention
	HYPERTENSION
	HYPERGLYCAEMIA inducing diabetes or
	  making diabetic control difficult
	IMMUNOSUPPRESSION leading to failure of
	  inflammatory response and reactivation
	  of some infection, e.g. tuberculosis
	OSTEOPOROSIS especially with long term use
	INCREASED CATABOLISM leading to wasting
	PEPTIC ULCERATION incidence increased
	ADRENAL SUPPRESSION which leads to a failure
	  to respond to stress
	CUSHINGS SYNDROME
	EUPHORIA and DEPRESSION
	HYPOTENSION, 'shock' or an exacerbation
	  of disease if STOPPED suddenly
	GROWTH RETARDATION in children
	MUSCLE WEAKNESS and ATROPHY
	SKIN ATROPHY and ECCHYMOSES
	CATARACT FORMATION
	
	NB: 0.7 mg EQUIVALENT to 5 mg of Prednisone
		ENHANCES HYPERGLYCAEMIC effect of THIAZIDES
		REDUCES effects of HYPOGLYCAEMIC agents
		REDUCES effects of SALICYLATES
		REDUCES effects of ANTICOAGULANTS
		RIFAMPICIN REDUCES effects due to enzyme
		  induction
		BARBITURATES REDUCE effects due to enzyme
		  induction
		PHENYTOIN REDUCES effects due to enzyme
		  induction

BETHANIDINE Adrenergic Neurone blocker Antihypertensive Agent Esbatal Esbaloid	POSTURAL and EXERCISE HYPOTENSION DIARRHOEA GIT UPSETS BRADYCARDIA DYSPNOEA OEDEMA IMPOTENCE, MYALGIA, BLURRING OF VISION *All of which are due to autonomic blockade*	ENHANCES effects of other ANTIHYPERTENSIVE agents AMPHETAMINES etc. cause SEVERE HYPERTENSION TRICYCLIC ANTIDEPRESSANTS, CHLORPROMAZINE, and HALOPERIDOL stop the HYPOTENSIVE effect. BARBITURATES and some anaesthetics potentiate the HYPOTENSIVE effect.

Drug	Major Side Effects	Interactions
BISACODYL Purgative Dulcodos Laco Dulcolax Contalax Anan Durolax Satolax-lo Laxbene Bicol Megalax Biscolax Oralax Theralax Toilax Bisacolax	COLIC DIARRHOEA HYPOKALAEMIA	None significant reported
BLEOMYCIN Cytotoxic Agent Blenoxane	RASH ORAL ULCERATION BONE MARROW DEPRESSION – mild and rare PULMONARY FIBROSIS FEVER *NB*: DO NOT EXCEED total dose of 300 mg	None significant reported
BROMHEXINE Sputum liquifying agent Bisolvon	GIT DISTURBANCE	None significant reported
BROMOCRIPTINE Dopaminergic Receptor Stimulant Parlodel	GIT DISTURBANCE VERTIGO POSTURAL DIZZINESS Are less frequent if you start with a small dose at night. Slowly increase and take with food.	None significant reported

Drug	Major Side Effects	Interactions
BORIC ACID ointment Mild disinfectant	RASH POISONING with vomiting of blue/green vomit. SHOCK COMA and DEATH – In children when applied to large areas of denuded skin in high concentration	None significant reported
BUMETANIDE Diuretic – potent loop Burinex	HYPOKALAEMIA HYPOTENSION in large doses HYPERURICAEMIA may precipitate GOUT HYPERGLYCAEMIA making diabetic control difficult HEARING is affected in large doses MUSCLE CRAMPS especially in high doses	ENHANCES NEPHROTOXIC effects of CEPHALOSPORINS ENHANCES DIGOXIN TOXICITY ENHANCES effects of ANTIHYPERTENSIVE agents ENHANCES OTOTOXICITY of AMINOGLYCOSIDES.
	NB: ONE OF THE MORE RECENTLY INTRODUCED DIURETICS THEREFORE ALL EFFECTS ARE NOT FULLY ESTABLISHED.	
BUSULPHAN Alkylating Agent Anti neoplastic Myleran Misulban	BONE MARROW DEPRESSION GIT DISTURBANCE PULMONARY FIBROSIS PIGMENTATION AMENORRHOEA	ADDITIVE BONE MARROW DEPRESSION with other BONE MARROW DEPRESSANTS.
CALAMINE Mild Astringent	None significant reported	None significant reported
CALCIUM GLUCONATE Inotropic agent Element Sandocal Calcium Juva Glucal Rectocalcium	CARDIAC ARRHYTHMIAS in large doses CONSTIPATION	ENHANCES TOXIC effects of DIGOXIN

Drug	Major Side Effects	Interactions
CALCIUM HYDROXIDE Alkali	None significant reported	None significant reported
CALCIUM LACTATE	CONSTIPATION HYPERCALCAEMIA	May INDUCE ARRHYTHMIAS with DIGOXIN
CARBACHOL Parasympathomimetic Carbyl Doryl Miostat Mistura C	GIT DISTURBANCE BRADYCARDIA	None significant reported
CARBENOXOLONE Anti Peptic ulcer Biogastrone Bioralgel Bioral Pellets Duogastrone	SALT and WATER RETENTION HEARTBURN MYOGLOBINURIA MYASTHENIA	SPIRONOLACTONE BLOCKS effects THIAZIDES ENHANCE HYPOKALAEMIA
CARBAMAZEPINE Anticonvulsant Anti trigeminal neuralgia Tegretol	GIT DISTURBANCE CNS DISTURBANCE – dose related RASH BONE MARROW DEPRESSION – rare HYPONATRAEMIA – water intoxication	REDUCES effects of WARFARIN REDUCES effects of PHENYTOIN REDUCES effects of TETRACYCLINES
CARBIMAZOLE Antithyroid Agent Neo Mercazole Carbazole Neo Mopphazole Neo Thyreostat	GIT Upsets RASHES Rarely AGRANULOCYTOSIS (usually early in treatment and preceded by a sore throat) LUPUS ERYTHEMATOSIS ARTHRALGIA *ALL less frequent than with thiourea group.* *NB*: CROSSES PLACENTA	None significant reported

H

Drug	Major Side Effects	Interactions
CARMUSTINE (BCNU) Cytotoxic Agent	GIT disturbance ORAL ULCERATION BONE MARROW DEPRESSION – delayed HEPATOTOXICITY NEPHROTOXICITY	ADDITIVE BONE MARROW DEPRESSION with other BONE MARROW DEPRESSANTS
ß CAROTENE Vitamin A Precursor	None significant reported	None significant reported
CASTOR OIL Purgative Neoloid Recifruit Unisoil	NAUSEA VOMITING SEVERE PURGATION	None significant reported
CELLULOSE PHOSPHATE Calcium binding Agent	None significant reported	None significant reported
CEPHALORIDINE Antibiotic Ceporin Ceporan Keflodin Refspor Loridine	RASH is common NEPHROTOXIC INCREASED PROTHROMBIN TIME – occasionally	ENHANCED nephrotoxicity with FRUSEMIDE, BUMETANIDE and ETHACRYNIC ACID ENHANCED Nephrotoxicity with GENTAMICIN Shared SENSITIVITY with PENICILLIN in SOME patients

Drug	Major Side Effects	Interactions
CEPHALOTHIN Antibiotic Keflin Cefalotine Cepovenin	RASH NEPHROTOXIC – less than Cephaloridine INCREASED PROTHROMBIN TIME – occasionally PAINFUL i.m.	ENHANCED nephrotoxicity with FRUSEMIDE, ETHACRYNIC ACID and BUMETANIDE ENHANCED NEPHROTOXICITY with GENTAMICIN SHARED SENSITIVITY with PENICILLIN in some patients.
CETRIMIDE Disinfectant Ceanel Cetavlon P.C. Collone QA Crodex C Cycloton A Cycloton V Morphan CHSA Seboderm Silquat C100 Vesogex	HYPERSENSITIVITY – RARE REPEATED applications cause excess dryness	None significant reported
CHENODEOXYCHOLIC ACID Bile acid Chendol	DIARRHOEA	None significant reported

Drug	Major Side Effects	Interactions
CHLORAL HYDRATE Hypnotic Noctec Aquachloral Felsules Kessodrate Rectules Chloradorm Chloralate Chloralix Dormel Eudorm Lanchloral Chloraldurat Chloralex Chloralixier Cloralvan Chloratol Nigracap Novochlorhydrate	GIT DISTURBANCE RASHES	ENHANCES CNS DEPRESSION with ALCOHOL INDUCES VASODILATATION with ALCOHOL ENHANCES effects of WARFARIN by displacement from plasma proteins, in the short term.
CHLORAMBUCIL Alkylating Agent Antineoplastic Leukeran Chloraminophene	BONE MARROW DEPRESSION GIT DISTURBANCE	ADDITIVE BONE MARROW DEPRESSION with other BONE MARROW DEPRESSANTS.

Drug		Major Side Effects	Interactions
CHLORAMPHENICOL		GIT disturbance	ENHANCES effects of WARFARIN
Antimicrobial		BONE MARROW DEPRESSION – reversible	REDUCES effects of IRON
Chloromycetin	Sintomicetine	APLASTIC ANAEMIA – irreversible	REDUCES effects of CYANOCOBALAMIN
Kemicetine	Solnicol	'GREY SYNDROME' in NEONATES	ENHANCES effects of HYPOGLYCAEMIC AGENTS
Econochlor	Tifomycine	NEURITIS – OPTIC & PERIPHERAL	ENHANCES effects of PHENYTOIN
Aquamycetin	Amphicol	STEVENS-JOHNSON SYNDROME	
Catilan	Antibiopto		
Bipimycetin	Ophthoclor		
Chloramphycin	Chloramsaar		
Chlomin	Gotimycin		
Chloramol	Kamaver		
Chloramex	Leukomycin		
Chlorfen	Nevimycin		
Jatcetin	Oleomycetin		
Lennacol	Pantovernil		
Chlornicin	Paraxin		
Enicol	Chloramphycin		
Fenicol	Opclor		
Mycinol	Chloroptic		
Novochlorocap	Chlorcol		
Pentamycetin	Chlornicol		
Paraxin	Troymycetin		
Succinat A			

Drug	Major Side Effects	Interactions
CHLORAMPHENICOL EYE DROPS Antibiotic for local use Chloroptic Chloromycetin redidrops Mycetin-ophthiole Spersanicol Minims chloramphenicol Opulets chloramphenicol Chloromin Chloromycetin Eye Drops (Opclor) Chloromycetin ophthalmic Chlorsig	APLASTIC ANAEMIA – rare RASHES *NB:* RARE WITH THIS PREPARATION AS ABSORPTION VARIABLE	ENHANCES effects of WARFARIN ENHANCES effects of TOLBUTAMIDE ENHANCES effects of PHENYTOIN
CHLORDIAZEPOXIDE Tranquilliser Calmoden Novopoxide Librium Protensin Tropium Relaxil Chemdipoxide Solium Corax Trilium C-Tran Via-Quil Diapax Elenium Medilium Libritabs Nack Risolid	DROWSINESS ATAXIA HYPOTENSION – uncommon GIT disturbance	ENHANCES the effects of TRICYCLIC ANTIDEPRESSANTS ENHANCES the effects of PHENYTOIN
CHLORHEXIDINE Disinfectant Bactigras Hexol Demofax Hygicreme Hibiscrub Hibitan Hibitane Rctersept Sterets H Carsodyl Cetal	LOCAL REACTION – rare OTOTOXICITY	REACTS with LABSTIX urine test for protein REACTS with ALBUSTIX urine test

Drug	Major Side Effects	Interactions
CHLORMETHIAZOLE	GIT DISTURBANCE	ENHANCES CNS DEPRESSION with other CNS
Hypnotic	DEPRESSION – in manic depressives	DEPRESSANTS.
Sedative	RESPIRATORY DEPRESSION	PHENOTHIAZINES ENHANCE effects.
Heminevrin	SNEEZING and conjunctival irritation	BUTYROPHENONES ENHANCE effect.
Distraneurin		
Hemineurin		
CHLOROQUINE	RETINAL reaction – usually IRREVERSIBLE	ENHANCED HEPATOTOXICITY with HEPATOTOXIC
Anti Malarial	CORNEAL reaction – usually REVERSIBLE	agents
Anti Rheumatic	PERIPHERAL NEUROPATHY – Rare	
Avloclor Chlorquin	LEUCOPENIA	
Resochin Malaquin	RASHES	
Malarivon Malarex		
Aralen Siragan	*NB*: REGULAR OPHTHALMIC TESTING IS MANDATORY	
Arachin Tresochin		
CHLORPHENIRAMINE	SEDATION	REDUCES ABSORPTION OF PAS
Antihistamine	DRY MOUTH	INCREASED CNS DEPRESSION with other CNS
Allerbid Allergex	GIT DISTURBANCE	DEPRESSANTS
Haynon Allergisan	CNS DEPRESSION	
Piriton Allerhist		
Allertab Chlorohist		
Antagonate Chlortrimeton		
Chlormene Chloramin		
Chloroton Histaids		
Drize Piranex		
Histadur Teledrin		
Histaspan Chlor-Trimeton		
Histol Chlor-Tripolon		
Lorphen Chlortone		
Niratron Histaspan		
Histalon		
Teldrin		

Drug	Major Side Effects	Interactions
CHLORPROMAZINE Tranquilliser Amargyl — Thoradex Chloractil — Thorazine Largactil — Hibernal Chlor-promaryl — Klorpromex Chlorprom-Ez-Ets — Korazin Elmarine — Megaphen Onazine — Plegomazine Promosol — Prccalm Chlor-PZ — Promadcid Promarchel — Protren Promarchlor — Serazone Promapar	DROWSINESS DRY MOUTH HYPOTENSION JAUNDICE – reversible AGRANULOCYTOSIS – rare EXTRAPYRAMIDAL DYSFUNCTION – usually reversible SKIN SENSITIVITY REACTION IRRITATION at injection site	ADDITIVE CNS DEPRESSION with ALCOHOL and other CNS DEPRESSANTS. ANTACIDS reduce ABSORPTION REDUCES effects of LEVODOPA REDUCES effects of GUANETHIDINE etc. ANTICHOLINERGICS reduce effects ENHANCES effects of PHENYTOIN ENHANCES side effects of TRICYCLIC ANTIDEPRESSANTS MAY REDUCE CONVULSION THRESHOLD
CHLORPROPAMIDE Sulphonylurea Diabinese Melitase Chloromide Novopropamide Stabinol Chloronase Diabetoral Diabetal Diabines	HYPOGLYCAEMIA – may be profound and prolonged in the elderly may present as a 'CVA' WATER INTOXICATION and HYPONATRAEMIA GIT disturbance BLOOD DYSCRASIA – rare RASHES JAUNDICE – usually within 6 weeks APPETITE increased	ASPIRIN ENHANCES effects PHENYLBUTAZONE ENHANCES effects SULPHONAMIDES ENHANCE effects ANTICOAGULANTS ENHANCE effects PROBENECID ENHANCES effects BETA BLOCKERS ENHANCE effects MAOI ENHANCE effects ALCOHOL INDUCES DISULFIRAM REACTION – common CORTICOSTEROIDS REDUCE effects ORAL CONTRACEPTIVES REDUCE effects THIAZIDES REDUCE effects 'LOOP' DIURETICS REDUCE effects

Drug	Major Side Effects	Interactions
CHLORPROTHIXENE Tranquilliser Taractan Tarasan Truxal Truxalleten	CNS DISTURBANCE DRY MOUTH JAUNDICE – REVERSIBLE DROWSINESS HYPOTENSION AGRANULOCYTOSIS – rare EXTRA PYRAMIDAL DYSFUNCTION – usually reversible SKIN SENSITIVITY REACTION IRRITATION at injection site	ADDITIVE CNS DEPRESSION with ALCOHOL and other CNS DEPRESSANTS ANTACIDS REDUCE ABSORPTION PHENOBARBITONE REDUCES effects REDUCES effects of LEVODOPA REDUCES effects of GUANETHIDINE ANTICHOLINERGICS REDUCE effects ENHANCES effects OF PHENYTOIN ENHANCES effects of TRICYCLIC ANTIDEPRESSANTS
CHLORTETRACYCLINE Antibiotic Aureomycin Aureomycine Chlortet Topmycin	GIT DISTURBANCE CANDIDA OVERGROWTH INCREASED URAEMIA if renal IMPAIRMENT PERMANENT DISCOLOURATION OF TEETH – if given during pregnancy or during first 8 years of life.	MILK REDUCES ABSORPTION ALKALIS REDUCE ABSORPTION ALUMINIUM HYDROXIDE REDUCES ABSORPTION CALCIUM REDUCES ABSORPTION IRON REDUCES ABSORPTION MAGNESIUM REDUCES ABSORPTION
CHLOROTHIAZIDE Thiazide diuretic Moderately potent Saluric Diurilix Flumen Minzil Saluren Salisan Yadalan	GIT disturbance ACUTE PANCREATITIS HYPERGLYCAEMIA – making diabetic control difficult RASH HYPERURICAEMIA – may precipitate acute GOUT HYPOKALAEMIA – especially with prolonged use	ENHANCES effects of LITHIUM REDUCES effects of HYPOGLYCAEMIC agents CHLORPROPAMIDE ENHANCES HYPONATURAEMIC effect CORTICOSTEROIDS increase POTASSIUM loss ENHANCES effects of ANTIHYPERTENSIVE agents
CHOLESTYRAMINE Chelating agent Cuemid Questran Quantalan	GIT disturbances, which are mild and TRANSIENT STEATORRHOEA in high dosage necessitating supplementation of the diet with Vitamins A, D, and K. INCREASED incidence of GALL STONES	REDUCES effects of WARFARIN REDUCES effects of DIGOXIN REDUCES absorption of VITAMINS A, D, K. CHELATES ACIDIC DRUGS in the GIT therefore do not give any other drugs for at lease ONE HOUR after any dose.

Drug	Major Side Effects	Interactions
CHLORTHALIDONE Moderately potent diuretic, similar to the thiazide diuretics Hygroton Igroton Uridon	GIT disturbance ACUTE PANCREATITIS HEPATIC COMA can be precipitated in patients with hepatic disease HYPERGLYCAEMIA may make diabetic control difficult. HYPERURICAEMIA may precipitate acute GOUT HYPOKALAEMIA especially with long term use.	REDUCES effects of HYPOGLYCAEMIC agents POTENTIATES effects of ANTIHYPERTENSIVE agents INCREASED DIGOXIN toxicity if HYPOKALAEMIA.
CHORIONIC GONADOTROPHIN Mainly lutenising hormone Trophic hormone Gonadotraphon LH Pregnesin Pregnyl Coriantin Antvitrin S Follutein APL Harvatropin Choragen Gonadex Predalon Primogonyl	OEDEMA due to salt and water retention *NB:* HYPER STIMULATION SYNDROME may occur with nausea, vomiting, abdominal pain and 'shock' due to ascites and pleural effusion formation.	None significant reported
CIMETIDINE H2 Antagonist Tagamet	RASH GIT DISTURBANCE HEPATIC NECROSIS ELEVATED CREATININE ONLY RECENTLY INTRODUCED THEREFORE ALL EFFECTS NOT ESTABLISHED	None significant reported
CINNARIZINE Antihistamine Stugeron: Apomiteril Glanil Corathiem Midronal Roin Stugeron	GIT DISTURBANCE SEDATION – not marked	ADDITIONAL CNS DEPRESSION with other CNS depressants

Drug	Major Side Effects	Interactions
CLINDAMYCIN Antibiotic Dalacin C Cleocin Sobelin	GIT DISTURBANCE PSEUDOMEMBRANOUS COLITIS	None significant reported
CLIOQUINOL Amoebicide Antiseptic for Topical use Iodochlorhydroxyquin Entero-Valodon Entero-Vioform Budoform Cremo-quin Enerto-quin Enteritan Vioform	Local irritation	None significant reported
CLOFAZIMINE Anti Leprotic Lamprene	GIT DISTURBANCE RED PIGMENT in skin and urine	None significant reported
CLOFIBRATE Cholesterol lowering agent Atromid S Liprinal Aterosol Atromibin Recolip Atheromide Atheropront Regelan N Skleromexe Lipavlon Claresan	GIT disturbance REVERSIBLE MYALGIA especially in patients with Nephrotic syndrome INCREASED MORTALITY in long term usage	ENHANCES effects of WARFARIN necessitating reduction of dose to ½ or a third. ENHANCES effects of FRUSEMIDE in the nephrotic syndrome. ENHANCES the effects of TOLBUTAMIDE

Drug	Major Side Effects	Interactions
CLOMIPHENE Inducer of Ovulation Clomid Clomivid Dynergic	BLURRED VISION GIT DISTURBANCE HOT FLUSHES BREAST DISCOMFORT WEIGHT GAIN DEPRESSION	None significant reported
CLONAZEPAM Anticonvulsant Rivotril Clonopin Ictorivil	CNS DISTURBANCE	ALCOHOL ENHANCES effects
CLONIDINE Anti migraine Dixarit	GIT DISTURBANCE CNS DISTURBANCE RASH – rare	? TRICYCLIC ANTIDEPRESSANTS REDUCE effects ? DIURETICS ENHANCE effects
	NB: VERY SMALL DOSE cf DOSE USED IN HYPERTENSION ∴ SIDE EFFECTS DOUBTFUL	
CLONIDINE Hypotensive Agent Catapres Catapressan Catapresan Isoglaucon	GIT DISTURBANCE CNS DISTURBANCE PAROTID PAIN IMPOTENCE POSTURAL HYPOTENSION – uncommon RASH – rare	TRICYCLIC ANTIDEPRESSANTS REDUCE effects DIURETICS ENHANCE effects
	NB: SUDDEN STOPPING CAUSES SEVERE REBOUND HYPERTENSION	
CLOTRIMAZOLE Antifungal Agent Trichomonacide Canesten Lotrimin	GIT DISTURBANCE LOCAL IRRITATION	None significant reported

Drug	Major Side Effects	Interactions

CLOXACILLIN
Antibiotic
(Penicillinase resistant)
  Orbenin
  Austrastaph
  Clocillin
  Cloxypen
  Orbenine
  Staphybiotic
  Ekvacillin
  Prostaphlin A
  Staphobristol
  Tegopen
	HYPERSENSITIVITY – Rare
	GIT disturbances
	RASHES
		PROBENECID REDUCES renal EXCRETION

COAL TAR (prepared)
Antipruritic ointment
  Carbo-cort
  Carbo-dome
  Cor-Tar-Quin
  Genisol
  Pologal picis
  Psoriderm
  Psorox
  Tarcortin
	LOCAL IRRITATION
	PHOTOSENSITIVITY
		None significant reported

COBALT EDETATE Anti-Cyanide Kelocyanor	NAUSEA VOMITING CARDIAC ARRHYTHMIAS ANGINA RASH	None significant reported
CODEINE Narcotic Analgesic	GIT disturbance DROWSINESS – common CONSTIPATION – common DEPENDENCE – with prolonged use	ENHANCED RESPIRATORY DEPRESSION with other respiratory depressing agents. ENHANCED SEDATION with other sedatives.

Drug	Major Side Effects	Interactions
CODEINE PHOSPHATE Narcotic Analgesic Anti-diarrhoeal Cough suppressant Codicept Tricodeine Codlin Paveral Histadyl Kaodene Tercolix	CONSTIPATION CNS DISTURBANCE GIT DISTURBANCE DEPENDENCE of the Morphine type	None significant reported
COLCHICINE Anti-gout agent Colcin Colgout Coluric Colchicine Aqua-Colchin Colchineos	DIARRHOEA GIT disturbance RASHES BONE MARROW DEPRESSION – with prolonged treatment	None significant reported

COMBINED ORAL CONTRACEPTIVES
Demulen 50   Norlestrin
Demulen 50   Orlest 21
Ovulen   Microgynon 30
Ovulen 50   Eugynon 30
Norinyl 1   Minilyn
Ortho-Novin   Norinyl 1/28
  1/50   Conova 30
Ovysmen   Brevinor
Anovlar 21   Ovran
Gynovlar 21   Ovran 30
Loestrin 20   Ovranette
Minovlar
	THROMBO–EMBOLISM
	HYPERTENSION
	DEPRESSION
	WEIGHT GAIN
	GIT DISTURBANCE
	LIVER DYSFUNCTION
		REDUCES effects of WARFARIN
		REDUCES effects of ANTIDIABETIC AGENTS
		RIFAMPICIN REDUCES effects by enzyme induction
		PHENOBARBITONE REDUCES effects by enzyme
		  induction
		PHENYTOIN REDUCES effects by enzyme induction

Drug	Major Side Effects	Interactions
COPPER SULPHATE Emetic Antiphosphorous agent Astringent	GIT DISTURBANCE	None significant reported
CORTICOSTEROID Eye and ear drops or ointment	LOSS OF SKIN COLLAGEN SUBCUTANEOUS ATROPHY INCREASED RISK OF INFECTION and AS FOR PREDNISONE – if enough absorbed.	As for prednisone if enough absorbed
CORTICOSTEROID AND ANTIBIOTIC Eye and ear drops or ointment Many different preparations	As for each component	As for each component
CO TRIMOXAZOLE Antimicrobial Mixture Bactrim Septrin Eusaprin Septra Septran Trib Trimetoprim-Sulpha	GIT disturbance SKIN rash – which may be severe MEGALOBLASTIC ANAEMIA – folic acid deficiency BONE MARROW DEPRESSION AVOID in PREGNANCY	BLOCKS FOLIC ACID METABOLISM ENHANCES anti folate effects of METHOTREXATE. CROSS SENSITIVITY with SULPHONAMIDES.
CROTAMITON Antipruritic ointment Eurax Teevex Bestloid Euraxil	Local reaction	None significant reported
CRYOPRECIPITATE Blood Fraction	AS FOR ALL BLOOD PRODUCTS	None specific reported

Drug	Major Side Effects	Interactions
CYCLIZINE Antihistamine used mainly as an anti-emetic Marzine Valoid Marezine	SEDATION worse initially	ADDITIVE CNS DEPRESSION with other CNS depressant drugs, e.g. ALCOHOL
CYCLOFENIL Inducer of Ovulation Ondonid Fertodur Ondogyne Sexovid	GIT DISTURBANCE HOT FLUSHES – rare JAUNDICE – less common than with Clomiphene	None significant reported
CYCLOPENTHIAZIDE Thiazide diuretic Moderately potent Navidrex	GIT disturbance ACUTE PANCREATITIS HEPATIC COMA can be precipitated in patients with hepatic disease HYPERGLYCAEMIA – making diabetic control difficult HYPERURICAEMIA may precipitate acute gout. HYPOKALAEMIA especially with long term use.	REDUCES effects of HYPOGLYCAEMIC agents. POTENTIATES effects of ANTIHYPERTENSIVE agents. INCREASED DIGOXIN TOXICITY IF HYPOKALAEMIA.
CYCLOPENTOLATE Cyclopegic and Mydriatic Mydrilate Ciclolux Cyclogyl Cyclopen Cyplegin Cyclopezic Mydplegic Zyklolat	GLAUCOMA CNS Disturbance – in repeated dosage	None significant reported

Drug	Major Side Effects	Interactions
CYCLOPHOSPHAMIDE Anti neoplastic agent Endoxana Genoxal Cytoxan Procytox Endoxan Sendoxan Enduxan	ALOPECIA – usually transient and common LEUCOPENIA – mainly neutrophils and reversible. NAUSEA and VOMITING CYSTITIS – often haemorrhagic OVARIAN and TESTICULAR suppression *NB*: LESS EFFECTIVE IN PRESENCE OF LIVER DISEASE	BARBITURATES MAY ENHANCE effects CORTICOSTEROIDS MAY ENHANCE effects
CYCLOPROPANE Anaesthetic	Post Anaesthetic HEADACHE Post Anaesthetic HYPOTENSION	ENHANCES effects of CATECHOLAMINES
CYSTEAMINE (Mercaptamine)	NAUSEA AND VOMITING	None significant reported
CYTARABINE Anti-neoplastic agent Stops DNA synthesis Anti-viral Agent Cytosine Arabinoside Ara C. Cytosar Alexan Aracytine	GIT disturbance BONE MARROW DEPRESSION HEPATOTOXICITY – Rare	ADDITIVE BONE MARROW DEPRESSION with other BONE MARROW DEPRESSANTS.
DACARBAZINE Cytotoxic Agent Dtic-Dome	GIT DISTURBANCE 'FLU LIKE SYNDROME ALOPECIA BONE MARROW DEPRESSION	ADDITIVE BONE MARROW DEPRESSION with other BONE MARROW DEPRESSANTS
DANAZOL Gonadotrophin inhibitor Danol Danatrol	WEIGHT GAIN RASHES GIT DISTURBANCE VIRILISM ATROPHIC VAGINITIS	None significant reported

Drug	Major Side Effects	Interactions
DANTHRON Purgative Dordane Modane	Causes RED/BROWN URINE	None significant reported
DANTHRON with Poloxamer 188 Purgative Dorbanex	Causes RED/BROWN URINE	None significant reported
DANTROLENE Muscle Relaxant Dantrium	GIT disturbance CNS disturbance RASH JAUNDICE	INCREASED CNS DEPRESSION with other CNS DEPRESSANTS
DAPSONE Anti Leprotic Anti Dermatitis Herpetiformis Avlosulfon	ALLERGIC DERMATITIS GIT DISTURBANCE CNS DISTURBANCE TACHYCARDIA ANAEMIA HEPATITIS AGRANULOCYTOSIS	PROBENECID ENHANCES effects
DAUNORUBICIN Cytotoxic Agent Cerubidin Daunoblastin Daunoblastina Ondena	GIT DISTURBANCE CARDIOTOXICITY if TOTAL DOSE EXCEEDS 20 mg/kg (or 550 mg/m^2) ALOPECIA RASH BONE MARROW DEPRESSION	ADDITIVE BONE MARROW DEPRESSION with other BONE MARROW DEPRESSANTS
DEHYDROEMETINE Amoebicide Dametine Mebadin	CARDIOTOXICITY HEPATOTOXICITY NEPHROTOXICITY GIT DISTURBANCE *All seen with excess dosage but less severe than with EMETINE.*	None significant reported

Drug	Major Side Effects	Interactions
DEMECARIUM BROMIDE Irreversible cholinesterase inhibitor Tosmilen Humorsol	ACUTE GLAUCOMA GIT DISTURBANCE CNS DISTURBANCE May be prolonged	None significant reported
DEMECLOCYCLINE (de-methyl-chlortetracycline) Antibiotic. 'Anti ADH' Ledermycin Declomycin Mexocine	GIT DISTURBANCE INCREASED UREAMIA if RENAL IMPAIRMENT PERMANENT DISCOLOURATION OF TEETH if given DURING PREGNANCY or FIRST 8 years OF LIFE. ALLERGIC REACTIONS	MILK REDUCES ABSORPTION ALKALIS REDUCE ABSORPTION ALUMINIUM HYDROXIDE REDUCES ABSORPTION CALCIUM REDUCES ABSORPTION IRON REDUCES ABSORPTION MAGNESIUM REDUCES ABSORPTION
DE-NOL Bismuth antacid	? CNS DISTURBANCE	None significant reported
DEOXYCORTONE ACETATE Natural corticosteroid (Mineralocorticoid) Cortiron Doca Percorten Syncorta Syncortyl	Common especially in LONG TERM USE SALT and WATER retention HYPERTENSION Side effects similar to those of Prednisone, can occur with prolonged high dosage, but do not occur with normal use. *NB:* 1. RARELY USED NOW 2. INJECTABLE, IMPLANTABLE MINERALOCORTICOID 3. ONE FIFTH AS ACTIVE AS ALDOSTERONE	ENHANCES HYPERGLYCAEMIC effect of THIAZIDE REDUCES effects of HYPOGLYCAEMIC agents REDUCES effects of SALICYLATES REDUCES effects of ANTICOAGULANTS RIFAMPICIN REDUCES effects due to enzyme induction. BARBITURATES REDUCE effects due to enzyme induction. PHENYTOIN REDUCES effects due to enzyme induction.
DESFERRIOXAMINE (deferoxamine) Iron chelating agent Desferal	ALLERGIC REACTIONS GIT DISTURBANCE	None significant reported

Drug	Major Side Effects	Interactions
DESMOPRESSIN Synthetic Posterior Pituitary Hormone DDAVP Minirin	No significant side effects	None reported

DEXAMETHASONE
Corticosteroid
(Anti inflammatory)
Decadron   Isopto-Maxidrex
Oradexon   Decaesadril
Aeroseb D   Decasterolone
Decaderm   Decofluor
Dexameth   Desacort
Dexone   Desacortone
Cammacorten   Desalark
Miral   Desameton
Carulon   Deseronil
Corson   Fluormone
Dectan   Fluorocort
Dethamedin   Luxazone
Metasolon   Deronil
Moco   Dexamethadrone
Orgadrone   Dexmethsone
Savosone   Hexadrol
Cortisumman   Spersodex
Dexamed
Dexa-Scheroson
Dexa-sine
Deximolone
Fortecortin
Millicorten
Predni-F
Decacort
Dexacortal
	COMMON ESPECIALLY IN LONG TERM USE
	SALT and WATER RETENTION
	HYPERTENSION
	HYPERGLYCAEMIA inducing diabetes or making
	  control difficult
	IMMUNOSUPPRESSION leading to failure of
	  inflammatory response and reactivation of
	  some infection, e.g. tuberculosis
	OSTEOPOROSIS especially with long term
	  therapy.
	INCREASED CATABOLISM leading to wasting
	PEPTIC ULCERATION incidence increased
	ADRENAL SUPPRESSION which leads to a failure
	  to respond to stress.
	CUSHINGS SYNDROME
	EUPHORIA and DEPRESSION
	HYPOTENSION, 'shock' or an exacerbation of
	  disease if stopped suddenly.
	GROWTH RETARDATION in children
	MUSCLE WEAKNESS and ATROPHY
	SKIN ATROPHY and ECCHYMOSES
	CATARACT FORMATION
	
	NB: 0.75 mg EQUIVALENT to 5 mg of Prednisone
		ENHANCES HYPERGLYCAEMIC effects of THIAZIDE
		REDUCES effects of HYPOGLYCAEMIC agents
		REDUCES effects of SALICYLATES
		REDUCES effects of ANTICOAGULANTS
		RIFAMPICIN REDUCES effects due to enzyme
		  induction.
		BARBITURATES REDUCE effects due to enzyme
		  induction.
		PHENYTOIN REDUCES effects due to enzyme
		  induction.

Drug	Major Side Effects	Interactions
DEXTRAN 40 Plasma expander Gentran 40 Lomodex 40 Perfudex Rheomacrodex L.M.D. Perfadex	ANAPHYLACTIC SHOCK HEART FAILURE RENAL DAMAGE MAY cause BLEEDING TENDENCY	None significant reported
DEXTROMORAMIDE Narcotic Analgesic Palfium Jetrium	GIT DISTURBANCE CNS DISTURBANCE CONSTIPATION – less than Morphine RESPIRATORY DEPRESSION – more than Morphine	ADDITIVE RESPIRATORY DEPRESSION with other RESPIRATORY DEPRESSANTS MAOI may INDUCE a SEVERE REACTION
DEXTROSE 10% Hypertonic Solution	none significant reported	None significant reported AVOID ADDING DRUGS
DEXTROSE 50% Markedly Hypertonic Solution	OSMOTIC DIURESIS LOCAL VEIN DAMAGE	None significant reported AVOID ADDING DRUGS
DIAMORPHINE Narcotic analgesic	ADDICTIVE EXCEPT when used for severe acute pain NAUSEA and VOMITING less common than with MORPHINE. RESPIRATORY DEPRESSION and coma MORE SEVERE THAN with MORPHINE. PULMONARY OEDEMA occurs with OVERDOSE CARE with DOSE in the ELDERLY, PATIENTS with HEPATIC DISEASE and INFANTS. LESS CONSTIPATION than with MORPHINE.	ADDITIVE RESPIRATORY DEPRESSION with other RESPIRATORY DEPRESSIVE drugs.
DIAMTHAZOLE Antifungal agent Asterol	LOCAL IRRITATION	None significant reported

Drug	Major Side Effects	Interactions

DIAZEPAM
Tranquilliser
Atensine
Tensium
Valium
Apozepam
Stesolid
E – Pam
Paxel
Serenak
Vival
Relanium
	FATIGUE ATAXIA and RESPIRATORY
	  DEPRESSION dose related
	HYPOTENSION – rarely with i.v.
	PARADOXICAL EXCITEMENT – rare
	
	ALL ARE RARE
		ADDITIVE CNS DEPRESSION with ALCOHOL
		  and other CNS DEPRESSANTS
		REDUCES effects of LEVODOPA.

DIAZOXIDE
Antihypertensive
Insulin secretion suppressor.
Eudemine
Hyperstat
Proglicem
	HYPERGLYCAEMIA
	GIT disturbance
	HYPERTRICHOSIS – common after some months
	  of oral use.
	HYPERURICAEMIA
	HYPOTENSION – care in patients with coronary
	  insufficiency.
	FLUID RETENTION
	STOPS LABOUR – should be avoided in
	  Pregnancy.
	ANOREXIA
	NAUSEA and VOMITING
	OEDEMA
		ENHANCES effects of WARFARIN
		ENHANCES effects of PROPRANOLOL
		THIAZIDES ENHANCE effects
		METARAMINOL REDUCES HYPOTENSIVE effects

DICHLORALPHENAZONE Hypnotic Paedo-sed Welldorm Chloralol Restwel Bonadorm Dormwell	GIT DISTURBANCE RASHES AGRANULOCYTOSIS – rare	ADDITIVE CNS DEPRESSION with other CNS DEPRESSANTS MAOI ENHANCE effects ENHANCES or REDUCES effects of WARFARIN

Drug	Major Side Effects	Interactions
DIENOESTROL Oestrogen Hormofemin Cycladiene Estraguard Farmacyrol	WEIGHT GAIN SALT AND WATER RETENTION THROMBO-EMBOLISM	REDUCES effects of WARFARIN REDUCES effects of PHENYTOIN REDUCES effects of ANTIDIABETIC AGENTS RIFAMPICIN REDUCES effects due to enzyme induction PHENOBARBITONE REDUCES effects due to enzyme induction.
DIETHYLCARBAMAZINE Antihelmintic Banocide Hetrazan Carbilazine Wotezine	GIT DISTURBANCE CNS DISTURBANCE ALLERGY – to the worm protein	None significant reported
DIGOXIN Cardiac glycoside Lanoxin Cardiox Dialoxin Digolan Fibroxin Natigoxin Prodigox Coragoxine Digoxine Davoxin Digacin Lanicor Lanatoxin Novodigal Lanacrist Natigoxine Rougoxin Wjnoxin	NAUSEA and VOMITING ANOREXIA CARDIAC ARRHYTHMIA both supraventricular and ventricular. GYNAECOMASTIA YELLOW VISION – rare CNS disturbance	ENHANCED toxicity with POTASSIUM losing agents. CALCIUM SALTS ENHANCE effects. CHOLESTYRAMINE REDUCES effects.

The Therapeutic ratio of Digoxin is small so that the toxic dose is close to the therapeutic dose. In elderly patients and in those with renal or hepatic impairment the dose needs to be reduced as excretion is reduced.
There are many different regimes for digitalising a patient, and in most cases it is best to do so slowly using a regime with which you are familiar, e.g. 0.5mg stat, then 0.25mg 6 hourly for 24 hours, then 0.25mg 12 hourly, then adjust as necessary.
As a general rule with supraventricular arrhythmias – if the patient is on Digoxin when the arrhythmias start then stop the drug. If not then start it.

Drug	Major Side Effects	Interactions
DIHYDROCODEINE Moderate analgesic DF. 118 Paracodin Tuscodin Fortuss Rikodeine	CONSTIPATION DEPENDENCE of MORPHINE TYPE GIT disturbance	None significant reported
1:25 DIHYDROXYCHOLECAL- CIFEROL Vitamin D Metabolite	None significant reported ONLY RECENTLY AVAILABLE AND THEREFORE EFFECTS ARE NOT FULLY ESTABLISHED	None significant reported
DIHYDROTACHYSTEROL Vitamin D Metabolite At. 10. Atecen Dygratyl Calcamine Hytakerol	GIT disturbance POLYURIA ECTOPIC CALCIFICATION *All due to overdose*	None significant reported
DI-IODOHYDROXYQUINOLINE Amoebicide Diodoquin Embequin Floraquin Direxiode Florequin Gynovules Ioquin Moebiquin Vaam-DHQ	GIT DISTURBANCE POSSIBLY OPTIC NEURITIS and ATROPHY	None significant reported
DILOXANIDE Amoebicide Furamide	GIT DISTURBANCE RASHES	None significant reported

Drug	Major Side Effects	Interactions
DIMERCAPROL (BAL) Chelating Agent	GIT disturbance BURNING SENSATIONS EXCESS LACHRYMATION and SALIVATION FEVER *ALL USUALLY TRANSIENT* *NB*: USE WITH CAUTION IF RENAL DAMAGE	None significant reported
DIMETHYL SULPHOXIDE Solvent Used to carry other drugs, e.g. Idoxuridine Increases penetration DMSO	LOCAL DISCOMFORT and IRRITATION GARLIC like ODOUR on BREATH	MAY ENHANCE TOXICITY of drugs DISSOLVED in it
DIOCTYL Surface tension lowering Agent. Wax softener Faecal softener Audinorm Condanol Emcal Manoxol Molcer Siponol-O-100 Soliwax Waxsol Adjust Bantex Constiban Octyl softener Regulex	Bu-lax Comfolax Dilax Colace Diomedicone Disonate Ilozoft Provilax Coloxyl Kylx Dioctyl forte Dioctyl medo D-S-S	None significant reported

Drug	Major Side Effects	Interactions
DIOCTYL SODIUM SULPHOSUCCINATE Surface tension lowering Agent. Wax softener. Audinorm, Condanol, Dioctyl, Emcal, Manoxol, Molcer, Normax, Siponolo, Soliwax, Waxsol, Adjust, Bantex, Constiban, Octyl softener, Regulex, Bu-lax, Comfolax, Dilax, DioMedicone, Disonate, Doxinate, Ilozoft, Provilax, Colace, Coloxyl, Klyx	None significant reported	None significant reported
DIPHENHYDRAMINE Antihistamine Benadryl, Benafed, Benzlets, Benylin, Caladryl, Guanar, Histalix, Ticipeet, Alergicap, Bidramine, Benhydramil, Dabylen, Dihydral, Dihydramine, Desentol, Lensen	SEDATION DRY MOUTH	REDUCES ABSORPTION OF PAS INCREASES CNS DEPRESSION of CNS DEPRESSANTS
DIPHENOXYLATE with ATROPINE Narcotic Anti-diarrhoea Lomotil, Reasec, Diarsed, Retardin	As for MORPHINE, but rare in usual dosage.	ADDITIVE RESPIRATORY DEPRESSION with other RESPIRATORY DEPRESSANTS MAOI may INDUCE A SEVERE REACTION

Drug	Major Side Effects	Interactions
DIPIPANONE Narcotic Analgesic Diconal Wellconal	GIT DISTURBANCE CNS DISTURBANCE CONSTIPATION – less than Morphine RESPIRATORY DEPRESSION – more than Morphine	ADDITIVE RESPIRATORY DEPRESSION with other RESPIRATORY DEPRESSANTS MAOI may INDUCE a SEVERE REACTION
DIPTHERIA antitoxin Antitoxin	ANAPHYLAXIS SERUM SICKNESS PYROGENIC reaction	None significant reported
DIPYRIDAMOLE Antiplatelet agent Persantin Anginal Persantine	GIT disturbance RASH HEADACHE	ENHANCES effects of WARFARIN
DISODIUM CROMOGLYCATE 'Stabilises' mast cells Intal Aarane Inostral Lomudal Rynacron Nasmil	BRONCHOSPASM – transient when powder inhaled.	None significant reported
DISOPYRAMIDE Antiarrhythmic agent Norpace Rhythmodan	GIT disturbance DRY MOUTH VENTRICULAR ARRHYTHMIAS URINARY RETENTION	None significant reported
DITHRANOL ointment Antipsoriatic Fungicide Dithrolan Lasan Stie-Lasan Batidol Lasan Pomade Dermaline Anthra-Derm Anthralin	STAINS CLOTHES (remove with Acetone) STAINS SKIN (remove with Chlorinated lime solution) LOCAL IRRITATION *AVOID IN RENAL DISEASE*	None significant reported

Drug	Major Side Effects	Interactions
DOMIPHEN Disinfectant Bradosol	None significant reported	None significant reported
DOXAPRAM Respiratory Stimulant Dopram	CNS STIMULATION HYPERTENSION TACHYCARDIA	MAOI ENHANCE HYPERTENSIVE effects SYMPATHOMIMETIC AGENTS ENHANCE HYPERTENSIVE effects.
DOXORUBICIN (Adriamycin) Cytotoxic Agent Adriblastina Farmiblastina Adriacin	CARDIOTOXICITY IF TOTAL dose of 550 mg/m² EXCEEDED GIT DISTURBANCE ALOPECIA RED URINE – OCCASIONALLY BONE MARROW DEPRESSION	ADDITIVE BONE MARROW DEPRESSION with other BONE MARROW DEPRESSANTS
DYDROGESTERONE Progestagen Duphaston Dufaston Gynorest	RASHES WEIGHT GAIN GIT DISTURBANCE CHANGE IN LIBIDO LIVER DAMAGE	May REDUCE effects of WARFARIN May REDUCE effects of PHENYTOIN May REDUCE effects of ANTI DIABETIC AGENTS RIFAMPICIN REDUCES effects by enzyme induction PHENOBARBITONE REDUCES effect by enzyme induction
ECOTHIOPATE Irreversible cholinesterase inhibitor Phospholine Iodide	ACUTE GLAUCOMA GIT DISTURBANCE CNS DISTURBANCE *May be prolonged*	None significant reported
EDROPHONIUM CHLORIDE Short acting anticholinesterase Tensilon	MIOSIS EXCESS SALIVATION URINARY and FAECAL INCONTINENCE BRADYCARDIA BRONCHOSPASM	None significant reported

Drug	Major Side Effects	Interactions
EMEPRONIUM BROMIDE Anticholinergic Agent Cetiprin	DRY MOUTH DILATATION OF PUPIL BRADYCARDIA and TACHYCARDIA VESICAL ATONY GIT ATONY LOCAL IRRITATION	TRICYCLIC ANTI-DEPRESSANTS ENHANCE effects.
EMETINE Amoebicide	CARDIOTOXICITY HEPATOTOXICITY NEPHROTOXICITY GIT DISTURBANCE *All seen with excess dosage*	None significant reported
EOSIN Mild disinfectant	LOCAL REACTION	None significant reported
EPHEDRINE Sympathomimetic Spaneph	PALPITATIONS TREMOR INSOMNIA DIFFICULTY with MICTURITION ANXIETY	REDUCES EFFECTS OF BETHANIDINE and GUANETHIDINE MAOI ENHANCE effects.
ERGOTAMINE TARTRATE Antimigraine agent Femergin Exmigra Lingraine Exmigrex Medihaler Gynergen Ergotamine Lingran Ergomar Lingrene Ergotart Etin	NAUSEA and VOMITING ARTERIAL CONSTRICTION	POSSIBLE ADDITIVE VASOCONSTRICTION effect with PROPRANOLOL

Drug	Major Side Effects	Interactions
ERYTHROMYCIN Antibiotic Erycen Ethrilk Erythrocin Ilotycin Erythromid Gluceptate Erythroped Kesso-mycin Ilosone Pfizer E Ilotycin QIDmycin Retcin SK Erythromycin Abboject EMU-V Eromel E-Mycin Rythrocaps Eratrex Abboticin Eromycin Propiocine Erostin Bistamycin Ethryn Chemthromycin Erycinum Emcinka Neo-Erycinum Erythromyctine Prediathrocin Novorythro Erythro ST Dowmycin E Pediamycin Erypar Robimycin	RASHES – uncommon LIVER DAMAGE – Estolate GIT disturbance	REDUCES effects of PENICILLIN REDUCES effects of LINCOMYCIN COMPETES for BINDINGS SITES with CLINDAMYCIN
ERYTHROMYCIN EYE DROPS/ OINTMENT Local Antibiotic	None significant reported	None significant reported
ETHACRYNIC ACID Diuretic – potent loop Edecrine Crinuryl Edercril Hydromedin	GIT Disturbance HEPATIC COMA can be precipitated in patients with hepatic disease. HYPERGLYCAEMIA may precipitate diabetes or make diabetic control difficult. HYPERURICAEMIA may precipitate acute gout. HYPOKALAEMIA especially with long term use. OTOTOXICITY may occur with large doses.	REDUCES effects of HYPOGLYCAEMIC agents. INCREASES NEPHROTOXICITY OF AMINO-GLYCOSIDE, antibiotics and probably CEPHALOSPORINS. INCREASED DIGOXIN toxicity if HYPOKALAEMIC. POTENTIATES effects of ANTIHYPERTENSIVE agents.

Drug	Major Side Effects	Interactions
ETHAMBUTOL Anti-tuberculous agent Myambutol Dexambutol Etibi Miambutol	RETROBULBAR NEURITIS – central scotoma and loss of green and red vision. Usually REVERSIBLE and RARE at 15 mg per kilogram per day.	None significant reported.
ETHAMBUTOL & ISONIAZID Anti-tuberculous combination Mynah	PERIPHERAL NEUROPATHY – pyridoxine responsive. RETROBULBAR NEURITIS – central scotoma and loss of green and red vision. RARE with dose of ISONIAZID less than 350 mg per day and dose of ETHAMBUTOL 15 mg per kg per day	ENHANCES plasma level of PHENYTOIN in slow acetylators ENHANCED HEPATOTOXICITY with RIFAMPICIN especially in slow acetylators. ALUMINIUM HYDROXIDE GEL REDUCES ABSORPTION.
ETHINYLOESTRADIOL Synthetic Oestrogen Lynoral Etivex Dyloform Linoral Edral Feminone Ertonyl Menolyn Estigyn Novestrol Primogyn C Gynolett Primogyn M Progynon C Estinyl Progynon M	WEIGHT GAIN SALT and WATER RETENTION THROMBOEMBOLISM	REDUCES effects of WARFARIN REDUCES effects of PHENYTOIN REDUCES effects of ANTIDIABETIC AGENTS RIFAMPICIN REDUCES effects due to enzyme induction PHENOBARBITONE REDUCES effects due to enzyme induction.
ETHOSUXIMIDE Anticonvulsant Emeside Zarontin Epileo Petit-mal Petnidan Pyknolepsinum Suxinutin	GIT disturbance CNS disturbance ANTI NUCLEAR ANTIBODIES – doubtful significance	None significant reported

Drug	Major Side Effects	Interactions
ETHYNODIOL Progestogen Femulen	RASHES GIT DISTURBANCE WEIGHT GAIN JAUNDICE – rare VIRILISES A FEMALE FETUS	REDUCES effects of WARFARIN REDUCES effects of PHENYTOIN REDUCES effects of ANTIDIABETIC AGENTS RIFAMPICIN REDUCES effects due to enzyme induction PHENOBARBITONE REDUCES effects due to enzyme induction.
EUSOL Antiseptic	LOCAL IRRITATION	None significant reported
FENOPROFEN Analgesic. Antipyretic. Anti-inflammatory. Fenopron	GIT disturbance RASH	May ENHANCE effects of WARFARIN
FERROUS SULPHATE Haematinic Factor Feospan Haemofort Ferro-Gradumet So-bifer Slow-Fe Ferr-O$_2$ Toniron Ferro 66 Duroferon Ferrophor-Dragees Feosol Resoferix Mol-Iron Ferosan-Tydales Fer-In-Sol Ferofor Feritard Novoferrosulfa Fespan	GIT DISTURBANCE	ANTACIDS REDUCE ABSORPTION REDUCES ABSORPTION of TETRACYCLINES
FLUCLOXACILLIN Antibiotic Floxapen Heracillin Staphylex	GIT disturbance SKIN RASH	PROBENECID ENHANCES blood level by blocking renal excretion. CROSS SENSITIVITY with other PENICILLINS.

Drug	Major Side Effects	Interactions
FLUDROCORTISONE Synthetic corticosteroid (Mineralocorticoid) Florinef Astonin H Scherofluron Cortineff	Common especially in long term use: SALT and WATER retention HYPERTENSION MYOPATHY – more common than with most other corticosteroids SIDE EFFECTS similar to those of PREDNISONE can occur with prolonged high dosage but do not occur with normal dosage. *NB:* EFFECTS ARE ¾ THAT OF ALDOSTERONE	ENHANCES HYPERGLYCAEMIC effects of THIAZIDES REDUCES effects of HYPOGLYCAEMIC agents REDUCES effects of SALICYLATES REDUCES effects of ANTICOAGULANTS RIFAMPICIN REDUCES effects due to enzyme induction BARBITURATES REDUCE effects due to enzyme induction. PHENYTOIN REDUCES effects due to enzyme induction.
FLUOCINOLONE Synthetic Corticosteroid for Topical use Synalar Synandone Flucort Fluonid Synemol Jellin Localyn Synamol	LOSS OF SKIN COLLAGEN SUBCUTANEOUS ATROPHY INCREASED RISK OF INFECTION and AS FOR PREDNISONE – if enough absorbed.	AS FOR PREDNISONE IF ENOUGH ABSORBED
FLUFENAMIC ACID Analgesic Anti inflammatory Anti pyretic Arlef Reumajust A Ansatin Saal-F Flufacid Surika Lanceat Orphyrin Nichisedan	GIT DISTURBANCE RASH ASTHMA with ASPIRIN sensitive patients	None significant reported

Drug	Major Side Effects	Interactions
FLUOROURACIL Cytotoxic Agent Anti-metabolite Efudix Fluoroplex	BONE MARROW DEPRESSION GIT DISTURBANCE ALOPECIA RASH	ADDITIVE BONE MARROW DEPRESSION with other BONE MARROW DEPRESSANTS
FLUOXYMESTERONE Anabolic Hormone Ultandren Halotestin Ora-Testryl Oratestin	JAUNDICE in prolonged use	ENHANCES effects of WARFARIN REDUCES effects of HYPOGLYCAEMIC agents PHENOBARBITONE REDUCES effects
FLUPENTHIXOL Tranquilliser Depixol Fluanxol Emergil	RESTLESSNESS PARKINSONS SYNDROME WEIGHT GAIN DROWSINESS DRY MOUTH BLURRED VISION ILEUS URINARY RETENTION VENTRICULAR TACHYCARDIA RETINAL PIGMENTATION	INCREASED CNS DEPRESSION with CNS DEPRESSANTS ANTACIDS REDUCE ABSORPTION ANTICHOLINERGICS REDUCE ABSORPTION ANTICHOLINERGICS ENHANCE side effects PHENOBARBITONE REDUCES effects ENHANCES effects of PHENYTOIN ENHANCES effects of TRICYCLIC ANTIDEPRESSANTS REDUCES effects of GUANETHIDINE etc. REDUCES effects of LEVODOPA
FLUPHENAZINE Tranquilliser Modecate Pacinol Moditen Siqualone Anatensol Permitil Dapotum Prolixin Lyogen Sevinol Omca	DROWSINESS PARKINSONS Syndrome – Akathasia – Tardive dyskinesia (may be irreversible) DRY MOUTH BLURRED VISION ILEUS URINARY RETENTION VENTRICULAR TACHYCARDIA RETINAL PIGMENTATION	INCREASED CNS DEPRESSIONS with CNS DEPRESSANTS ANTACIDS REDUCE ABSORPTION ANTICHOLINERGICS REDUCE ABSORPTION ANTICHOLINERGICS ENHANCE SIDE EFFECTS PHENOBARBITONE REDUCES effects ENHANCES effects of PHENYTOIN ENHANCES effects of TRICYCLIC ANTIDEPRESSANTS REDUCES effects of GUANETHIDINE etc. REDUCES effects of LEVODOPA

Drug	Major Side Effects	Interactions
FOLIC ACID Haematinic Cytofol Folettes Folsan Millafol Folacin Foldine Folasic Folvite	None significant reported *NB*: MAY PRECIPITATE NEUROLOGICAL DEFICIT IF GIVEN TO PATIENTS WITH PERNICIOUS ANAEMIA UNLESS ACCOMPANIED BY AN ADEQUATE SUPPLY OF HYDROXOCOBALAMIN.	None significant reported REDUCES effects of FOLIC ACID ANTAGONISTS
FOLINIC ACID Folic Acid Metabolite Leucovorin Lederfoline	None significant reported	
FORMALDEHYDE Disinfectant Preservative Dowling's wart paint Pict's solution Emoform Veracur Lysoform	LOCAL REACTION GIT DISTURBANCE	None significant reported
FOSFESTROL (diethyl Stilboestrol) Oestrogen Honvan Honvol ST-52 Stilphostrol	GIT DISTURBANCE FLUID RETENTION GYNAECOMASTIA PAIN at the site of BONY SECONDARIES and PERINEUM	None significant reported
FRAMYCETIN eye drops/ointment ear drops/ointment Topical Antibiotic Framygen Soframycin	HYPERSENSITIVITY (may be masked by corticosteroids in combined medication)	None significant reported

Drug	Major Side Effects	Interactions
FRESH FROZEN PLASMA Blood Fraction	AS FOR ALL BLOOD PRODUCTS	None specific reported
FRUSEMIDE Diuretic – potent loop Dryptal Frusid Lasix Arasemide Franyl Impugan Lasilix Seguril	HYPOKALAEMIA HYPOTENSION in large doses HYPERURICAEMIA may precipitate acute gout. HYPERGLYCAEMIA making diabetic control difficult. HEARING may be affected in large doses. RASH DIARRHOEA PANCREATITIS – uncommon	ENHANCES NEPHROTOXIC effects of CEPHALOSPORINS. ENHANCES DIGOXIN toxicity ENHANCES effects of ANTIHYPERTENSIVE agents ENHANCES OTOTOXICITY of AMINOGLYCOSIDES CLOFIBRATE ENHANCES effects in the NEPHROTIC syndrome
GAMMA BENZENE HEXACHLORIDE Insecticide Larvicide Acaricide Derbac Soap Lorexane Quellada Aphtiria Elentol Jacutin Kwell Kwellada	LOCAL IRRITATION CNS disturbance GIT disturbance Only seen with overdose.	INDUCES LIVER ENZYMES
GAVISCON Antacid Mixture	DIARRHOEA CONSTIPATION	REDUCES effects of ASPIRIN REDUCES effects of TETRACYCLINES REDUCES effects of PHENOTHIAZINES REDUCES effects of ISONIAZID REDUCES effects of DIGOXIN REDUCES effects of IRON (All due to reduced absorption)

Drug	Major Side Effects	Interactions
GELATIN EYE LAMELLAE Gelfilm ophthalmic	None significant reported	None significant reported
GENTAMICIN Antibiotic Cidomycin Genticin Garamycin Garamycina Gentalline Geomycine Refobacin Sulmycin	OTOTOXICITY – vestibular greater than acoustic. NEPHROTOXICITY – care with dose in patients with renal impairment *AVOID IN PREGNANCY*	CEPHALORIDINE ENHANCES NEPHROTOXICITY FRUSEMIDE, BUMETANIDE, and ETHACRYNIC ACID ENHANCE OTOTOXICITY and NEPHROTOXICITY.
GENTIAN VIOLET Disinfectant GVS Genapax	GIT disturbance HEADACHE LOCAL REACTION	None significant reported
GLIBENCLAMIDE Sulphonylurea Hypoglycaemic agent Daonil Euglucon Glutril Diabeta	HYPOGLYCAEMIA – less than Chlorpropramide GIT disturbance RASHES BLOOD DYSCRASIA – rare APPETITE – increased	ANTICOAGULANTS ENHANCE effects PHENYLBUTAZONE ENHANCES effects SULPHONAMIDES ENHANCE effects BETA BLOCKERS ENHANCE effects PROBENECID ENHANCES effects MONOAMINE OXIDASE INHIBITORS ENHANCE effect ALCOHOL ENHANCES effects ALCOHOL INDUCES DISULPHIRAM REACTION – rare CORTICOSTEROIDS REDUCE effect ORAL CONTRACEPTIVES REDUCE effects THIAZIDES REDUCE effects 'LOOP' DIURETICS REDUCE effects.
GLYCEROL Hygroscopic Agent Osmotic diuretic Laxative	HEADACHE THIRST GIT disturbance	None significant reported

Drug	Major Side Effects	Interactions
GLUCAGON Hyperglycaemic Agent Glucagon Novo	GIT disturbance HYPERSENSITIVITY HYPOKALAEMIA Severe HYPERTENSION in patients with PHAEOCHROMOCYTOMA	ENHANCES effects of WARFARIN (in prolonged use) INHIBITS effects of ANTIDIABETIC AGENTS
GLYCEROL EYE DROPS Osmotic Agent	None significant reported	None significant reported
GLYCERYL TRINITRATE Artery dilator	HEADACHE, which can be limited by discarding the tablet when the chest pain is relieved. HYPOTENSION	None significant reported

GLYCERYL TRINITRATE
Artery dilator

Nitrocontin	Lenitral
Sustac	Nitora
Anginine	Nitro-bid
Triagin	Nitrolar
Vasitrin	Nitrolex T
Angised	Nitropin
Gilucor nitro	Nitro S.A.
Klavikondal-Retard	Nitrospan
Nitrangin	Nitroglyn
Nitrolingual	Nitrol
Nitro Mack Retard	Nitrostat
Nitrorectal	Nitrong
Nitrozell Retard	Nitroretard
Glynite	Nitrostabilin

Drug	Major Side Effects	Interactions
GOLD (Sodium Aurothiomalate) Anti-rheumatic agent Myocrisin Myochrysine Tauredon	Common RASHES STOMATITIS PROTEINURIA BLOOD DYSCRASIA (often dose related) – may be of SUDDEN ONSET – can be BE PERMANENT APLASTIC ANAEMIA *NB:* START WITH TEST DOSE	INCREASED RISK of BLOOD DYSCRASIA with other BONE MARROW DEPRESSANTS: e.g. Phenylbutazone. ? PENICILLAMINE REDUCES effects

Drug	Major Side Effects	Interactions
GRISEOFULVIN Systemic Fungicide Fulcin Gis-Peg Grisovin Grisefuline Fulvicin-U/F Lamoryl Grisactin Likuden Grifulvin-V	RASH GIT disturbance – mild HEADACHE – mild SEVERE RASHES – rare LEUCOPENIA – rare PROTEINURIA	ENHANCES effects of ALCOHOL. REDUCES effects of WARFARIN by enzyme induction BARBITURATES REDUCE effects
GROWTH HORMONE Hormone Crescormon Somacton	ANTIBODY FORMATION HYPERCALCURIA REDUCED radio iodine uptake by the thyroid *NB*: SPECIES SPECIFIC (One pituitary gland equivalent to one dose of growth hormone)	MAY ENHANCE effects of MORPHINE

GUANETHIDINE
Adrenergic Neurone Blocker
Antihypertensive Agent
Ismelin
	POSTURAL and EXERCISE HYPOTENSION
	DIARRHOEA and GIT upsets
	BRADYCARDIA, dyspnoea and oedema
	IMPOTENCE, myalgia, blurring of
	   vision, all of which are due to
	   autonomic blockade
	PAROTID PAIN and SWELLING
	NASAL STUFFINESS
		ENHANCES effects of other ANTIHYPER-
		   TENSIVE agents.
		AMPHETAMINES, etc. cause severe
		   HYPERTENSION.
		BARBITURATES and some anaesthetics
		   potentiate the HYPOTENSIVE effect.
		TRICYCLIC ANTIDEPRESSANTS, Chlor-
		   promazine and Haloperidol stop the
		   HYPOTENSIVE effect.

GUANETHIDINE EYE DROPS Adrenergic Neurone blocker Ismelin	SUPERFICIAL PUNCTATE KERATOSIS	None significant reported with eye drops
GUANIDINE	BONE MARROW depression CNS disturbance GIT disturbance CARDIAC ARRHYTHMIAS	None significant reported

Drug	Major Side Effects	Interactions
HALOPERIDOL Tranquilliser Haldol Serenace	GIT disturbance DROWSINESS EXTRA PYRAMIDAL DYSFUNCTION HYPOTENSION – rare RASHES JAUNDICE BLOOD DYSCRASIA – rare	ADDITIONAL CNS DEPRESSION with ALCOHOL and other CNS DEPRESSANTS ENHANCES effects of TRICYCLIC ANTIDEPRESSANTS
HEPARIN Anticoagulant Calcium Heparin Hamocura Heparin Injection Liquemin Weddel Norheparin Heparin Retard Thrombophob Minihep Thrombo-Vetren Pularin Vetren Depo-Heparin Hepalean Heprinar Hepathrom Disebrin Pan Heprin	BLEEDING anywhere ALLERGIC REACTIONS – rare	ASPIRIN and DIPYRIDAMOLE INCREASE the risk of BLEEDING.
HERPES ZOSTER IMMUNOGLOBULIN	Anaphylaxis in sensitive patients	None significant reported
HEXACHLOROPHANE Disinfectant E-Z Scrub Gamophen Phiso-med Orahex Steridermis Gill liquid Ster-Zac Hexacreme Zalpon Hexaklen Dermohex Kalacide Hexachlorone Sapoderm Hexaphen-yl Soy-dome Surgiderm	CNS disturbance PHOTOSENSITIVITY SENSITISATION EFFECTS WORSE IN INFANTS	None significant reported

Drug	Major Side Effects	Interactions
HOMATROPINE Cycloplegic Mydriatic SNP Homatropine Osopto homatropine Omatropina lux	GLAUCOMA SYSTEMIC EFFECTS IN INFANTS	None significant reported
HUMAN ANTITETANUS IMMUNOGLOBULIN Humotet Pro-Tet Ar-tet Hypertet Gamatet Tetagam Homo-tet Tetanobulin Gamulin T Tetabullin Hu-tet Tetaglobuline Immu-Tetanus	ALLERGIC REACTION – rare	NEUTRALISIED by TETANUS TOXOID injected at the same site.
HYCANTHONE Schistosomicide Etrenol	GIT disturbance – common CNS disturbance – common EPILEPSY may occur HEPATIC DAMAGE – rare but serious	ENHANCES TOXIC effects of PHENOTHIAZINE
HYDRALLAZINE Antihypertensive Apresoline Aprelazine Hyperazin Lopress	TACHYCARDIA, SEVERE HEADACHE anorexia, nausea, vomiting and POSTURAL HYPOTENSION. (Most of these are transient and are prevented by the simultaneous use of beta blockers). DISSEMINATED LUPUS like syndrome which appears to be DOSE RELATED	ENHANCES the effect of other ANTIHYPERTENSIVE agents. NEUROLEPTICS increase adverse CARDIOVASCULAR effects. Many SIDE EFFECTS PREVENTED by BETA BLOCKERS.

Drug	Major Side Effects	Interactions
HYDRARGAPHEN Trichomonacide Anti-bacterial Anti-fungal Conotrane Penotrane Versotrane	None significant reported	None significant reported

HYDROCHLORTHIAZIDE
Thiazide Diuretic
Moderately potent
Direma
Esidrex
HydroSaluric
Chemhydrazide
Diuchlor H
Hydrazide
Hydrid
Hydro-Aquil
Hydrodiuretex
Hydrosaluret
Neo-Codema
Novo hydrazide
Urozide
Diucen H
Hyeloril
Lexxor
Loqua
Mictrin
Oretic
Thiuretic
Hydrozide
Neoflumen
	GIT disturbance
	ACUTE PANCREATITIS
	HEPATIC COMA can be precipitated in patients
	  with hepatic disease
	HYPERGLYCAEMIA making diabetes difficult to
	  control. (Only mild effect)
	HYPERURICAEMIA may precipitate acute gout
	HYPOKALAEMIA especially with long term use
	RASH – occasionally Stevens-Johnson Syndrome
		REDUCES effects of HYPOGLYCAEMIC agents
		POTENTIATES effects of ANTIHYPERTENSIVE
		  agents.
		INCREASED DIGOXIN toxicity if HYPOKALAEMIA.
		ENHANCES effects of LITHIUM
		CHLORPROPAMIDE ENHANCES HYPONATURAEMIC
		  effect
		CORTICOSTEROIDS INCREASE POTASSIUM LOSS.

Drug	Major Side Effects	Interactions
HYDROCORTISONE ACETATE Natural corticosteroid Used in ointments and for local therapy Colifoam Cortril Efcortelan Dermacort Hydrocortistab Hydrosone Acticort Hysone A Cortomister Sigmacort Cortamed Siguent Hycor Conticreme Squibb H.C. Novohydrocort Ficortril Wincort Acetate Hydrocortal Cortef Idrocortisone Cortifoam Litraderm Pramosone Scheroson F.	The same side effects as seen with all corticosteroid's can occur (see Prednisone) but at the dosage usually used are rare.	ENHANCES HYPERGLYCAEMIC effects of THIAZIDES REDUCES effects of HYPOGLYCAEMIC AGENTS REDUCES effects of ANTICOAGULANTS RIFAMPICIN REDUCES effects due to enzyme induction. BARBITURATES REDUCE effects due to enzyme induction. PHENYTOIN REDUCES effects due to enzyme induction
HYDROCORTISONE SODIUM SUCCINATE Corticosteroid for injection and Pellets for local use. Corlan Nordicort Efcortelan Venocort Flebocortid Solu-Glye Intracort	CARDIOVASCULAR COLLAPSE – with rapid injection Other side effects as for other cortico-steroids, but rare as only used for short time. 20mg Is EQUIVALENT to 5mg of Prednisone.	ENHANCES HYPERGLYCAEMIC effects of THIAZIDES REDUCES effects of HYPOGLYCAEMIC AGENTS REDUCES effects of ANTICOAGULANTS RIFAMPICIN REDUCES effects due to enzyme induction. BARBITURATES REDUCE effects due to enzyme induction. PHENYTOIN REDUCES effects due to enzyme induction
HYDROCORTISONE EYE DROPS Local anti-inflammatory agent Hydrocortistab Hycor eye drops Hydrosone Scherosan F. Ophthalmicum Siguent Hycor (eye)	GLAUCOMA UVEITIS CATARACTS FLAIR UP of VIRAL INFECTION Other effects as for systemic corticosteroids occur rarely.	None significant reported

Drug	Major Side Effects	Interactions
HYDROCORTISONE/SULPHUR Ointment Mild Antiseptic Mild Anti inflammatory	AS FOR EACH COMPONENT	AS FOR EACH COMPONENT
HYDROXOCOBALAMIN Haematinic Neo-cytamen Hydroxobase Alpharedisol Dehepan novum Alpha-Ruvite Hapagon novum Hydroxo-B12 Oxobemin Neo-Betalin 12 Docelan Rubesol-LA Hydroxo Sytobex-H Novobedouze Aqo-cytobion Neo-Benol Axlon Vibeden Berubi-long Cobalparen-Depot Docivit	RASH ALLERGY – rare	None significant reported
HYDROXYCHLOROQUINE Anti-malarial Anti-rheumatic Plaquenil Ercoquin Plaquinol Quensyl	RETINAL REACTION – usually irreversible CORNEAL REACTION – usually reversible PERIPHERAL NEUROPATHY – rare LEUCOPENIA RASHES *NB*: REGULAR OPHTHALMIC TESTING IS MANDATORY	ENHANCED HEPATOTOXICITY with Hepatotoxic Agents.

Drug	Major Side Effects	Interactions
HYDROXYPROGESTERONE Progestogen Primolut.-Depot Delalutin Estralutin Hyproval PA Lutate Luteocrin Depot Progesterone – Retard Pharlon Proluton Depot	RASHES GIT disturbances WEIGHT GAIN JAUNDICE – in previously sensitized patients. VIRILISES a female fetus	REDUCES effects of WARFARIN REDUCES effects of PHENYTOIN REDUCES effects of ANTIDIABETIC AGENTS RIFAMPICIN REDUCES effects due to enzyme induction PHENOBARBITONE REDUCES effects due to enzyme induction
1α HYDROXYCHOLECALCIFEROL Vitamin D. Metabolite One Alpha	HYPERCALCAEMIA ONLY RECENTLY AVAILABLE. THEREFORE EFFECTS NOT FULLY ESTABLISHED	None significant reported
HYDROXYUREA Cytotoxic Agent Hydrea Litalir	GIT disturbance RASH ALOPECIA BONE MARROW DEPRESSION	ADDITIVE BONE MARROW DEPRESSION with other BONE MARROW DEPRESSANTS
HYOSCINE Anti-cholinergic Agent Scopolamine	DRY MOUTH DILATATION OF THE PUPIL CONSTIPATION URINARY RETENTION GLAUCOMA DROWSINESS	AMANTADINE ENHANCES effects TRICYCLIC ANTIDEPRESSANTS ENHANCE effects REDUCES ABSORPTION of LEVODOPA
IBUPROFEN Anti-inflammatory Analgesic Anti-pyretic Brufen Motrin	RASHES GIT disturbance (less than others in the group) ASTHMA with ASPIRIN sensitive patients	None significant reported

Drug	Major Side Effects	Interactions
ICHTHYOL (Ichthammol)	None significant reported	None significant reported
IDOXURIDINE Anti viral agent (Blocks DNA synthesis) Dendrid Herpid Kerecid Ophthalmadine Herpidu Herplex Iduridin Iduviran Stoxil Synmiol Virunguent	LOCAL STINGING LOCAL PRURITIS LOCAL OEDEMA PHOTOPHOBIA – Rare GIT disturbance – systemic use BONE MARROW DEPRESSION – systemic use HEPATOTOXICITY – systemic use	None significant reported
IMIPRAMINE Tricyclic Antidepressant Berkomine Somipra Dimipressin Chemipramine Norpramine Impranil Oppanyl Impril Praminil Novopramine Tofranil Imavate Censtim Janimine Imiprin Presamine Iramil S-K-Pramine Melipramine Panpramine Prodepress Thymorpramine	DRY MOUTH BLURRED VISION CONSTIPATION etc due to PARASYMPATHOLYTIC ACTION CARDIAC ARRHYTHMIAS CHOLESTATIC JAUNDICE AGRANULOCYTOSIS – rare RASHES WEIGHT GAIN	BARBITURATES REDUCE effects except in OVERDOSE when they ENHANCE SIDE EFFECTS ENHANCES effects of ALCOHOL ENHANCES effects of WARFARIN ENHANCES effects of SYMPATHOMIMETIC DRUGS REDUCES effects of BETHANIDINE, GUANETHIDINE and DEBRISOQUINE. SEVERE REACTION may occur with MAOI

Drug	Major Side Effects	Interactions
IMMUNE SERUM GLOBULIN	ALLERGY	None significant reported
Allergobuline Gammapovit		
Diammaglobuline Igege		
Gamma Rhodiglobin		
Beriglobin Gamma-Venin		
Gamastan Gammar		
Gamma Veinine Immunglobin		
Gammagee Gamulin		
Gammabyk Immu-G		
Intraglobin		
INDOMETHACIN	GIT disturbance – may induce ulcers	PROBENECID ENHANCES serum levels.
Anti-inflammatory	HEADACHE AND DIZZINESS are common initially	
Analgesic	and may persist.	
Antipyretic	AGRANULOCYTOSIS – very rare	
Imbrilon Indocin	SKIN RASHES – rare	
Indocid Indomee	FLUID RETENTION – may cause cardiac failure	
Amuno Infrocin		
Confortid Metindol		
Inacid Mezolin		
Indacin		
INSULIN	HYPOGLYCAEMIA	ANABOLIC STEROIDS may INCREASE effects
Hormone	FAT ATROPHY at site of INJECTION	ALCOHOL may INCREASE effects
	FAT HYPERTROPHY at site of INJECTION	β BLOCKERS REDUCE SYMPTOMS of
	ANTIBODY formation	HYPOGLYCAEMIA
		CORTICOSTEROIDS DECREASE effects
		THIAZIDES DECREASE effects
		'LOOP' DIURETICS DECREASE effects
	SEE TABLE OVERLEAF.	DIAZOXIDE DECREASES effects
		ORAL CONTRACEPTIVES may DECREASE effects

Type of Insulin	Duration of Effect (hours)	Strength Available (units/ml)	Source	Trade Names
SOLUBLE				
Acid	5–7	20,40,80,320	Beef	Endopancrine
Neutral	5–7	40,80	Pork	Regular Iletin
ACTRAPID MC (Mono Component Neutral Soluble)				
SEMI LENTE (Zinc suspension Amorphous)	10–15	40,80	Beef	
SEMI TARD MC (Monocomponent Semi Lente)	10–15	40,80	Pork Beef	Semi Lente Iletin
GLOBIN ZINC	12–18	40,80		
ISOPHANE (NPH)	18–24	40,80	Beef	Endopancrine Zinc Protamine
LEO RETARD (Rarely Immunogenic Isophane)	18–24	40,80	Pork	Protamine Zinc and Iletin
LENTE (Zinc suspension 30% amorphous 70% crystalline)	18–24	40,80	Beef	Lente Iletin
MONOTARD MC. (Monocomponent (Lente))	14–22	40,80	Pork	
ULTRA LENTE (Zinc suspension Crystalline)	24–36	40,80	Beef	Ultra Lente Iletin
PROTAMINE ZINC	24–36	40,80	Beef	
ULTRATARD M.C. (Monocomponent Ultralente)	24–36	40,80	Beef	

NB CHANGING TO MONOCOMPONENT or RARELY IMMUNOGENIC INSULIN may necessitate a reduction in dosage

Further details in Yue & Turtle (1977) *Diabetes* **26** 341

Drug	Major Side Effects	Interactions
IODINE Element	RASH Occasionally HYPOTHYROIDISM Rarely HYPERTHYROIDISM – (Jod-Basedow Hypersensitivity reaction – rare phenomenon)	May be SYNERGISTIC with LITHIUM causing HYPOTHYROIDISM
RADIOACTIVE IODINE Radioactive element	HYPOTHYROIDISM – 100% incidence if patient lives long enough. (50% at 10 years) HYPOPARATHYROIDISM – rare and usually not clinically significant. NEOPLASIA – very rare HYPOGONADISM	ENHANCES SUSCEPTIBILITY to IODINE induced HYPOTHYROIDISM
IPECACUANHA Emetic	GIT disturbance ALBUMINURIA CARDIAC ARRHYTHMIAS	None significant reported
IRON DEXTRAN Haematinic Imferon Direx Imferdex Niferex Ironorm Iron Hy-Dex	LOCAL skin staining ALLERGIC REACTION – rare PAIN WITH INJECTION ARTHRALGIA	None significant reported
IRON SORBITOL Haematinic Jectofer	METALLIC TASTE GIT disturbance ALLERGIC REACTION – rare	CONCOMITANT ORAL IRON THERAPY MAY CAUSE A REACTION
ISONIAZID Anti-tuberculous agent Rimifon Niconyl Cedin Nydrazid Isozid Panazid Neoteben Isobicina Tb-Pholgin Isotamine Hydronsan Isotinyl INH Tibinide	PERIPHERAL NEUROPATHY – pyridoxine responsive LIVER DAMAGE - rare HYPERSENSITIVITIES – rare FITS AND PSYCHOSES – rare *ALL RARE with doses LESS THAN 350 mg per day*	ENHANCES plasma level of PHENYTOIN in slow acetylators due to reduced hepatic metabolism. ENHANCED HEPATOTOXICITY with RIFAMPICIN especially in slow acetylators ALUMINIUM HYDROXIDE GEL REDUCES ABSORBTION.

Drug	Major Side Effects	Interactions
ISOPRENALINE Sympathomimetic Alendrin Isovan Saventrine Isolin Suscardia Isuprel Aludrin Neo-Epinine Ingelan Novisodrine Erydin Luf-Iso Isopropydrin Prcternal Iso-Intanefrin Vapo-N-Iso	TACHYCARDIA – dose related VENTRICULAR FIBRILLATION	ENHANCES effect of other SYMPATHOMIMETIC drugs.
ISPAGHULA HUSK Bulk Laxative Fybogel Isogel Vi-Siblin Ispaghul Osmolax Spagulax	None significant reported	None significant reported
KAOLIN ET MORPHINE MIXTURE Anti-diarrhoeal	None significant reported	REDUCES ABSORPTION of LINCOMYCIN
LASSARS PASTE Dermatological mixture Astringent Skin protective Vehicle	None significant reported	None significant reported
LEAD Astringent	GIT disturbance ANAEMIA CNS DISTURBANCE PERIPHERAL NEUROPATHY LEAD LINE *ALL RARE unless prolonged use over large area of skin*	CORTICOSTEROIDS CAN PRECIPITATE SEVERE SYMPTOMS WITH OVERDOSE OF LEAD

Drug	Major Side Effects	Interactions
LEVODOPA (+ Decarboxylase inhibiter) Antiparkinsonian (mixture) Berkdopa Emeldopa Larodopa Helfo-dopa Levopa Ledopa Brocadopa Sobiodopa Veldopa Sepciodopa Bendopa Syndopa Dopar Sinemet Dopastral Madopar Parkidopa	GIT disturbance POSTURAL HYPOTENSION – less than with Levodopa alone. PSYCHIATRIC DISTURBANCES – dose dependent DYSKINESIA – dose dependent ABNORMAL INVOLUNTARY MOVEMENTS – dose dependent ON OFF EFFECT	ANTACIDS INCREASE absorption ANTICHOLINERGICS REDUCE absorption MAOI INDUCES SEVERE HYPERTENSION PHENOTHIAZINES REDUCE effect PYRIDOXINE REDUCES effects AMANTADINE ENHANCES effects ANTICHOLINERGICS ENHANCE effects AMPHETAMINE ENHANCES effects ENHANCES HYPOTENSIVE effects of GUANETHIDINE
LIGNOCAINE Antiarrhythmic, local anaesthetic Xylocard	HYPOTENSION, which is uncommon CONFUSION and fits in overdose	None reported
LIO THYRONINE Hormone (T_3) Tertroxin Cynomel Cytomel Trithyrone Triiodothyronine	PALPITATIONS ANGINA more often than with L. Thyroxine	ENHANCES effects of WARFARIN ENHANCES effects of TRICYCLIC ANTIDEPRESSANTS PHENYTOIN can ENHANCE effects CHOLESTYRAMINE REDUCES absorption KETAMINE induces HYPERTENSION AND TACHYCARDIA
LIQUID PARAFFIN Laxative	LOCAL GRANULOMATA REDUCES ABSORPTION of FAT SOLUBLE VITAMINS. LIPOID PNEUMONIA – when inhaled	None significant reported in short term use

Drug	Major Side Effects	Interactions
LITHIUM Tranquilliser Camcolit 250 Phasal Priadel Carbolith Lithocarb Eskalith Lithonate Lithotabs Hypnorex Lithium duriles Lithane Lithicarb Lithionit Lithium Oligosol Neurolithium Maniprex Quilonum	GIT disturbance TREMOR NEPHROGENIC DIABETES INSIPIDUS, WITH EXCESS DOSAGE DROWSINESS ATAXIA DYSARTHRIA CONFUSION CONVULSIONS COMA HYPOTHYROIDISM	ACETAZOLAMIDE REDUCES effects AMINOPHYLLINE REDUCES effects DIURETICS ENHANCE effects by reducing RENAL EXCRETION SODIUM SALTS REDUCE effects by INCREASING RENAL EXCRETION
LOMUSTINE (CCNU) Cytotoxic Agent	GIT disturbance ORAL ULCERATION BONE MARROW DEPRESSION – delayed HEPATOTOXICITY	ADDITIVE BONE MARROW DEPRESSION with other BONE MARROW DEPRESSANTS
LOPERAMIDE Antidiarrhoeal Imodium	DRY MOUTH CNS disturbance RASH GIT disturbance	None significant reported
LUCANTHONE Schistosomicide Nilodin Miracil D	GIT disturbance – Common CNS disturbance – Common EPILEPSY may occur	ENHANCES toxic effects of PHENOTHIAZINES

Drug	Major Side Effects	Interactions
LYSINE VASOPRESSIN Synthetic Posterior Pituitary Hormone Syntopressin Lypressin Diapid Prostacton	INTESTINAL CRAMPS – diarrhoea UTERINE CRAMPS PALLOR CORONARY ARTERY CONSTRICTION BRONCHOCONSTRICTION NASAL IRRITATION	None significant reported
MAGENTA PAINT (Castellanis paint) Mild disinfectant	None significant reported	None significant reported
MAGNESIUM HYDROXIDE Antacid Mild Laxative Aquamag Chlorumagene	PURGATION	None significant reported
MAGNESIUM SULPHATE Saline Purgative Addex-Magnesium Chronicystine Manor Magnoplasm	None significant unless Renal Impairment	None significant reported
MAGNESIUM TRISILICATE Antacid Magsorbent Nulacin Trisillac Neutrasil Novasorb Trisil Rolo Trisomin	DIARRHOEA	None significant reported

Drug	Major Side Effects	Interactions
MALATHION Insecticide Derbac Liquid Co Prioderm	GIT disturbance CNS disturbance – only seen with overdose. LOCAL IRRITATION – rare	None significant reported
MANNITOL Osmotic diuretic Osmitrol Manicol Osmosol	CIRCULATION OVERLOAD INTRA CELLULAR DEHYDRATION GIT disturbance NB: DO NOT MIX WITH BLOOD	None significant reported
MEDIUM CHAIN TRIGLYCERIDES Alembicol D MCT oil Miglyols Portagen Neobee O	COLIC DIARRHOEA	None significant reported
MEDROXYPROGESTERONE Hormone Provera Depo Provera Amen Clinovir Farlutal Gestapuran	GIT disturbance SALT and WATER retention	None significant reported
MELPHALAN Alkylating Agent Antineoplastic Alkeran	BONE MARROW DEPRESSION GIT disturbance ALOPECIA	ADDITIVE BONE MARROW DEPRESSION with other BONE MARROW DEPRESSANTS

Drug	Major Side Effects	Interactions
MENOPAUSAL URINARY GONADOTROPHIN (Both follicular stimulating and lutenising hormones) Trophic Hormone Pergonal Homogonal Uumegon	MULTIPLE PREGNANCIES ASCITES in overdose NB: HYPER-STIMULATION SYNDROME May occur with nausea, vomiting, abdominal pain and 'shock' due to ascites and pleural effusion formation	None significant reported
MENTHOL Antipruritic ointment	LOCAL IRRITATION	None significant reported
MEPACRINE Antimalarial Antineoplastic Atabrine Tenicridine	GIT disturbance HEADACHE MALAISE PYREXIA	ALCOHOL may induce a DISULFIRAM LIKE REACTION
6-MERCAPTOPURINE Antineoplastic Puri-Nethol	BONE MARROW DEPRESSION GIT disturbance LIVER DAMAGE	ALLOPURINOL ENHANCES effects, therefore, reduce dose of 6-Mercaptopurine TO 25% ADDITIVE BONE MARROW DEPRESSION with other BONE MARROW DEPRESSANTS.
MESTRANOL Oestrogen	WEIGHT GAIN SALT AND WATER RETENTION THROMBO-EMBOLISM	REDUCES effects of WARFARIN REDUCES effects of ANTIDIABETIC AGENTS RIFAMPICIN REDUCES effects due to enzyme induction PHENOBARBITONE REDUCES effects due to enzyme induction
METARAMINOL Sympathomimetic Aramine	HYPERTENSION LOCAL NECROSIS	MAOI ENHANCE effects GUANETHIDINE ENHANCES effects RESERPINE ENHANCES effects

Drug	Major Side Effects	Interactions
METFORMIN Biguanide Glucophage Metiguanide Diabex SR Diabexyl Haurymellin	GIT disturbance – less than PHENFORMIN LACTIC ACIDOSIS – less than PHENFORMIN	ENHANCES effects of WARFARIN ALCOHOL increases risk of LACTIC ACIDOSIS CHLORPROPRAMIDE increases risk of LACTIC ACIDOSIS
METHADONE Narcotic Analgesic Physeptone Dolophine Westadone L. Polamidon	GIT disturbance CNS disturbance CONSTIPATION – less than morphine RESPIRATORY DEPRESSION – more than morphine	ADDITIVE RESPIRATORY DEPRESSION with other RESPIRATORY DEPRESSANTS MAOI MAY INDUCE SEVERE REACTION
L METHIONINE Amino–Acid Meonine Ninol Unihepa Pedameth Lobamine Uracid Methnine Uranap	NAUSEA and VOMITING	None significant reported
METHISAZONE Antiviral Smallpox prophylactic Marboran	GIT disturbance FLUID RETENTION – short lived	ALCOHOL ENHANCES EFFECTS
METHOTREXATE Cytotoxic Agent (Folic Acid Antagonist) Methotrexate Ledertrexate	GIT disturbance BONE MARROW depression LIVER DAMAGE GIT BLEEDING LUNG damage – usually self limiting	SALICYLATES ENHANCE effects TETRACYCLINES ENHANCE effects PHENYTOIN ENHANCES effects SULPHONAMIDES ENHANCE effects PARA-AMINOBENZOIC ACID ENHANCES effects ALCOHOL ENHANCES HEPATO-TOXICITY

Drug	Major Side Effects	Interactions
METHOXSALEN (Methoxypsoralen) Pigmenting agent Meladinine Oxsoralen Soloxsalen	NAUSEA – common CNS disturbance – less common LOCAL BURNS AVOID in: Diabetes Mellitus Liver Disease Lupus erythematosis Porphyria	ENHANCES effects of PHOTOSENSITIVITY drugs e.g. Chlorpromazine Nalidixic Acid
METHYL CELLULOSE Hygroscopic material Bulk Laxative Celacolm Cellothyl Celevac Hydrolose Cellucon Syncelose Cologel Cellulone Methocel A Genazell Nilstim	None significant reported	None significant reported
METHYLCELLULOSE EYE DROPS (Hypromellose) Artificial Tears Lubricating Agent Celacol HPM Isopto Alkaline Iospto Plain Methocel H.G. Contactisol Isopto-tears Lacril Isopto-Fluid Methopt	None significant reported	

Drug	Major Side Effects	Interactions
METHYLDOPA antihypertensive Aldomet Co Caps Methyldopa Dopamet Medomet Aldometil Presinol Sembrina Hyperpexa Methoplain	SEDATION, drowsiness, nasal stuffiness and dry mouth – which are common, especially early in treatment and when there is a change in dosage. POSTURAL and exercise HYPOTENSION Change in bowel habit IMPOTENCE ALLERGIC REACTION POSITIVE COOMBS TEST in 2-25% of patients after 6 months treatment, which is reversible. HAEMOLYTIC ANAEMIA – rare and reversible. POSITIVE L.E. CELLS found in the blood. DEPRESSION, which is not as common as with Reserpine. HEPATITIS, which is rare but may be severe.	ENHANCES the effects of BARBITURATES ENHANCES the effects of HALOPERIDOL. ENHANCES effects of other ANTI-HYPERTENSIVE agents. REDUCES effects of LEVODOPA. TRICYCLIC ANTIDEPRESSANTS stop the HYPOTENSIVE effect. Care with HALOTHANE because of possible hepato-toxicity.
METHYLENE BLUE Desmoid pillen M-B tabs Urolene blue	GIT disturbance CNS disturbance LOCAL ABSCESS FORMATION GREEN URINE	None significant reported
METHYLPENTYNOL Hypnotic Insomnol Oblivon Allotropal	GIT disturbance *NB*: USE WITH CARE IN CAR DRIVERS	ADDITIVE CNS DEPRESSION with other CNS DEPRESSANTS MAOI ENHANCE EFFECTS ENHANCES effects of WARFARIN
METHYSERGIDE Antimigraine Serotonin Antagonist Deseril Desernil Sansert	GIT disturbance CNS disturbance CVS disturbance RETROPERITONEAL FIBROSIS with long term use STOP USE FOR 1-2 MONTHS EVERY 6 months	None significant reported

Drug	Major Side Effects	Interactions
METOCLOPRAMIDE Peristaltic Stimulant Maxolon Primperan Donopon-6P Metoclol Moriperan Maxeran Paspertin Reglan	DROWSINESS – rare EXTRA PYRAMIDAL SYNDROME RASHES GIT disturbance	REDUCES ABSORPTION of DIGOXIN ENHANCES PARKINSONIAN side effects of PHENOTHIAZINE ANTICHOLINERGICS REDUCE effects

METOPROLOL
Cardioselective ß blocker
Betaloc
Lopresor
Seloken
	GIT upsets
	SLEEP disturbance
		ENHANCES hypoglycaemia of INSULIN
		   and SULPHONYLUREAS.
		ENHANCES cardiac depressive effects
		   of many ANAESTHETICS.
		ATROPINE reverses effect.
		May cause ASYSTOLE with VERAPAMIL.
		Beta-adrenergic stimulators reduce effects

METRIPHONATE Anti Protozoan Insecticide Antihelmintic Bi Larcil	GIT DISTURBANCE CNS disturbance	ATROPINE REVERSES side effects
METRONIDAZOLE Anti Protozoal Anti bacterial Flagyl Neo-tric Clont Novonidazol Entizol Trichazol Elyzol Trikacide Meronidal Trikamon Nida Sanatrichom	GIT disturbance CNS disturbances – UNCOMMON LEUCOPENIA – TRANSIENT	ALCOHOL INDUCES DISULFIRAM LIKE REACTION

Drug	Major Side Effects	Interactions
METYRAPONE Blocker of corticosteroid Synthesis (11β hydroxylase) Metopirone	GIT disturbance ADRENAL INSUFFICIENCY	PHENYTOIN HALVES effects of ORAL DOSE
MEXENONE Sunscreen Uvistat Uvicone	None significant reported	None significant reported
MEXILITINE Anti-arrhythmic Mexitil	GIT upsets even when given i.v. DROWSINESS ATAXIA, etc. when given i.v. HYPOTENSION when given i.v.	None significant reported
MICONAZOLE Antifungal Agent Daktarin Dermonistat GynoDaktarin Monistat Micatin	LOCAL IRRITATION	None significant reported
MIST. POTASSIUM CITRATE Urinary alkalising agent Kajos K-lyte	None significant reported	None significant reported
MITOTANE (O^1 P^1 DDD) Blocker of corticosteroid synthesis Lysodren	GIT disturbance CNS SYMPTOMS – PERMANENT brain damage with prolonged use. ADRENAL INSUFFICIENCY	None significant reported

Drug	Major Side Effects	Interactions
MONOBENZONE ointment Depigmenting agent Aloquin Benoquin Depigman	LOCAL IRRITATION	None significant reported
MORPHINE Potent Narcotic analgesic Nepenthe Duna-phorine	ADDICTIVE except when used for severe acute pain. NAUSEA and VOMITING are common CONSTIPATION is common. RESPIRATORY DEPRESSION and coma. CARE with DOSE in ELDERLY patients, patients with hepatic disease and in INFANTS.	ADDITIVE RESPIRATORY DEPRESSION with other RESPIRATORY DEPRESSING drugs. MAOI MAY INDUCE SEVERE REACTION
MUSTINE Anti-neoplastic Caryolysine Mustargen	GIT disturbance BONE MARROW depression AMENORRHOEA ALOPECIA	ADDITIVE BONE MARROW DEPRESSION with other BONE MARROW DEPRESSANTS
NALORPHINE Narcotic Antagonist Lethidrone	CNS DISTURBANCE BRADYCARDIA WITHDRAWAL SYMPTOMS (if dependant on narcotics)	None significant reported
NALOXONE Narcotic Antagonist Narcan	WITHDRAWAL SYMPTOMS (if dependant on narcotics) OTHERS – rare	None significant reported
NANDROLONE DECANOATE Androgen Anabolic Steroid Deca-Durabolin Abolon Deca-Durabol	VIRILISM	None significant reported

Drug	Major Side Effects	Interactions
NANDROLONE PHENYLPROPIONATE Androgen Anabolic steroid Durabolin Durabol	VIRILISM	None significant reported
NAPROXEN Antipyretic Analgesic Antiinflammatory Naprosyn Naxen Proxen	GIT disturbance RASH CNS disturbance	May ENHANCE effects of WARFARIN
NEOMYCIN eye drops/ointment ear drops/ointment Topical antibiotic Maxitrol Necsporin Neobacrin Nivemycin Neocortef Otosporin	HYPERSENSITIVITY (May be masked by corticosteroids in combined medication). OTOTOXICITY	None significant reported
NEOMYCIN Antibiotic for local and oral use Mycifradin Neocin Myciguent Neobiotic Neomin Otobiotic Nivemycin Neobram Bykomycin Neomate Myacyne NeoMorrhuol Emelmycin Neopt Neopan Neosulf Herisan	DEAFNESS – dose related RENAL DAMAGE – rare with local use GIT disturbance LOCAL ALLERGY MALABSORPTION	ENHANCES effects of WARFARIN - when taken orally DIMETHYL SULFOXIDE enhances absorption and therefore TOXICITY

Drug	Major Side Effects	Interactions
NEOSTIGMINE Anticholinesterase Parasympathomimetic Prostigmin Juvastigmin Synstigmin	MIOSIS EXCESS SALIVATION URINARY AND FAECAL INCONTINENCE BRADYCARDIA BRONCHOSPASM CHOLINERGIC CRISIS (excess dose in Myasthenia)	REDUCES EFFECTS OF LEVODOPA ANTAGONISES TRICYCLIC ANTIDEPRESSANTS ANTAGONISES ANTICHOLINERGICS

NICOTINIC ACID
Lipid lowering agent
Acidemel   Nicospan
Diacin   Nictinex
Efacin   Vasotherm
Niac   Wampocap
Nico-400 Nicangin
Nicobid   Niconacid
Nicolar   Nicyl
	COMMON in dose needed to lower cholesterol.
	GIT disturbances which settle
	   on continuing treatment
	FLUSHING
	VASODILATATION
		REDUCES effects of INSULIN after
		   long term use.
		POSSIBLY ENHANCES the effects of
		   ANTIHYPERTENSIVE agents.

NIFURATEL Trichomonacide Inimur Macmiror Omnes Polmiror	GIT disturbance RASHES	None significant reported
NIKETHAMIDE Respiratory Stimulant Analeptic Coramine Cardiamide Cormed Juvacor Kardonyl Cordiaminum	GIT disturbance CNS stimulation Tachycardia	None significant reported

Drug	Major Side Effects	Interactions
NIMORAZOLE Trichomonacide Acterol Forte Naxogin Naxogyn Nulogyl	GIT disturbance RASH HYPERSENSITIVITY AVOID IN PATIENTS WITH CNS DISEASE, NURSING MOTHERS AND EARLY PREGNANCY	ALCOHOL my induce DISULFIRAM REACTION
NIRIDAZOLE Schistosomicide Ambilhar	GIT disturbance CARDIOTOXICITY NEUROPSYCHIATRIC REACTION EPILEPSY – Rare Side effects worse if associated LIVER DISEASE Side effects STOP when Treatment Stops.	Reacts with ISONIAZID, therefore avoid simultaneous use
NORETHISTERONE Progestogen Micronor Micronovum Noriday Norfcr Primulut N Norluten Micronett Norlutin Mini Pe Nor QD	RASHES GIT disturbance WEIGHT GAIN JAUNDICE – rare VIRILISES a FEMALE FETUS	REDUCES effects of WARFARIN REDUCES effects of PHENYTOIN REDUCES effects of ANTIDIABETIC AGENTS RIFAMPICIN REDUCES effects due to enzyme induction PHENOBARBITONE REDUCES effects due to enzyme induction.
NORGESTREL Progestogen Neogest Ovrette Follistrel Microlution Microlut Mikro-30	RASHES GIT disturbance WEIGHT GAIN JAUNDICE – rare VIRILISES A FEMALE FETUS	REDUCES effects of WARFARIN REDUCES effects of PHENYTOIN REDUCES effects of ANTIDIABETIC AGENTS RIFAMPICIN REDUCES effects due to enzyme induction PHENOBARBITONE REDUCES effects due to enzyme induction.

Drug	Major Side Effects	Interactions

K NOXYTHIOLIN
Antiseptic
  Gynaflex
  Noxyflex
  NSB
	Local irritation	None significant reported

NYSTATIN
Anti fungal agent
  Nystan   Diastatin
  Candio-Hermal Korostatin
  Moronal   Mycostatin
  Canstat   Mycostatine
  Fungalex   Nilstat
  Fungistatin
	GIT disturbance – mild and reversible	None significant reported

OESTRADIOL VALERATE
Oestrogen
  Primogyn Depot
  Progynova
  Delestragen
  Estratab
  Femogex
  Prognyon-Depot
	WEIGHT GAIN
	NAUSEA
	JAUNDICE
	SALT and WATER retention
	THROMBOEMBOLISM
	BREAST TENDERNESS
	HEADACHE
	GYNAECOMASTIA
		REDUCES effects of WARFARIN
		REDUCES effects of PHENYTOIN
		REDUCES effects of ANTIDIABETIC AGENTS
		RIFAMPICIN REDUCES effects due to enzyme induction
		PHENOBARBITONE REDUCES effects due to enzyme induction.

OESTRIOL
Oestrogen
  Ovestin
  Hemostyptanon
  Synapause
  Horin
  Hormomed
  Orgestyptin
  Ovesterin
  Triodurin
  Triovex
	WEIGHT GAIN
	NAUSEA
	JAUNDICE
	SALT and WATER retention
	THROMBOEMBOLISM
	BREAST TENDERNESS
	HEADACHE
	GYNAECOMASTIA
		REDUCES effects of WARFARIN
		REDUCES effects of PHENYTOIN
		REDUCES effects of ANTIDIABETIC AGENTS
		RIFAMPICIN REDUCES effects due to enzyme induction
		PHENOBARBITONE REDUCES effects due to enzyme induction.

Drug	Major Side Effects	Interactions

OESTROGENS – Conjugated
Oestrogen
Premarin SKoestrogens
Amnestrogen Tab 39
Ces Trocosone
Conest Zeste
Conestron Climestrone
Conjes Est-omed
Estratab Femacoid
Estropan Menotrol
Evex Neo-Estrone
Femest Novoconestrone
Femogen Oestrilin
Geneake Ecuigyne
Genisis Oestro-feminal
Glyestrin Oestropak
Menest morning
Menogen Presomen
Msmed Transannon
Par Estro Promarit
	WEIGHT GAIN
	SALT and WATER RETENTION
	THROMBOEMBOLISM
	NAUSEA
	JAUNDICE
	BREAST TENDERNESS
	HEADACHE
	GYNAECOMASTIA
		REDUCES effects of WARFARIN
		REDUCES effects of PHENYTOIN
		REDUCES effects of ANTIDIABETIC AGENTS
		RIFAMPICIN REDUCES effects due to enzyme
		  induction
		PHENOBARBITONE REDUCES effects due to enzyme
		  induction.

OLIVE OIL Softening agent Emollient Purgative	None significant reported	None significant reported

ORCIPRENALINE
β stimulator
Alupent
Metaprel
Novasmasol
	TREMOR which is common
	HEADACHE
	TACHYCARDIA
	GIT disturbance
		PROPRANOLOL (non-selective beta blocker)
		  REDUCES effect.
		METOPROLOL (selective beta blocker) causes
		  less REDUCTION IN EFFECTS.

Drug	Major Side Effects	Interactions
ORPHENADRINE Anti Parkinsonian Disipal Mephenamin Orpadrex	DRY MOUTH DILATED PUPIL CONSTIPATION URINARY RETENTION TACHYCARDIA RASH	None significant reported
OXPRENOLOL Beta blocker Trasicor	GIT disturbance – common BAD DREAMS PARAESTHESIA BRADYCARDIA – which may be profound after i.v. injection ASTHMA CARDIAC FAILURE	ENHANCES HYPOGLYCAEMIA OF HYPOGLYCAEMIC agents ENHANCES CARDIAC DEPRESSION of many ANAESTHETICS ENHANCES effects of HYPOTENSIVE agents ENHANCES ANTI-TREMOR effects OF L-DOPA ATROPINE REVERSES effect VERAPAMIL HAS BEEN REPORTED TO CAUSE ASYSTOLE DIURETICS ENHANCE effects BETA ADRENERGIC STIMULATORS REDUCE effects
OXYCODONE Narcotic Analgesic Proladone Pancodone	CONSTIPATION VOMITING RESPIRATORY DEPRESSION	ADDITIONAL RESPIRATORY DEPRESSION with other RESPIRATORY DEPRESSANTS ADDITIONAL CNS DEPRESSION WITH other CNS DEPRESSANTS MAOI MAY INDUCE SEVERE REACTION
OXYGEN	PULMONARY DAMAGE after 100% for 24 hours. RETROLENTAL FIBROPLASIA in premature infants. HYPERCAPNIA in patients having hypoxia as a respiratory drive.	None significant reported.

Drug	Major Side Effects	Interactions
OXYMETAZOLINE Nasal decongestant Sympathomimetic Iliadin-mini Afrin Drixine Hazol Nafrine Nasivin Nezeril	LOCAL BURNING REBOUND CONGESTION with CHRONIC use.	None significant reported
OXYMETHOLONE Androgen Anabolic Steroid Anapolon Anadrol Anasteron Nastenon	ACNE VIRILISM CRAMP JAUNDICE	May ENHANCE WARFARIN effects.
PADIMATE A Sunscreen ointment Escalol 506 Spectraban Pabafilm Phiasol AS Uvosan Lotion	None significant reported	None significant reported

Drug

PARACETAMOL
Analgesic
Antipyretic

Ceetanol	Lyteca
Napamol	Nebbs
Panado	Neopap
Pandel	Phendex
Pyralen	Proval
Repamol	SK-apap
Tempra	Tapar
Valadol	Temlo
Calpol	Atasol
Centramol	Campain
Centamol	Chemcetaphen
Clonamol	Pediaphen
Panadol	Rounox
Panasorb	Ben-U-Ron
Ticelgesic	Ceetmol
Salzone	Dolamin
Parmol	Dymadon
Alvedon	Nevrol
Panodil	Paracet
Termidor	Parasin
Anuphen	Parmol
Apamide	Placemol
Capital	Cetamol
Cen-apap	Doliprane
Dolanex	Napamol
Febrigesic	Restin Elixir
Febrogesic	Pacemol
Korum	Tylenol
Liquiprin	

Major Side Effects

SKIN RASHES
LIVER DAMAGE – FREQUENTLY FATAL in
    overdose
GIT disturbance
ASTHMA – sensitivity response – uncommon

Interactions

None significant reported

Drug	Major Side Effects	Interactions
PARALDEHYDE Hypnotic Sedative Paral	GASTRIC IRRITATION RASH ABSCESS with INTRAMUSCULAR INJECTION CNS DEPRESSION in OVERDOSE	DISULFIRAM ENHANCES effects ENHANCES CRYSTALLURIA with SULPHONAMIDES ENHANCES CNS DEPRESSION with other CNS DEPRESSANTS
PANCREATIN Pancreatic enzyme Combizym Zypanar Cotazym Elzyme Cotazym B Pentazyme Enzypan Nucleoton Nutrizym Pankreon Panar Panteric Pancrex Trypsogen Pancrex V Vickase Pancreatin	ULCERATION either oral or anal ALLERGY – not a major problem	ACID in STOMACH REDUCES effects.

PENICILLAMINE
Chelating Agent
Cuprimine
Depamine
Distamine
Cuprenil
D-Penamine
Metalcaptase
Trolovol
	OCCUR IN 20-30% of PATIENTS:
	ACUTE HYPERSENSITIVITY
	AUTO IMMUNE REACTIONS, e.g. SLE
	RENAL diease – Proteinuria – common
	                    Nephritis – less common
	                    Nephrotic syndrome
	BONE MARROW DEPRESSION
	GIT disturbance
	IMPAIRED COLLAGEN SYNTHESIS
	PENICILLIN SENSITIVE PATIENTS MAY
	    REACT ADVERSELY
		IRON REDUCES EFFECTS BY REDUCING ABSORPTION
		GOLD ENHANCES ADVERSE effects
		ANTIMALARIALS ENHANCE ADVERSE effects

Drug

PENICILLIN V
Antibiotic

Apsin VK	Roscopenin
Co Caps Peni-	Tixacillin
cillin VK	Arcasin
C.V.K (Compo-	Beromycin
cillin VK)	Isocillin
Crystapen V	Ispenoral
Distaquaine VK	Dowpen
Econocil VK	Kesso-Pen-VK
G.P.V.	Paclin VK
ICIPEN 300	Penapar VK
Stabillin VK	Pfizerpen VK
V-Cil-K	QID pen VK
Abbocillin VK	Robicillin VK
Adacillin	Uticillin VK
Bramcillin	V-cillin
Cilicaine V	Veetids
Falcopen V	Calcipen
Lanpen	Rocilin
LPV	Compocillin VK
PVK	Corcillin V
PVO	Darocillin
Pen-cillin-V	Deltacillin
Pfipen V	Diacipen VK
Caps-Pen-V	Jatcillin
Cillaphen	Nutracillin
Pancillen	Orapen
Peni-vee	Veekay
Viraxacillin V	Vikacillin
Alocillin	Fenoxicillin
Apopen	Fenoxypen
Calciopen	Hi-Pen
Kavepenin	Nadopen-V
Meropenin	Novopen-V

Major Side Effects

GIT disturbance
RASH – common
ANAPHYLACTIC COLLAPSE and
HYPOTENSION – rare

Interactions

PROBENECID REDUCES RENAL EXCRETION
NEOMYCIN REDUCES ABSORPTION

Drug	Major Side Effects	Interactions
PENICILLIN V (contd.) Pen-Vee PVF-K VC-K500 Win-V-K Ledercillin VK Oracilline Orvepen Ospen Pen-vee-K V-cillin K		
PENICILLIN EYE DROPS/ OINTMENT Local Antibiotic	As for Penicillin *NB*: 1. Local Allergy 2. Sensitivity Reaction	As for Penicillin
PENTAZOCINE Potent Analgesic Fortral Fortalgesic Fortralin Sosegon Talwin	SEDATION NAUSEA PSYCHOTOMIMETIC effects HYPOTENSION RESPIRATORY DEPRESSION DEPENDENCE	None significant reported
PENTOLINIUM Ganglion blocking antihypertensive Ansolysen	POSTURAL and EXERCISE HYPOTENSION CONSTIPATION, PARALYTIC ILEUS or diarrhoea TACHYCARDIA, dyspnoea and oedema. IMPOTENCE, myalgia, blurring of vision, all of which are due to autonomic blockade.	ENHANCES effects of other ANTI- HYPERTENSIVE agents. AMPHETAMINES, etc. cause severe HYPERTENSION. TRICYCLIC ANTIDEPRESSANTS, Chlorpro- mazine, Haloperidol, stop the HYPOTENSIVE effect. BARBITURATES and some anaesthetics potentiate the HYPOTENSIVE effect.

Drug	Major Side Effects	Interactions

PETHIDINE
Potent narcotic analgesic
Demerol
Dolantin
Dolosal
Suppolosal
Pethoid
Phytadon
	ADDICTIVE
	NAUSEA and VOMITING, which are more
	  common than with morphine.
	RESPIRATORY depression
	SLIGHTLY ANTISPASMODIC
	CONSTIPATION and URINARY RETENTION
	  less frequent than with morphine.
		ENHANCES RESPIRATORY DEPRESSION of
		  other RESPIRATORY DEPRESSING agents.
		MONOAMINOXIDASE INHIBITORS induce a
		  MARKED REACTION in SOME PATIENTS.

PHENETURIDE Anticonvulsant Benuride Trinuride	GIT disturbance RASH BONE MARROW DEPRESSION	PHENYTOIN ENHANCES effects
PHENFORMIN Biguanide Dibotin Dipar Metral D.B. Retard D.B.I. Dibein Glucopostin Insoral	GIT disturbance LACTIC ACIDOSIS if predisposing conditions – HIGH mortality	ENHANCES effects of WARFARIN ALCOHOL INCREASES risk of LACTIC ACIDOSIS
PHENOL Disinfectant (in weak solution) Antipruritic ointment	LOCAL IRRITATION	None significant reported

Drug	Major Side Effects	Interactions

PHENOBARBITONE
Cerebral depressant
Anti-convulsant
  Gardenal   PEBA
  Luminal   Phenbar
  Phenomet   Phen-o-caps
  Ensobarb   Sedebar
  Phenased   Luminaletten
  Epilol   Phenaemal
  Epsylone   Phenamaletten
  Eskabarb   Seda-Tablinen
  Hypnolone Solfoton
  Novo-pheno Stertal
	Rare in normal dosage	REDUCES effects of WARFARIN
		ENHANCES CNS DEPRESSION due to ALCOHOL
		  and all other CNS DEPRESSANTS
		*REDUCES effects of ORAL CONTRACEPTION
		*REDUCES effects of CORTICOSTEROIDS
		ENHANCES effects of CYCLOPHOSPHAMIDE
		ENHANCES OR REDUCES effects of PHENYTOIN
		REDUCES effects of GRISEOFULVIN
		REDUCES effects of TETRACYCLINE
		REDUCES effects of RIFAMPICIN
		SODIUM VALPROATE INCREASES effects
		ENHANCES TOXIC effects of TRICYCLIC
		  ANTIDEPRESSANTS
		*due to enzyme induction

PHENOXYBENZAMINE
Alpha adrenergic blocker
  Dibenyline
  Dibenzyline
	FAILURE OF EJACULATION
	POSTURAL HYPOTENSION
	GIT disturbance
	SEDATION
	NASAL STUFFINESS
	SKIN SENSITIVITY in HANDLERS
		None significant reported

PHENTOLAMINE
Alpha adrenergic blocker
  Rogitine
  Regitine
  Regitine
	POSTURAL HYPOTENSION
	GIT disturbance
	NASAL STUFFINESS
	TACHYCARDIA & ARRHYTHMIAS
		None significant reported

Drug

PHENYLBUTAZONE
Anti-inflammatory analgesic

Butacote	Atrizin	
Butazolidin	Atropan	
Butazone	Diossidone	
Flexazone	Kadol	
Ethibute	Ticinil	
Oppazone	Azolid	
Tetnor	Butacal	
Algoverine	Butalan	
Butagesic	Butalgin	
Chembutazone	Butaphen	
Ecobutazone	Butarex	
Eributazone	Butoroid	
Intrabutazone	Butoz	
Malgesic	Buzon	
Merizone	Phenybute	
Nadozone	Butapirazol	
Neo-Zoline	Butina	
Novophenyl	Butozone	
Phenbutazol	Butrex	
Phylbetazone	Panazone	
Tazone	Elmedal	
Wescozone	Praecirhevmin	

Major Side Effects

GIT disturbance – may induce ulceration
FLUID RETENTION – causing cardiac failure
or hypertension.
SKIN RASH which can be SEVERE
SORE THROAT – STOP DRUG AT ONCE
AGRANULOCYTOSIS, which is less common with
a dose below 400 mg per day. More common
in elderly or after prolonged treatment.
SALIVARY GLAND enlargement – rare
RENAL IMPAIRMENT
LIVER DAMAGE
GOITRE FORMATION
EPIDERMAL NECROLYSIS – rare

Interactions

*ENHANCES effect of WARFARIN
*ENHANCES effect of TOLBUTAMIDE
*ENHANCES effect of CHLORPROPAMIDE
*ENHANCES effect of PHENYTOIN
§REDUCES effect of THIAZIDE DIURETIC
§REDUCES effect of GUANETHIDINE

*due in part to displacement from plasma
proteins
§due to fluid retention

Drug	Major Side Effects	Interactions
PHENYLEPHRINE Sympathomimetic Agent	LOCAL REACTION HYPERTENSION	MAOI INDUCES HYPERTENSION GUANETHIDINE ENHANCES effects METHYLDOPA ENHANCES effects TRICYCLIC ANTIDEPRESSANTS ENHANCE effects

Isopto Frin Mistura-D
Biomydrin Deca Nephrine
Fenox Degest
Hayphryn I-Care
Narex Mistol Mist
Neophryn Phenephrin
Nez Isonefrine
Uniflu Isotropina
Vibrocil Isophrin
Coryban-D

| **PHENYLPROPANOLAMINE** Nasal decongestant Sympathomimetic | SYMPATHETIC OVERACTIVITY HYPERTENSION | MAOI INDUCE HYPERTENSIVE CRISIS REDUCES effects of BETHANIDINE |

Eskornade Triotussic
Totolin Propradrine
Rinurel Rhindecon
Triogesic Tepanil
Triominic

| **PHENYTOIN** Membrane Stabiliser Anticonvulsant | GIT diturbance NYSTAGMUS with ataxia and diplopia GUM HYPERTROPHY MEGALOBLASTIC ANAEMIA due to folic acid deficiency BONE MARROW DEPRESSION | PHENYLBUTAZONE ENHANCES effects PAS ENHANCES effects CHLORAMPHENICOL ENHANCES effects ALCOHOL REDUCES effects COMPLEX INTERACTION with WARFARIN PHENOBARBITONE ENHANCES and REDUCES effects |

Epanutin Dilabid
Dantoin Ekko
Diphentyn Ilessodanten
Divulsan Dilantin
Novodiphenyl Ditoin
Difhydan Phentoin
Fenantoin Phenhydan
Di-Hydan Zentropil
Pyoredol Toin Unicelles
Solantyl

Phenytoin dose is best monitored by measuring the serum level which in most cases should be maintained between 10-20 µg/ml.

Drug	Major Side Effects	Interactions
PHOLCODINE Cough suppressant Adaphol Pholtussin Duro-Tuss Sed Linctus Lantuss Sednaco Pectolin Sednine Pholcolin Tussinol Pholevan Folcodan Pholtrate Tussokon	GIT diturbance CNS disturbance	None significant reported
PHYSOSTIGMINE Anticholinesterase Parasympathomimetic Antilirium Fisostin Isopto-Eserine	MIOSIS EXCESS SALIVATION URINARY AND FAECAL INCONTINENCE BRADYCARDIA BRONCHOSPASM More severe than with Neostigmine	REDUCES effects of LEVODOPA ANTAGONISES TRICYCLIC ANTIDEPRESSANTS ANTAGONISES ANTICHOLINERGICS
PILOCARPINE Parasympathomimetic Isopto Carpine Nova Carpine Adsorbo Carpine Pilocarpina lux Mi-Pilo Pilopt Mistura P PV Carpine Pilocar Spersacarpine Mio-Carpine- SMP	TACHYCARDIA HYPERTENSION GIT disturbance	None significant reported

PIPERAZINE OESTRONE
SULPHATE
Synthetic Oestrogen
Harmogen
Ogen
	WEIGHT GAIN
	SALT AND WATER RETENTION
	THROMBOEMBOLISM
		REDUCES effects of WARFARIN
		REDUCES effects of PHENYTOIN
		REDUCES effects of ANTIDIABETIC AGENTS
		RIFAMPICIN REDUCES effects due to enzyme
		   induction
		PHENOBARBITONE REDUCES EFFECTS due to
		   enzyme induction

Drug	Major Side Effects	Interactions
PITRESSIN TANNATE Posterior Pituitary Hormone	INTESTINAL CRAMPS – diarrhoea UTERINE CRAMPS PALLOR CORONARY ARTERY CONSTRICTION BRONCHOCONSTRICTION ALLERGY	None significant reported
PIZOTIFEN Antimigraine Serotonin Antagonist Sanomigran Sandomigran Sandomigrin	WEIGHT GAIN GIT disturbance CVS disturbance	None significant reported
PODOPHYLLIN PAINT Anti mitotic Posalfilin Vericap PLL	LOCAL IRRITATION *AVOID IN PREGNANCY*	None significant reported
POLYMYXIN eye drops/ointment ear drops/ointment Local antibiotic Aerosporin Otopol Ototrips Polmix Polyfax	ALLERGIC RESPONSE OTOTOXICITY – if applied to middle ear. Therefore avoid if ear drum perforated.	ENHANCES effects of MUSCLE RELAXANTS

POLYTHIAZIDE
Thiazide diuretic
Moderately potent
Nephril
Drenusil
Renese
	GIT disturbance
	ACUTE PANCREATITIS
	HEPATIC COMA can be precipitated in
	  patients with hepatic disease.
	HYPERGLYCAEMIA may make diabetic
	  control difficult
	HYPERURICAEMIA may precipitate acute gout.
	HYPOKALAEMIA especially with long term use.
		REDUCES effects of HYPOGLYCAEMIC
		  agents.
		POTENTIATES effects of ANTIHYPERTENSIVE
		  agents.
		INCREASED DIGOXIN toxicity if
		  HYPOKALAEMIA.

Drug	Major Side Effects	Interactions
POTASSIUM IODIDE Vehicle for Iodine Pima SSKI Solvejob	Occasionally HYPOTHYROIDISM Rarely HYPERTHYROIDISM (Jod Basedow Phenomenon) HYPERSENSITIVITY reaction – rare	May be SYNERGISTIC with LITHIUM causing HYPOTHYROIDISM
POTASSIUM SUPPLEMENTS Element Katorin Kalipor K-Contin Kalitabs Leo-K Duretter Sando-K Mikalyt Slow-K Kalinor Kay-Cee-L Rekawon Kloref Kaochlor Camcopot Kayliel Chlorvescent Kato Klor-lyte K-lor K-son Pfiklol Span-K Rum K Klo Peterkal Kaleorid Potassion Kalilente	INTESTINAL ULCERATION especially with enteric coated potassium chloride.	ACCUMULATES in presence of SPIRONOLACTONE, AMILORIDE or TRIAMTERENE.
POTASSIUM PERCHLORATE Anti-thyroid Agent Peroidin Thyronorman	AGRANULOCYTOSIS PANCYTOPENIA RASH GIT disturbance	IODINE REDUCES EFFECTS
POTASSIUM PERMANGANATE Peroxide Astringent	LOCAL IRRITATION	None significant reported

Drug	Major Side Effects	Interactions
POVIDONE IODINE Antiseptic Betadine Disadine E-Z scrub Pevidine Bridine Proviodine Efodine Isodine Ultradine Providine K	None significant reported	ALKALIS reduce effects
PRACTOLOL Antiarrhythmic beta blocker Eraldin (Only available as injection)	SCLEROSING PERITONITIS with prolonged use. DRY EYE with prolonged use. PSORIASIFORM RASH with prolonged use. DLE with prolonged use.	ENHANCES effect of ANTIHYPERTENSIVE Agents ASYSTOLE has been reported when used with VERAPAMIL.

Drug

PREDNISONE
Synthetic steroid

De Cortisyl	Keteocort
Delta-cortone	Prednilonga
Di adreson	Predniment
Marsone	Predni-tablinen
Adasone	Rectodelt
Presone	Ultracorten
Propred	Dacortin
Sone	Nisone
Ancortone	Delcortin
Delta Cortene	Delta Dome
Delta-Prenovis	Lisacort
Prednital	Ovasone
Colisone	Prednium M
Wescopred	Servisone
Winpred	Deltasone
Contacyl	Deltison
Inocortyl	Encorton
Urtilove	Meticorten
Dabroson	Panafcort
Decortin	Parmenison
Erftopred	Predeltin
Hostacortin	Prednilong

Major Side Effects

COMMON ESPECIALLY IN LONG TERM USE
SALT and WATER retention
HYPERTENSION
HYPERGLYCAEMIA inducing diabetes or
    making diabetic control difficult.
IMMUNOSUPPRESSION leading to failure of
    inflammatory response and reactivation
    of some infections, e.g. tuberculosis
OSTEOPOROSIS especially with long term
    therapy.
INCREASED CATABOLISM leading to wasting.
PEPTIC ULCERATION incidence increased
ADRENAL SUPPRESSION which leads to a
    failure to respond to stress.
CUSHINGS SYNDROME
EUPHORIA and DEPRESSION
HYPOTENSION, 'shock' or an exacerbation
    of disease IF STOPPED SUDDENLY.
GROWTH RETARDATION in children
MUSCLE WEAKNESS and ATROPHY
SKIN ATROPHY and ECCHYMOSES
CATARACT FORMATION

The coticosteroid drugs are potent agents.
They have many side effects, many of which are dose related.
The lowest possible dose should be used.
To achieve this in most cases treatment is started with between 40 and 60 mg/day
and then slowly reduced to the lowest dose which is still effective.
Repeated attempts should be made to stop steroid therapy and to do this the dose should be reduced slowly.
After prolonged therapy this may include reduction as small as 1 mg a week, otherwise the disease process may
'flare up' and the patient develop symptoms.

Interactions

ENHANCES HYPERGLYCAEMIC effect of THIAZIDES
REDUCES effects of HYPOGLYCAEMIC agents
REDUCES effects of SALICYLATES
REDUCES effects of ANTICOAGULANTS
RIFAMPICIN REDUCES effects due to enzyme
    induction
BARBITURATES REDUCE effects due to enzyme
    induction.
PHENYTOIN REDUCES effects due to enzyme
    induction.

Drug	Major Side Effects	Interactions
PRIMAQUINE Anti-Malarial	GIT disturbance BONE MARROW DEPRESSION – Rare METHAEMAGLOBINAEMIA – Rare HAEMOLYTIC ANAEMIA *ALL MORE FREQUENT with G6PD deficiency*	MEPACRINE ENHANCES effects ENHANCED BONE MARROW DEPRESSION with BONE MARROW DEPRESSANTS
PRIMIDONE Anticonvulsant Mysoline Elmidone Midone Liskantin	MEGALOBLASTIC ANAEMIA – Rare GIT disturbance	PHENYTOIN ENHANCES level of PHENOBARBITONE in blood.
PROBENECID Uricosuric Agent Benemid Panuric Proben Benacen Probenid Probexin Urecid	HEADACHE GIT disturbance RASHES ACUTE GOUT	SALICYLATES reduce EFFECTS THIAZIDES reduce EFFECTS INCREASES effects of CHLORPROPAMIDE INCREASES level of PARAAMINOSALICYLIC ACID INCREASES level of CEPHALORIDINE INCREASES level of PENICILLINS INCREASES level of INDOMETHACIN
PROCAINAMIDE Antiarrhythmic Pronestyl Novocamid Procapan	SLE can be induced. HYPOTENSION when given i.v. VENTRICULAR FIBRILLATION and ASYSTOLE if given quickly i.v.	MAY ENHANCE effects of HYPOTENSIVE AGENTS

Drug	Major Side Effects	Interactions
PROCAINE PENICILLIN Medium acting Penicillin Bicillin Viraxacillin Depocillin Ayercillin Almopen Francacilline Hostacillin Ibacillin-Aqeous Novocillin Therapen i.m. Procillin Crystacillin a.s. Aquacaine G Pentids-P a.s. Aquacillin Pfizerpen a.s. Cilicaine Duracillin a.s. Evacilin Wycillin Megacilin Flocilline Megapen Suspenine	GIT disturbance RASH which is COMMON ANAPHYLACTIC COLLAPSE and HYPOTENSION which is RARE.	PROBENECID REDUCES renal EXCRETION
PROCAINE PENICILLIN with Aluminium Sterate Sustained action Penicillin PAM	GIT disturbance RASH – common ANAPHYLACTIC COLLAPSE HYPERTENSION – rare	PROBENECID REDUCES RENAL EXCRETION
PROCARBAZINE Cytotoxic Agent Natulan Matulane Natulanar	GIT disturbance RASH BONE MARROW DEPRESSION	ADDITIVE BONE MARROW DEPRESSION with other BONE MARROW DEPRESSANTS ENHANCES effects of CENTRAL NERVOUS SYSTEM DEPRESSANTS DISULPHIRAM LIKE REACTION WITH ALCOHOL IS AN MAOI THEREFORE reacts with CHEESE etc and SYMPATHOMIMETIC DRUGS
PROCHLORPERAZINE Anti-emetic Phenothiazine Stemetil Compazine Vertigon Tementil Antinavs	DROWSINESS POSTURAL HYPOTENSION TACHYCARDIA EXTRA PYRAMIDAL SIGNS	ENHANCES effects of CNS DEPRESSANT drugs. ENHANCES effects of ATROPINE ENHANCES effects of ANTIHYPERTENSIVE agents. TRICYCLIC ANTIDEPRESSANTS ENHANCE ANTICHOLINERGIC effects

Drug	Major Side Effects	Interactions
PROCYCLIDINE Anticholinergic Kemadrin Osnervan	DRY MOUTH FIXED DILATED PUPILS TACHYCARDIA ACUTE URINARY RETENTION – if prostate enlarged HALLUCINATIONS *AVOID IN CLOSED ANGLE GLAUCOMA*	ENHANCES effects of other ANTICHOLINERGIC drugs
PROGUANIL Anti-malarial Paludrine Paludrinol	GIT disturbance *Safest anti-Malarial Available*	None significant reported
PROMAZINE Tranquilliser Sparine Promezerine Liranol Pro-Tran Atarzine Eliranol Intrazine Prazine Promanyl Protactyl Promazettes	DROWSINESS DRY MOUTH HYPOTENSION JAUNDICE – reversible AGRANULOCYTOSIS – rare EXTRA PYRAMIDAL DYSFUNCTION – usually reversible SKIN SENSITIVITY REACTION IRRITATION AT INJECTION SITE	ADDITIVE CNS DEPRESSION with ALCOHOL and other CNS DEPRESSANTS ANTACIDS reduce ABSORPTION REDUCES effects of LEVODOPA REDUCES effects of GUANETHIDINE ANTICHOLINERGICS reduce effects ENHANCES effects of PHENYTOIN ENHANCES effects of TRICYCLIC ANTIDEPRESSANT ANTICHOLINERGICS enhance SIDE EFFECTS
PROMETHAZINE HYDROCHLORIDE Antihistamine Phenergan Histatil Atosil Lenazine Ganphen Lergigan Lemprometh Meth-zine Promethapar Progan Quadnite Prothazine Remsed Zipan	DROWSINESS DRY MOUTH HYPOTENSION JAUNDICE – reversible AGRANULOCYTOSIS – rare EXTRA PYRAMIDAL DYSFUNCTION – usually reversible SKIN SENSITIVITY REACTION IRRITATION AT INJECTION SITE	ADDITIVE CNS DEPRESSION with ALCOHOL and other CNS DEPRESSANTS ANTACIDS reduce ABSORPTION REDUCES effects of LEVODOPA REDUCES effects of GUANETHIDINE ANTICHOLINERGICS reduce effects ENHANCES effects of PHENYTOIN ENHANCES effects of TRICYCLIC ANTIDEPRESSANT ANTICHOLINERGICS enhance SIDE-EFFECTS

Drug	Major Side Effects	Interactions
PROMETHAZINE THEOCLATE Antihistamine Avomine	SEDATION DRY MOUTH AGRANULOCYTOSIS – rare JAUNDICE – rare EXTRAPYRAMIDAL reaction – rare	ENHANCES CNS DEPRESSION due to other CNS DEPRESSANTS
PROPANTHELINE Anticholinergic Pro-Banthine Neo Banex Banlin Pantheline Ercotina Prodixamon	DRY MOUTH FIXED DILATED PUPILS TACHYCARDIA ACUTE URINARY RETENTION if prostate enlarged HALLUCINATIONS *AVOID in CLOSED ANGLE GLAUCOMA*	ENHANCES effects of other ANTICHOLINERGIC DRUGS

PROPRANOLOL
Beta Adrenergic Blocker
Inderal
Dociton
Herzul
Kemi
	GIT upsets: common
	BAD DREAMS
	PARAESTHESIA
	BRADYCARDIA which may be profound
	  after i.v. injection
	ASTHMA
	CARDIAC FAILURE
	CNS disturbance
		ENHANCES hypoglycaemia of INSULIN
		  and HYPOGLYCAEMIC agents.
		ENHANCES cardiac depression of many
		  ANAESTHETICS.
		ENHANCES effect of HYPOTENSIVE agents.
		ENHANCES anti-tremor effects of L-DOPA.
		ATROPINE reverses effects.
		VERAPAMIL has been reported to cause
		  ASYSTOLE.
		DIURETICS ENHANCE effects
		β ADRENERGIC STIMULATORS REDUCE effects

PROPYLTHIOURACIL Antithyroid	RASH GIT upsets ARTHRALGIA Rarely AGRANULOCYTOSIS (usually early in treatment and preceded by a sore throat) LUPUS ERYTHEMATOSIS BLEEDING – rare *ALL more frequent than with Carbimazole* *NB: CROSSES PLACENTA*	None significant reported

Drug	Major Side Effects	Interactions
PROTAMINE SULPHATE Anti heparin	FLUSHING with HYPOTENSION rapid BRADYCARDIA i.v. injection	None significant reported

PROTRIPTYLINE
Antidepressant
Concordin
Maximed
Triptil
Vivactil
	DRY MOUTH
	BLURRED VISION
	CONSTIPATION etc due to PARASYMPATHO-
	    LYTIC ACTION
	CARDIAC ARRHYTHMIAS
	CHOLESTATIC JAUNDICE
	AGRANULOCYTOSIS – rare
	RASHES
	WEIGHT GAIN
		BARBITURATES REDUCE effects except in
		    OVERDOSE when they ENHANCE SIDE EFFECTS
		ENHANCES effects of ALCOHOL
		ENHANCES effects of WARFARIN
		ENHANCES effects of SYMPATHOMIMETIC DRUGS
		REDUCES effects of BETHANIDINE, GUANETHI-
		    DINE and DEBRISOQUINE.

PSEUDO-EPHEDRINE Sympathomimetic Actifed Besan Emprazil D-feda Extil Novafed Linctifed Sudabid Paragesic Tussaphed Sudafed	PALPITATIONS ANXIETY TREMOR DIFFICULTY with MICTURITION in MEN	MAOI INDUCES HYPERTENSION GUANETHIDINE REDUCES effects METHYLDOPA REDUCES effects TRICYCLIC ANTIDEPRESSANTS ENHANCE effects
PYRIDOSTIGMINE Anticholinesterase Mestinon Regonal	MIOSIS EXCESS SALIVATION URINARY AND FAECAL INCONTINENCE BRADYCARDIA BRONCHOSPASM CHOLINERGIC CRISIS (excess dosage in Myasthenia)	None significant reported

Drug	Major Side Effects	Interactions
PYRIMETHAMINE Anti-Malarial Daraprim Chloridin Fansidar Erbaprelina Maloprim Malocide	BONE MARROW DEPRESSION – Rare in normal dosage, Reversible with Folinic Acid	FOLIC ACID REVERSES EFFECTS PARA-AMINO BENZOIC ACID REDUCES EFFECTS ? ENHANCES effects of QUININE SULPHONAMIDES ENHANCE effects
PYROGALLOL ointment Co (Pyrogallic acid) Antipsoriatic Fungicide	STAINS SKIN (remove with ammonium persulphate or 10% oxalic acid sol.) STAINS HAIR BLACK LOCAL IRRITATION CNS disturbance HAEMOLYSIS METHAEMAGLOBINAEMIA RENAL DAMAGE	None significant reported
P 32 Radioactive element	BONE MARROW DEPRESSION	None significant reported
QUINESTROL Oestrogen Estrovis	SALT and WATER RETENTION NAUSEA and VOMITING THROMBOSIS	REDUCES effects of WARFARIN REDUCES effects of PHENYTOIN REDUCES effects of ANTIDIABETIC AGENTS RIFAMPICIN REDUCES effects due to enzyme induction PHENOBARBITONE REDUCES effects due to enzyme induction.
QUININE Anti Malarial Bi-quinate Dentosel Quinbisan Quinate Quinsan	GIT disturbance CNS disturbance CINCHONISM BLACK WATER FEVER ALLERGY THROMBOCYTOPENIA ANAEMIA OPTIC NEURITIS	PYRIMETHAMINE ENHANCES effects

Drug	Major Side Effects	Interactions
RESERPINE Antihypertensive agent depletes catecholamine stores Serpacil Rau-sed Alserin Reserpoid Ebserpine Sandril Neo-serp Serpate Resercrine Serfin Reserpanca Vio-serpine Serpax Resedrex Serpone Ryser Sertina Serpiloid Eskaserp Tenserp Raurine Sedaraupin	DEPRESSION NASAL STUFFINESS GIT disturbance RASH HYPOTENSION	MAOI ENHANCE effects DIGOXIN ENHANCES DYSRHYTHMIAS INHIBITS effects of LEVODOPA
RIFAMPICIN Anti-tuberculous agent Rifadin Rimactane Rifa	HEPATOTOXICITY – rise in enzymes and possibly development of overt jaundice. Usually MILD and SETTLES with CONTINUED TREATMENT. GIT disturbance – common initially COLOURED URINE (red-yellow), SPUTUM AND TEARS. ENZYME INDUCTION. FLU – like syndrome with INTERMITTENT THERAPY SHOCK and RENAL FAILURE especially with RESTARTING THERAPY THROMBOCYTOPENIA	ENHANCED HEPATOTOXICITY with ISONIAZID PAS REDUCES plasma level due to reduced absorbtion. *PHENOBARBITONE REDUCES plasma level. PROBENECID REDUCES excretion. *REDUCES effects of WARFARIN *REDUCES effects of CORTICOSTEROIDS *REDUCES effects of ORAL CONTRACEPTIVES *due to enzyme induction.

Drug	Major Side Effects	Interactions
RIFAMPICIN PLUS INAH Anti-tuberculous combination Rifinah Rimactazid	HEPATOTOXICITY GREATER than with EITHER DRUG ALONE COLOURED URINE (red-yellow), SPUTUM and TEARS. PERIPHERAL NEUROPATHY – responds to pyridoxine	ENHANCES plasma level of PHENYTOIN in slow acetylators, due to changes in hepatic metabolism. ALUMINIUM HYDROXIDE GEL REDUCES ABSORBTION. PAS REDUCES plasma level due to reduced absorbtion. *PHENOBARBITONE REDUCES plasma level. PROBENECID REDUCES excretion. *REDUCES effects of WARFARIN *REDUCES effects of CORTICOSTEROIDS *REDUCES effects of ORAL CONTRACEPTIVES. *due to enzyme induction
SALBUTAMOL ß stimulator Ventolin Sultanol	TREMOR which is common HEADACHE TACHYCARDIA	PROPRANOLOL (non-selective beta blocker) REDUCES effect. METOPROLOL (selective beta blocker) causes less reduction in effects.
SALICYLIC ACID OINTMENT Keratolytic Bacteriostatic Sebaveen Acnaveen Shampoo Monphytol Batisal Phytodermine Egocappol Pragmatar Keralyt Salactol	DEPENDING ON AMOUNT ABSORBED – AS FOR ASPIRIN LOCAL IRRITATION	DEPENDING ON AMOUNT ABSORBED – as for ASPIRIN
SAVENTRINE Sympathomimetic Long Acting Isoprenaline	TACHYCARDIA – dose related ANXIETY ARRHYTHMIAS	ENHANCES effect of other SYMPATHOMIMETIC drugs.
SEMUSTINE (Methyl CCNU) Cytotoxic Agent	GIT disturbance BONE MARROW DEPRESSION – delayed	ADDITIVE BONE MARROW DEPRESSION with other BONE MARROW DEPRESSANTS.

Drug		Major Side Effects	Interactions
SENNA Purgative Senokot Bekunis Colonorm Palamkotta Senpurgin	Sennosides Senade Glysennid	None significant reported	None significant reported
SODIUM BICARBONATE LOTION Bathing solution		None significant reported	None significant reported
SODIUM BICARBONATE Alkali		HEART FAILURE – if excess volume	REDUCES EXCRETION of AMPHETAMINES INCREASE EXCRETION of LITHIUM REDUCES effects of METHENAMINE REDUCES EXCRETION of PROCAINAMIDE REDUCES EXCRETION of QUINIDINE
SODIUM CALCIUM EDETATE Chelating agent Ledclair Sequestrene NA2Ca		GIT disturbance REVERSIBLE RENAL DAMAGE RASHES	None significant reported
SODIUM CHLORIDE 0.9% Eye Lotion Washing Agent		None significant reported *DISCARD 24 HOURS AFTER OPENING CONTAINER*	None significant reported
SODIUM CHLORIDE 0.9% Isotonic Solution		Fluid overload	None significant reported
SODIUM CHLORIDE 0.45% Hypotonic Solution		WATER INTOXICATION	None significant reported AVOID ADDING DRUGS

Drug	Major Side Effects	Interactions
SODIUM FUSIDATE Antibiotic Fucidin Fucidina Fucidine	GIT disturbance SKIN RASH *USUALLY USED WITH ANOTHER ANTIBIOTIC ESPECIALLY AGAINST STAPHYLOCOCCI*	None significant reported
SODIUM NITRITE Anti Cyanide	NAUSEA VOMITING HYPOTENSION SHOCK	None significant reported
SODIUM THIOSULPHATE Chelating Agent Anti Cyanide Sodothiol Soufre Oligosol	None significant reported	None significant reported
SODIUM VALPROATE Anticonvulsant Epilim Depakene Depakine Ergenyl Urekene	GIT disturbance CNS disturbance ALOPECIA – transient	ENHANCES effects of PHENOBARBITONE ENHANCES effects of ANTIDEPRESSANTS
SPECTINOMYCIN Anti-microbial agent Anti-gonococcal Trobicin Stanilo	GIT disturbance CNS disturbance	None significant reported
SPIRAMYCIN Anti-microbial agent Rovamycin Selectomycin	GIT disturbance RASHES – Rare	None significant reported

Drug	Major Side Effects	Interactions

SPIRONOLACTONE
Diuretic
Aldosterone antagonist
    Aldactone
	HYPERKALAEMIA – especially if POTASSIUM
	    SUPPLEMENTS are also prescribed or in the
	    presence of RENAL FAILURE.
	HEADACHE and DROWSINESS in large doses.
	GYNAECOMASTIA
	MENSTRUAL IRREGULARITIES
		ASPIRIN blocks NATRIURESIS
		PREVENTS the action of CARBENOXOLONE
		    on ulcer healing.
		ENHANCES effects of HYPOTENSIVE agents

STIBOCAPTATE Schistosomicide Astiban	CARDIOTOXICITY ANAPHYLAXIS GIT disturbance ARTHRALGIA MYALGIA	None significant reported
STILBOESTROL Oestrogen Pabestrol Dicorvin Acnestrol Stilbetin Cyren-A Vagestral Oekolp Distilbene Oestromon Stilbium Desma Stilbol	NAUSEA JAUNDICE SALT and WATER retention THROMBOSIS BREAST TENDERNESS HEADACHE VAGINAL TUMOURS in daughters of patients given LARGE DOSES in PREGNANCY	None significant reported

STREPTOKINASE
Thrombolytic agent
    Kabikinase
    Streptace
	HAEMORRHAGE – may need EACA to stop
	FEVER – often suppressed by giving
	    corticosteroids
	ALLERGIC REACTION
	
	*NB: ANAPHYLAXIS – do NOT REPEAT course of
	treatment within THREE to SIX MONTHS.
	Avoid treatment if recent streptococcal
	infection.*
		HEPARIN ENHANCES HAEMORRHAGIC risk.

Drug	Major Side Effects	Interactions
STREPTOMYCIN Antibiotic Darostrep Novostrep Strepolin Strept-evanules Streptosol	OTOTOXICITY – mainly vestibular – partly reversible in young patients. SKIN rash – especially in those who HANDLE the DRUG. DRUG fever NEUROMUSCULAR blockade – which is like myasthenia gravis and reversed by Neostigmine or calcium. CIRCUMORAL PARAESTHESIAE – COMMON	FRUSEMIDE and ETHACRYNIC ACID ENHANCE OTOTOXICITY. CEPHALORIDINE ENHANCES NEPHROTOXICITY.
STREPTOZOTOCIN ß islet cell toxin	NAUSEA and VOMITING HYPOGLYCAEMIA RENAL FAILURE – diabetes insipidus BONE MARROW DEPRESSION	None significant reported
SULPHACETAMIDE EYE DROPS/OINTMENT Local sulphonamide Albucid Antebor Minims Bleph sulphacetamide Cetamide Ocusol Optiole S Sulfapred Sodium Sulamyd Sulfacalyrn Isopto-Cetamide Vasosulf Op-Sulfa Acetopt Sebizon Optamide Sulf-10	LOCAL BURNING AND STINGING	None significant reported
SULPHADIAZINE Sulphonamide Solu-Diazine	CRYSTALLURIA STEVENS-JOHNSON SYNDROME GIT disturbance BONE MARROW DEPRESSION	PARA-AMINO BENZOIC ACID REDUCES effects ENHANCES effects of SULPHONYLUREAS

Drug	Major Side Effects	Interactions

SULPHADIMIDINE
Sulphonamide
Sulphamethazine
Dimethazine + Merzin
Diminsul
S-Dimidine
Sulfadine
	GIT disturbance
	RASHES
	BONE MARROW DEPRESSION – Rare
	CNS disturbance
	HAEMOLYTIC ANAEMIA especially
	  with G.6.PD deficiency
		MAY ENHANCE effects of METHOTREXATE
		PARA-AMINO BENZOIC ACID REDUCES effects.
		MAY ENHANCE effects of WARFARIN
		ENHANCES EFFECTS of ORAL DIABETIC agents
		ENHANCES effects of PHENYTOIN
		METHENAMINE ENHANCES risk of
		  CRYSTALLURIA

SULPHAFURAZOLE Soluble Sulphonamide Gantrisin Sulagen Chemovag Sulfizole SK Soxazole US 67 Sosol Sulfagan Soxomide Sulfazole Sulfalar Sulfisin Gantrisine Urogan Novosoxazole Sulfasan	STEVENS JOHNSON SYNDROME BONE MARROW DEPRESSION GIT disturbance	ENHANCES effects of HYPOGLYCAEMIC AGENTS ENHANCES effects of PHENYTOIN ENHANCES effects of METHOTREXATE METHENAMINE ENHANCES risks of CRYSTALLURIA PARA-AMINOBENZOIC ACID REDUCES effects.
SULPHAMETHIZOLE Sulphonamide Proklar-M Methisul Ul-rasul Urolucosil Rufol Famet Salimol S-Methizole Urocydal Urolex Sulfametin Urolin Thiosulfil Uroz Lucosil	STEVENS JOHNSON SYNDROME BONE MARROW DEPRESSION GIT disturbance	ENHANCES effects of HYPOGLYCAEMIC agents ENHANCES effects of PHENTOIN ENHANCES effects of METHOTREXATE METHENAMINE ENHANCES risks of CRYSTALLURIA PARA-AMINOBENZOIC ACID REDUCES effects

Drug	Major Side Effects	Interactions

SULPHAPYRIDINE
Sulphonamide
  M&B 693
  Dagenan
  Eubasinum
  Septipulmon
	GIT disturbance
	STEVENS JOHNSON SYNDROME
	BONE MARROW DEPRESSION
		ENHANCES effects of HYPOGLYCAEMIC AGENTS
		ENHANCES effects of PHENYTOIN
		ENHANCES effects of METHOTREXATE
		METHENAMINE ENHANCES risks of CRYSTALLURIA
		PARA-AMINOBENZOIC ACID reduces effects

SULPHASALAZINE
Sulphonamide
Anticolitic
  Salazopyrin
  Azulfidine
  Rorasul
  Salazopyrine
  SAS-500
  Sulcolon
	GIT disturbance (dose related)
	RASHES
	ANAEMIA – rare
	AGRANULOCYTOSIS – rare
	FIBROSING ALVEOLITIS – rare
		None significant reported

SULPHATRIAD Sulphonamide mixture	STEVENS JOHNSON SYNDROME GIT disturbance BONE MARROW DEPRESSION CRYSTALLURIA – less than single sulphonamide	PARA-AMINOBENZOIC ACID reduces effects ENHANCES effects OF SULPHONYLUREAS
SULPHINPYRAZONE Uricosuric Agent Antiplatelet Agent Anturan	GIT disturbance ACUTE GOUT BLOOD DYSCRASIAS	SALICYLATES reduce effects THIAZIDES reduce effects
SULPHUR ointment Mild Antiseptic	None significant reported	None significant reported
SUN FLOWER SEED OIL Sunflo Oil	None significant reported	None significant reported

Drug	Major Side Effects	Interactions
TAMOXIFEN Oestrogen Antagonist Nolvadex	GIT disturbance THROMBOCYTOPENIA – transient VAGINAL BLEEDING OEDEMA	None significant reported
TERBUTALINE ß stimulator Bricanyl Filair Brethine Feevone	TREMOR which is common HEADACHE TACHYCARDIA	PROPRANOLOL (non-selective beta blocker) REDUCES effect. METOPROLOL (selective beta blocker) causes less reduction in effects.
TESTOSTERONE ENANTHATE Androgenic Anabolic Hormone Primoteston Depot Androtardyl Delatestryl Malogen LA Testate Testostroval-PA Malogex Testoviron – Depot	OEDEMA HYPERCALCAEMIA HYPERCHOLESTEROLAEMIA	ENHANCES effects of WARFARIN ENHANCES effects of HYPOGLYCAEMIC agents PHENOBARBITONE REDUCES effects
TESTOSTERONE PROPIONATE Androgenic Anabolic Hormone Virormone Paretest Malogen Sterandryl Testex Testine Neo Hombreol Testoviron Oreton Propionate	OEDEMA HYPERCALCAEMIA HYPERCHOLESTEROLAEMIA	ENHANCES effects of WARFARIN ENHANCE effects of HYPOGLYCAEMIC agents PHENOBARBITONE reduces effects

L

Drug	Major Side Effects	Interactions
TETANUS ANTITOXIN	ALLERGIC REACTION	NEUTRALIZED by TETANUS TOXOID if given at the same site.
TETANUS TOXOID Tetanol Tetatoxoid Tetavax T-Immun	LOCAL REACTIONS FEVER HYPERSENSITIVITY REACTION	CORTICOSTEROIDS REDUCE effects IMMUNOSUPRESSANTS reduce effects
TETRABENAZINE Antichorea Nitoman	DROWSINESS – dose related DEPRESSION – dose related	REDUCES effects of LEVODOPA REDUCES effects of RESERPINE
TETRACOSACTRIN Synthetic Corticotrophic Hormone Cortrosyn Depot Synacthen	HYPERPIGMENTATION CUSHINGS SYNDROME CATARACTS HYPERSENSITIVITY WITH INJECTIONS SALT and WATER retention HYPERTENSION HYPERGLYCAEMIA inducing diabetes or making control difficult IMMUNOSUPRESSION leading to failure of inflammatory response and reactivation of some infection, e.g. tuberculosis OSTEOPOROSIS especially with long term therapy. INCREASED CATABOLISM leading to wasting PEPTIC ULCERATION incidence increased EUPHORIA and DEPRESSION HYPOTENSION, 'shock' or an exacerbation of disease IF STOPPED SUDDENLY GROWTH RETARDATION in children MUSCLE WEAKNESS and ATROPHY SKIN ATROPHY and ECCHYMOSES	ENHANCES HYPERGLYCAEMIC effect of THIAZIDES REDUCES effects of HYPOGLYCAEMIC agents REDUCES effects of SALICYLATES REDUCES effects of ANTICOAGULANTS RIFAMPICIN REDUCES effects due to enzyme induction. BARBITURATES REDUCE effects due to enzyme induction. PHENYTOIN REDUCES effects due to enzyme induction.

Drug	Major Side Effects	Interactions
TETRACYCLINES Antimicrobial Agents	GIT disturbance CANDIDA OVERGROWTH Increase URAEMIA if renal impairment Permanent DISCOLOURATION of TEETH if given during PREGNANCY or during first 8 YEARS OF LIFE Acquired FANCONI SYNDROME – with old stock	Absorption REDUCED by MILK, ALKALIS, ALUMINIUM HYDROXIDE, CALCIUM, IRON and MAGNESIUM IONS.

Achromycin	Qudracyclin
Aureomycin	Quatrax
Berkmycen	Tetramykoin
Chymocyclar	Bristacycline
Clinimycin	Centet
Co Caps	Cylopar
Tetracycline	Derma
Econmycin	Kesso-tetra
Galenomycin	Lemtrex
Imperacin	Lexocycline
Mysteclin	Panmycin
Oxydon	QIDtet
Oxymycin	Retet
Steclin	Rexamycin
Stecsolin	Robitet
Sustamycin	Rocycline
Terramycin	U-tet
Tetrabid	Cefracycline
Tetrachel	Chemcycline
Tetracyn	Decabiotic
Tetrex	Decycline
Tetrex PMT	Gene-cycline
Totmycin	G.T.
Unimycin	Muracine
Ambramycin-B	Neo-tetrine
Capcyline	Novotetra
Fermentmycin	Pexobiotic
Phusmycine	Tetral
Riocyclin	Tetralean
Austramycin	Tetrosol
Hydracycline	Wintracin
Panmycin	Dumocyclin
Polycycline	Suedccyklin

Drug	Major Side Effects	Interactions
TETRACYCLINES (contd.) Tetradecin Florocycline Hexacycline Miriamycine Sanclomycine Sifacycline Hostacyclin Supramycin N Quaddcin		
TETRACYCLINE EYE DROPS Local antibiotic Achromycin	As for Tetracycline THE EXTENT OF THESE REACTIONS DEPEND ON THE AMOUNT ABSORBED, WHICH IS VARIABLE	As for Tetracycline
THIAMINE Aneurine Vitamin B₁ Aneurone Benerva Berin Betamin Beta-Sol Beta-Tabs Invite B₁ Vibex — Betabion Betaxin Thianeuron Vitobun Betalin S Betaxin Bevitine Bewon	None significant reported	None significant reported
THIETHYLPERAZINE Tranquillisers Antiemetic Torecan	DRY MOUTH HYPOTENSION JAUNDICE – reversible AGRANULOCYTOSIS – rare EXTRA PYRAMIDAL DYSFUNCTION SKIN SENSITIVITY IRRITATION at injection site CNS DISTURBANCE	ADDITIVE CNS DEPRESSION with other CNS DEPRESSANTS ANTACIDS REDUCE absorbtion PHENOBARBITONE REDUCES effects REDUCES effects of LEVODOPA REDUCES effects of GUANETHIDINE ANTICHOLINERGICS REDUCE absorption ANTICHOLINERGICS ENHANCE side effects ENHANCES effects of TRICYCLIC ANTIDEPRESSANTS

Drug	Major Side Effects	Interactions
THIOGUANINE Antineoplastic Lanvis	BONE MARROW DEPRESSION GIT disturbance LIVER DAMAGE	ADDITIVE BONE MARROW DEPRESSION with other BONE MARROW DEPRESSANTS
THIOPENTONE Anaesthetic Pentothal Nesdonal Trapanal Intraval	RESPIRATORY DEPRESSION Otherwise uncommon	None significant in acute usage.
THIOPROPAZATE Tranquilliser Dartalan Dartal	CNS cisturbance DRY MOUTH HYPOTENSION JAUNDICE – reversible AGRANULOCYTOSIS – rare EXTRAPYRAMIDAL DYSFUNCTION – usually reversible SKIN SENSITIVITY REACTION IRRITATION AT INJECTION SITE	ADDITIVE CNS DEPRESSION with ALCOHOL and other CNS DEPRESSANTS ANTACIDS REDUCE absorption PHENOBARBITONE REDUCES effect REDUCES effects of LEVODOPA REDUCES effects of GUANETHIDINE and similar drugs ANTICHOLINERGICS REDUCE absorption ANTICHOLINERGICS ENHANCE side effects ENHANCES effects of PHENYTOIN ENHANCES effects of TRICYCLIC ANTIDEPRESSANTS
THIORIDAZINE Tranquilliser Melleril Mallorol Mellaril Melleretten Novorediazine Thioril	DROWSINESS – uncommon PARKINSONS syndrome – rare DRY MOUTH BLURRED VISION ILEUS URINARY RETENTION VENTRICULAR TACHYCARDIA RETINAL PIGMENTATION OPTIC ATROPHY ANTERIOR CORTICAL LENS OPACITY FAILURE OF EJACULATION	INCREASED CNS DEPRESSION with CNS DEPRESSANTS ANTACIDS REDUCE absorption ANTICHOLINERGICS REDUCE absorption ANTICHOLINERGICS ENHANCE side effects PHENOBARBITONE REDUCES effects ENHANCES effects of TRICYCLIC ANTIDEPRESSANT REDUCES effects of GUANETHIDINE etc. REDUCES effects of LEVODOPA

Drug	Major Side Effects	Interactions
THIOTEPA Antineoplastic agent Tifosyl	BONE MARROW DEPRESSION – all cell types may be IRREVERSIBLE. GIT disturbance – less than with other neoplastic agents. ALOPECIA less common than with cyclophosphamide. HEADACHE	ENHANCES effects of SUXAMETHONIUM
THIOTHIXENE Tranquilliser Navane ß Orbinamon	DROWSINESS – uncommon PARKINSON syndrome DRY MOUTH BLURRED VISION ILEUS URINARY RETENTION VENTRICULAR TACHYCARDIA RETINAL PIGMENTATION	INCREASED CNS DEPRESSION with CNS DEPRESSANTS ANTACIDS REDUCE absorption ANTICHOLINERGICS REDUCE absorption ANTICHOLINERGICS ENHANCE side effects PHENOBARBITONE REDUCES effects ENHANCES effects of PHENYTOIN ENHANCES effects of TRICYCLIC ANTIDEPRESSANT REDUCES effects of GUANETHIDINE etc. REDUCES effects of LEVODOPA
TOLAZOLINE Arterial dilator α blocking agent Priscol Priscoline Zoline	APPREHENSION GIT disturbance	None significant reported
L. THYROXINE Hormone (T_4) Eltroxin Thyratabs Cytolen Oroxine Letter Thyrine Levoid Thyroxevan Synthroid Thyroxinal Euthyrox Percutacrine Levaxin Thyroxinique	PALPITATIONS ANGINA	ENHANCES effects of WARFARIN ENHANCES effects of TRICYCLIC ANTIDEPRESSANTS PHENYTOIN can ENHANCE effects CHOLESTYRAMINE REDUCES absorption KETAMINE INDUCES HYPERTENSION and TACHYCARDIA

Drug	Major Side Effects	Interactions
TOLBUTAMIDE Sulphonylurea Pramidex Mobenol Rastinon Neo-Dibetic Arcosal Novobutamide Artosin Oramide Dolipol Tolbutol Insilange-D Tolbutone Nigloid Wescotol Ipoglicone Orbetic Chembutamide Ovinase Mellitol	HYPOGLYCAEMIC – less than Chlorpropamide GIT disturbance BLOOD DYSCRASIA – rare RASHES JAUNDICE – usually within 6 weeks APPETITE – increased	ANTICOAGULANTS ENHANCE effects PHENYLBUTAZONE ENHANCES effects SULPHONAMIDES ENHANCE effects BETA BLOCKERS ENHANCE effects PROBENECID ENHANCES effects MONOAMINOXIDASE INHIBITORS ENHANCE effects ALCOHOL ENHANCES effects ALCOHOL INDUCES DISULFIRAM REACTION CORTICOSTEROIDS REDUCE effects ORAL CONTRACEPTIVES REDUCE effects THIAZIDES REDUCE effects 'LOOP' DIURETICS REDUCE effects
TOLNAFTATE Antifungal agent Tinaderm Sporiline Tinacidin Tinactin Tonoftal	LOCAL IRRITATION	None significant reported
TRETINOIN OINTMENT Vitamin A Acid (Retinoic Acid) Peeling ointment Retin-A Aberel Aberela Dermairol Eudyna	LOCAL REACTION	ENHANCES effect of other PEELING AGENTS

Drug	Major Side Effects	Interactions

TRIAMCINOLONE
Synthetic corticosteroid
(Anti-inflammatory)
Adcortyl
Ledercort
Aristocort
Delphicort
Volon
Kenacort
Triamcort
Sodutedarol
	COMMON ESPECIALLY IN LONG TERM USE
	MYOPATHY – more common than with other
	  corticosteroids.
	HYPERTENSION
	HYPERGLYCAEMIA inducing diabetes or
	  making diabetic control difficult.
	IMMUNOSUPPRESSION leading to failure of
	  inflammatory response and reactivation of
	  some infection, e.g. tuberculosis
	OSTEOPOROSIS especially with long term
	  therapy.
	INCREASED CATABOLISM leading to wasting.
	PEPTIC ULCERATION incidence increased
	ADRENAL SUPPRESSION which leads to a failure
	  to respond to stress
	CUSHINGS SYNDROME
	EUPHORIA and DEPRESSION
	HYPOTENSION 'shock' or an exacerbation
	  of disease if STOPPED SUDDENLY
	GROWTH RETARDATION in children
	MUSCLE WEAKNESS AND ATROPHY
	SKIN ATROPHY and ECCHYMOSES
	CATARACT FORMATION
	
	NB: 4 mg EQUIVALENT to 5 mg of Prednisone
		ENHANCES HYPERGLYCAEMIC effect of THIAZIDES
		REDUCES effects of HYPOGLYCAEMIC agents
		REDUCES effects of SALICYLATES
		REDUCES effects of ANTICOAGULANTS
		RIFAMPICIN REDUCES effects due to enzyme
		  induction.
		BARBITURATES REDUCE effects due to enzyme
		  induction
		PHENYTOIN REDUCE effects due to enzyme
		  induction.

TRICHLORETHYLENE Anaesthetic Trilene Anamenth	TACHYPNOEA BRADYCARDIA	ENHANCES effects of CATECHOLAMINES NEUROTOXICITY with SODA LIME

TRICLOFOS
Hypnotic
Tricloryl
Triclos
	GIT disturbance – less than with
	  Chloral Hydrate
	RASHES
		ENHANCES effects of WARFARIN by
		  displacement from plasma protein.
		INCREASED CNS DEPRESSION with CNS
		  DEPRESSANTS

Drug	Major Side Effects	Interactions
TRIFLUOPERAZINE Tranquilliser Amylozine Stelazine Calmazine Chemflurazine Clinazine Fluazine Novoflurazine Pentazine Solazine Trifluoper-Ez-Ets Triflurin Jatroneural Terfluzin	DROWSINESS PARKINSON syndrome DRY MOUTH BLURRED VISION ILEUS URINARY RETENTION VENTRICULAR TACHYCARDIA RETINAL PIGMENTATION ANTERIOR CORTICAL LENS OPACITIES POSTERIOR CORNEAL OPACITIES	INCREASED CNS DEPRESSION with CNS DEPRESSANTS ANTACIDS REDUCE absorption ANTICHOLINERGICS REDUCE absorption ANTICHOLINERGICS ENHANCE side effects PHENOBARBITONE REDUCES effects ENHANCES effects of PHENYTOIN ENHANCES effects of TRICYCLIC ANTIDEPRESSANTS REDUCES effects of GUANETHIDINE etc. REDUCES effects of LEVODOPA
TRIPLE SULPHA Antimicrobial Sultrin	RASHES GIT disturbance BONE MARROW DEPRESSION – rare CNS disturbance HAEMOLYTIC ANAEMIA especially with G6PD deficiency LOCAL IRRITATION	May ENHANCE effects of METHOTREXATE PARA-AMINO BENZOIC ACID REDUCES effects May ENHANCE effects of WARFARIN ENHANCES effects of oral HYPOGLYCAEMIC agents.
TRIPROLIDINE Long acting Antihistamine Actidil Pro-Actidil Actidilon Pro-Actidilon	SEDATION DRY MOUTH	INCREASES CNS DEPRESSION with other CNS DEPRESSANTS.
TROPICAMIDE Cyclopegic and Mydriatic Mydriacyl Myriaticum Mydriaticum	GLAUCOMA	None significant reported

Drug	Major Side Effects	Interactions
TROXIDONE Anticonvulsant Tridione Epidione Trimedone	PHOTOPHOBIA and DAY BLINDNESS – transient AGRANULOCYTOSIS and APLASTIC ANAEMIA – RARE NEPHROTIC SYNDROME – RARE STEVENS-JOHNSON SYNDROME – RARE ALOPECIA	None significant reported
VERAPAMIL Antiarrhythmic Cordilox Isoptin Vasolan	GIT disturbance HYPOTENSION with i.v. therapy	BETA BLOCKERS MAY INDUCE ASYSTOLE ADDITIVE effects with CARDIAC DEPRESSANTS
VIDARABINE Anti-Viral Agent Vira-A	Local IRRITATION LACRIMATION RECENTLY INTRODUCED AGENT, THEREFORE EFFECTS NOT FULLY ESTABLISHED.	None significant reported
VINBLASTINE Vinca Alkaloid Anti Neoplastic Velbe Velban	GIT disturbance ALOPECIA BONE MARROW DEPRESSION NEUROTOXICITY both CENTRAL AND PERIPHERAL	ADDITIVE BONE MARROW DEPRESSION with other BONE MARROW DEPRESSANTS

Drug	Major Side Effects	Interactions
VINCRISTINE Vinca Alkaloid Anti-neoplastic Oncovin	GIT disturbance ALOPECIA BONE MARROW DEPRESSION – rare NEUROTOXICITY both CENTRAL and PERIPHERAL *NB: DO NOT EXCEED 2 mg/cycle*	None significant reported
VITAMIN A Fat Soluble Vitamin Ro A Vit. Avita A313 Fab-A-Vit Avibon Arovit Halivite Ido A Alphalin Atamin A-Mulsin Carotin A-Vicotrat Oculotect Vogan Solatene Anatola Solu A Aquasol A V Doma A	TOXIC effects in large doses usually seen only after skin therapy, or eating fresh polar bear liver. Symptoms include skin rash, headache, bone and joint pain and GIT disturbance	CHOLESTYRAMINE REDUCES EFFECTS by reducing absorbtion.
VITAMIN D Calciferol Vitamin Sterogyl –15	HYPERCALCAEMIA ANOREXIA and NAUSEA POLYURIA – RENAL CALCIFICATION IRRITABILITY ALL due to overdose	CHOLESTYRAMINE REDUCES effects by REDUCING ABSORPTION

Drug	Major Side Effects	Interactions
VITAMIN K$_1$ Essential Clotting Factor Aquamephyton Kaywon Konakion Mephyton	ALLERGIC REACTION (i.v.)	REVERSES effects of WARFARIN

WARFARIN
Anticoagulant
Marevan
Coumadine
Panwarfin
Waran
Warfilone
Warnerin

GIT disturbance
BLEEDING – from anywhere
Other reactions are rare.

DRUGS WHICH POTENTIATE BLEEDING:

Alcohol	INAH
Anabolic steroids	Indomethacin
Antibiotics	Mefenamic Acid
Aminoglycosides	Phenylbutazone
Chloramphenicol	Salicylates
Clofibrate	Thyroid preparations
Disulfiram	Tolbutamide
Ethacrynic acid	Tricyclics
Glucagon	

DRUGS WHICH ANTAGONISE ANTICOAGULANTS:

Barbiturates	Haloperidol
Carbamazepine	Oral contraceptives
Cholestyramine	Rifampicin
Glutethimide	Thiazides
Griseofulvin	Vitamin K

COMPLEX INTERACTION WITH PHENYTOIN

WHEN ANY DRUG IS GIVEN TO A PATIENT ON WARFARIN THE PROTHROMBIN TIME SHOULD BE CHECKED MORE FREQUENTLY THAN USUAL AS IT IS LIKELY THAT REACTIONS, AS YET UNREPORTED WILL OCCUR.

Drug	Major Side Effects	Interactions
XYLOMETAZOLINE Nasal decongestant Sympathomimetic Otrivine Otriven Otrix	HEADACHE HYPERTENSION	MAOI INDUCE HYPERTENSION
YTTRIUM 90 Radioactive ß Emitter	HYPOPITUITARISM	None significant reported
ZINC SULPHATE element Zinofrin Zincomed Op-thal-min Orazinc Solvezink Zinkaps-220	GIT disturbance	None significant reported
ZINC & CASTOR OIL ointment Emollient Mild Astringent	None significant reported	None significant reported
ZINC OXIDE Astringent Skin Protective Multiple compound products	None significant reported	None significant reported

TO DETERMINE A GENTAMICIN DOSE SCHEDULE (Fig 2)

A. Patient not receiving dialysis treatment.

1. Join with a straight line the serum creatinine concentration appropriate to the sex on scale A and the age on scale B. Mark the point at which the straight line cuts line C.

2. Join with a straight line the mark on line C and the body weight on scale D. Mark the points at which this line cuts the dosage lines L and M.

3. The loading dose (mg) is written against the marked part of line L. The maintenance dose (mg) and the appropriate interval (hours) between doses are written against the marked part of line M.

4. The nomogram is designed to give serum concentrations of gentamicin with the range 3-10 mg/12 hours after each dose. In patients with renal insufficiency it is still desirable to perform check assays and to make appropriate dose adjustment.

Example

male, serum creatinine 0.40 mmol/l, 45 years, 55 kg: loading dose 120 mg, maintenance dose 40 mg, interval between doses 12 hours.

B. Patient receiving dialysis treatment.

5. When the patient is severely oliguric or anuric do not use the serum creatinine and age scales. To determine the dose schedule join with a straight line the bottom end of line C and the body weight on scale D.

6. Peritoneal dialysis. In addition to the dose schedule add gentamicin to the dialysis fluid. A concentration of 5 mg/l is suitable.

7. Haemodialysis. In addition to the dose schedule give a booster dose after dialysis. Half the loading dose is suitable after a 10 hour Kiill dialysis.

REFERENCE

Mawer, G.E., Admad, R., Dobbs, Sylvia M., McGough, J.G., Lucas, S.B. & Tooth, J.A., (1974) Prescribing aids for gentamicin. *Br. J. clin. Pharmac.* **1**, 45-50.

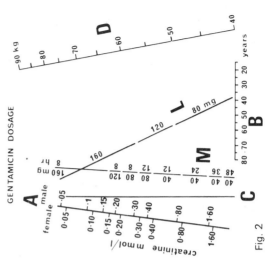

GENTAMICIN DOSAGE

Fig. 2

Section 3

Proprietary/Non-proprietary Drug Index

A 313	Vitamin A
Aarane	Disodium Cromoglycate
Abbocilin	Benzyl Penicillin
Abbocillin VK	Penicillin V
Abboject	Erythromycin
Abboticine	Erythromycin
Abbotiun	Erythromycin
Aberel	Tretinoin
Aberela	Tretinoin
Abolon	Nandrolone Decanoate
Acetophen	Aspirin
Acetopt	Sulphacetamide eye drops/ointment
Acetyl-Sal	Aspirin
Acetylin	Aspirin
Achromycin	Tetracycline
Acid mantle	Aluminium Acetotartrate
Acidemel	Nicotinic acid
A-cillin	Ampicillin
Acnaveen	Salicylic Acid
Acnestrol	Stilboestrol
Acocillin	Penicillin V
Acortan	A.C.T.H.
Acterol Forte	Nimorazole
Acthar	A.C.T.H.
Actidil	Triprolidine
Actidilon	Triprolidine
Actifed	Pseudoephedrine
Acton	A.C.T.H.
Adacillin	Penicillin V
Adagel	Aluminium Hydroxide
Adaphol	Pholcodine
Adasone	Prednisone
Adcortyl	Triamcinolone
Addex-Magnesium	Magnesium sulphate
Adjust	Dioctyl
Adjust	Dioctyl Sodium Sulphosuccinate
Adriamycin	Doxorubicin
Adrox	Aluminium Hydroxide
Adsorbo Carpine	Pilocarpine
Aeroseb D	Dexamethasone
Aerosporin	Polymyxin
Afrin	Oxymetazoline
Agrasol A	Vitamin A
Albyl-Selters	Aspirin

Albucid	Sulphacetimide eye drops/ointment
Aldactone	Spironolactone
Aldecin	Beclomethasone dipropionate
Aldocorten	Aldosterone.
Aldomet	Methyldopa
Aldometil	Methyldopa
Alergicap	Diphenhydramine
Aleudrin	Isoprenaline
Alexan	Cytarabine
Alfatrofin	A.C.T.H.
Algoverine	Phenylbutazone
Allerbid	Chlorpheniramine
Allergex	Chlorpheniramine
Allergisan	Chlorpheniramine
Allerglobuline	Immune serum globulin
Allerhist	Chlorpheniramine
Allertab	Chlorpheniramine
Allotropal	Methylpentynol
Almopen	Procaine penicillin
Aloquin	Monobenzone ointment
Alox	Aluminium Hydroxide
Alpen	Ampicillin
Alphalin	Vitamin A
Alpha-Ruvite	Hydroxocobalamin
Alpharedisol	Hydroxocobalamin
Alserin	Reserpine
Alsol	Aluminium Acetotartrate
Alucap	Aluminium Hydroxide
Aludrin	Isoprenaline
Aludrox	Aluminium Hydroxide
Alupent	Orciprenaline HCL
Alusorb	Aluminium Hydroxide
Alvedon	Paracetamol
Amargyl	Chlorpromazine
Ambilhar	Niridazole
Amblosin	Ampicillin
Ambramycin-ß	Tetracycline
Amcill	Ampicillin
Amcill-S	Ampicillin
Amen	Medroxyprogesterone
Amfipen	Ampicillin
Aminodur	Aminophylline
Aminophyl	Aminophylline
Amipenex	Ampicillin
Amizol	Amitriptyline
Ammonchlor S.S.W.	Ammonium Chloride
Amnestrogen	Oestrogens-Conjugated
Amoxil	Amoxycillin
Ampen	Ampicillin
Amperil	Ampicillin
Ampexin	Ampicillin
Amphicol	Chloramphenicol
Amphojel	Aluminium Hydroxide
Ampho-Moronal	Amphotericin B
Amphotabs	Aluminium Hydroxide
Ampilean	Ampicillin

Ampilum	Ampicillin
Ampilux	Ampicillin
Ampipenin	Ampicillin
A-Mulsin	Vitamin A
Amuno	Indomethacin
Amylozine	Trifluoperazine
Anadrol	Oxymetholone
Anamenth	Trichlorethylene
Anapolon	Oxymetholone
Anasteron	Oxymetholone
Anatensol	Fluphenazine
Anatola	Vitamin A
Ancasal	Aspirin
Ancortone	Prednisone
Andophyllin	Aminophylline
Androphyllin	Aminophylline
Androtardyl	Testosterone Enanthate
Aneurone	Thiamine
Anginal	Dipyridamole
Anginine	Glyceryl Trinitrate
Angised	Glyceryl Trinitrate
Annolytin	Amitriptyline
Anovlar 21	Combined Oral Contraceptives
Ansatin	Flufenamic acid
Ansolysen	Pentolinium
Antagonate	Chlorpheniramine
Antebor	Sulphacetamide eye drops/ointment
Anthra-derm	Dithranol ointment
Anthralin	Dithranol ointment
Antibiopto	Chloramphenicol
Antilirium	Physostigmine
Anti-naus	Prochlorperazine
Anti-spas	Benzhexol
Antitrem	Benzhexol
Anturan	Sulphinpyrazone
Antvitrin S	Chorionic Gonadotrophin
Anuphen	Paracetamol
Apamide	Paracetamol
Aparkane	Benzhexol
Apernyl	Aspirin
Aphtiria	Gamma Benzene Hexachloride
A.P.L.	Chorionic Gonadotrophin
Apomiteril	Cinnarizine
Apopen	Penicillin V
Apozepam	Diazepam
Aprelazine	Hydrallazine
Apresoline	Hydrallazine
Aprinox	Bendrofluazide
Aprinox M.	Bendrofluazide
Apsin VR	Penicillin V
Aquacaine G	Procaine penicillin
Aquachloral	Chloral Hydrate
Aquacillin	Procaine penicillin
Aqua-Colchin	Colchicine
Aquamag	Magnesuim hydroxide
Aquamephyton	Vitamin K,

Aquamycetine	Chloramphenicol
Aquaprin	Aspirin
Aquo-Cytobion	Hydroxocobalamin
ARA.C.	Cytarabine
Arachin	Chloroquine
Aracytine	Cytarabine
Aralen	Chloroquine
Aramine	Metaraminol
Arasemide	Frusemide
Arcasin	Penicillin V
Arcosal	Tolbutamide
Aristocort	Triamcinolone
Arlef	Flufenamic Acid
Arovit	Vitamin A
Artane	Benzhexol
Ar-tet	Human antitetanus immunoglobulin
Artrizin	Phenylbutazone
Artropan	Phenylbutazone
Artosin	Tolbutamide
A.S.A.	Aspirin
Ascabiol	Benzyl Benzoate
Asodrine	Aspirin
Aspasol	Aspirin
Aspegic	Aspirin
Aspergum	Aspirin
Aspirisucre	Aspirin
Aspisol	Aspirin
Asterol	Diamthazole
Astiban	Stibocaptate
Astonin H	Fludrocortisone
AT. 10.	Dihydrotachysterol
Atabrine	Mepacrine
Atamin	Vitamin A
Atarzine	Promazine
Atasol	Paracetamol
Atecen	Dihydrotachysterol
Atensine	Diazepam
Aterosol	Clofibrate
Atheromide	Clofibrate
Atheropront	Clofibrate
Atosil	Promethazine Hydrochloride
Atromid S	Clofibrate
Atromidin	Clofibrate
Atropinol	Atropine
Atropisol	Atropine
Atropt	Atropine eye drops
Atroptol	Atropine eye drops
Audinorm	Dioctyl
Audinorm	Dioctyl Sodium Sulphosuccinate
Aureomycin	Chlortetracycline
Aureomycin	Tetracycline
Aureomycine	Chlortetracycline
Austramycin	Tetracycline
Austrapen	Ampicillin
Austrastaph	Cloxacillin
Avibon	Vitamin A

A-Vicotrat	Vitamin A
Avita	Vitamin A
Avloclor	Chloroquine
Avlosulfon	Dapsone
Avomine	Promethazine Theoclate
Axlon	Hydroxocobalamin
Ayercillin	Procaine penicillin
Azolid	Phenylbutazone
Babiprin	Aspirin
Bactigras	Chlorhexidine
Bactrim	Co Trimoxazole
B.A.L.	Dimercaprol
Bamyl	Aspirin
Banlin	Propantheline
Bantex	Dioctyl
Bantex	Dioctyl Sodium Sulphosuccinate
Basoquin	Amodiaquine
Batidrol	Dithranol ointment
Batisal	Salicylic acid
B.C.N.U.	Carmustine
Beconase	Beclomethasone Dipropionate
Becotide	Beclomethasone Dipropionate
Bekunis	Senna
Benacen	Probenecid
Benadryl	Diphenhydramine
Benafed	Diphenhydramine
Bendopa	Levodopa
Benemid	Probenecid
Benerva	Thiamine
Benhydramile	Diphenhydramine
Benoquin	Monobenzone ointment
Benoxyl	Benzoxyl Peroxide
Ben P	Benzathine Penicillin
Bentelan	Betamethasone
Benuride	Pheneturide
Ben-U-Ron	Paracetamol
Benylin	Diphenhydramine
Benzagel	Benzoxyl peroxide
Benzlets	Diphenhydramine
Beriglobin	Immune Serum globulin
Berkdopa	Levodopa
Berkmycen	Tetracycline
Berkozide	Bendrofluazide
Beromycin	Penicillin V
Berubi-long	Hydroxocobalamin
Besan	Pseudoephedrine
Bestloid	Crotamiton
Betabion	Thiamine
Betadine	Povidone Iodine
Betalins	Thiamine
Betaloc	Metoprolol
Betamin	Thiamine
Beta-Sol	Thiamine
Betasolon	Betamethasone
Betaxin	Thiamine

Betnelan	Betamethasone
Betnesol	Betamethasone
Betneval	Betamethasone
Betnovat	Betamethasone
Betnovate	Betamethasone
Bevitine	Thiamine
Bewon	Thiamine
Bextasol	Betamethasone
Bicillin	Benzathine Penicillin
Bicillin	Procaine Penicillin
Bicillin L.A.	Benzathine Penicillin
Bidramine	Diphenhydramine
Bi-Larcil	Metriphonate
Binotal	Ampicillin
Biomydrin	Phenylephrine
Bipimycetin	Chloramphenicol
Bi-prin	Aspirin
Bi-Quinate	Quinine
Bisolvon	Bromhexine
Blenoxane	Bleomycin
Bleph	Sulphacetamide eye drops/ointment
Bleph-1C-Liquifilm	Sulphacetamide eye drops
Bleph-10-liquifilm	Sulphacetamide eye drops/ointment
Bloxanth	Allopurinol
Bonadorm	Dichloralphenazone
Bradosol	Domiphen
Bramcillin	Penicillin V
Breoprin	Aspirin
Brethine	Terbutaline
Brevinor	Combined Oral Contraceptives
Bricanyl	Terbutaline
Bridine	Povidone Iodine
Bristacycline	Tetracycline
Bristamycin	Erythromycin
Bristin	Ampicillin
Bristuric	Bendrofluazide
Brocadopa	Levodopa
Brufen	Ibuprofen
Budoform	Clioquinol
Bu-Lax	Dioctyl
Bu-Lax	Dioctyl Sodium Sulphosuccinate
Burinex	Bumetanide
Butaphen	Phenylbutazone
Butacal	Phenylbutazone
Butacote	Phenylbutazone
Butafesic	Phenylbutazone
Butalan	Phenylbutazone
Butalgin	Phenylbutazone
Butapirazol	Phenylbutazone
Butarex	Phenylbutazone
Butazolidin	Phenylbutazone
Butazone	Phenylbutazone
Butina	Phenylbutazone
Butoroid	Phenylbutazone
Butoz	Phenylbutazone
Butazone	Phenylbutazone

Butrex	Phenylbutazone
Buzon	Phenylbutazone
Bykomycin	Neomycin
Caladryl	Diphenhydramine
Calcamine	Dihydrotachysterol
Calciferol	Vitamin D
Calciopen	Penicillin V
Calcipen	Penicillin V
Calcium Heparin	Heparin
Calcium Juva	Calcium gluconate
Calmazine	Trifluoperazine
Calmoden	Chlordiazepoxide
Calpol	Paracetamol
Camcolit 250	Lithium
Camcopot	Potassium supplements
Campain	Paracetamol
Candio-Hermal	Nystatin
Canstat	Nystatin
Capcycline	Tetracycline
Capital	Paracetamol
Caprin	Aspirin
Caps-Pen-V	Penicillin V
Carbazole	Carbimazole
Carbo-cort	Coal tar
Carbo-dome	Coal Tar
Carbolith	Lithium
Carbyl	Carbachol
Cardiamide	Nikethamide
Cardiox	Digoxin
Cardophylin	Aminophylline
Cardophyline	Aminophylline
Carena	Aminophylline
Carene	Aminophylline
Carine	Aminophylline
Carotin	Vitamin A
Carsodyl	Chlorhexidine
Carulon	Dexamethasone
Caryolysine	Mustine
Castellanis Paint	Magenta Paint
Catapres	Clonidine
Catapresan	Clonidine
Catilan	Chloramphenicol
C.C.N.U.	Lomustine
Ceanel	Cetrimide
Cedin	Isoniazid
Ceetanol	Paracetamol
Ceetmol	Paracetamol
Cefalotine	Cephalothin
Cefracycline	Tetracycline
Celacol H.P.M.	Methyl cellulose eye drops
Celestan	Betamethasone
Celestene	Betamethasone
Celestoderm	Betamethasone
Celestoderm-V	Betamethasone
Celeston A	Betamethasone

Celestone	Betamethasone
Cen-apap	Paracetamol
Centamol	Paracetamol
Centet	Tetracycline
Centramol	Paracetamol
Centyl	Bendrofluazide
Ceporan	Cephaloridine
Ceporin	Cephaloridine
Cepovenin	Cephalothin
Ces	Oestrogens-conjugated
Cetal	Chlorhexidine
Cetamide	Sulphacetamide eye drops/ointment
Cetamol	Paracetamol
Cetasal	Aspirin
Cetavlon	Cetrimide
Cetiprin	Emepronium Bromide
Chembutamide	Tolbutamide
Chembutazone	Phenylbutazone
Chemcetaphen	Paracetamol
Chemcycline	Tetracycline
Chemflurazine	Trifluoperazine
Chemgel	Aluminium Hydroxide
Chemhydrazide	Hydrochlorthiazide
Chemdipoxide	Chlordiazepoxide
Chemovag	Sulphafurazole
Chemthromycin	Erythromycin
Chlomin	Chloramphenicol
Chloramex	Chloramphenicol
Chloractil	Chlorpromazine
Chloradorm	Chloral Hydrate
Chloralate	Chloral Hydrate
Chloraldurat	Chloral Hydrate
Chloralex	Chloral Hydrate
Chloralix	Chloral Hydrate
Chloralixier	Chloral Hydrate
Chloralol	Dichloralphenazone
Chloramin	Chlorpheniramine
Chlorammonic	Ammonium Chloride
Chloramol	Chloramphenicol
Chloramphycin	Chloramphenicol
Chloramsaar	Chloramphenicol
Chloratol	Chloral hydrate
Chlorcol	Chloramphenicol
Chloridin	Pyrimethamine
Chlormene	Chlorpheniramine
Chlornicin	Chloramphenicol
Chlornicol	Chloramphenicol
Chlorohist	Chlorpheniramine
Chloromide	Chlorpropamide
Chloromin	Chloramphenicol eye drops
Chloromycetin	Chloramphenicol
Chloromycetin eyedrops- (Opclor)	Chloramphenicol eye drops
Chloromycetin Ophthalmic	Chloramphenicol eye drops
Chloromycetin redidrops	Chloramphenicol eye drops
Chloronase	Chlorpropamide

Chloroptic	Chloramphenicol eye drops
Chloroton	Chlorpheniramine
Chlor-Promanyl	Chlorpromazine
Chlor-promaryl	Chlorpromazine
Chlorprom-ez-ets	Chlorpromazine
Chlor-PZ	Chlorpromazine
Chlorquin	Chloroquine
Chlorsig	Chloramphenicol eye drops
Chlortet	Chlortetracycline
Chlortone	Chlorpheniramine
Chlortrimeton	Chlorpheniramine
Chlor-Trimeton	Chlorpheniramine
Chlor-Tripolon	Chlorpheniramine
Chlortrone	Chlorpheniramine
Chlorumagene	Magnesium hydroxide
Chlorvescent	Potassium supplements
Choragen	Chorionic Gonadotrophin
Chronicystine Manor	Magnesium Sulphate
Chymocyclar	Tetracycline
Ciclolux	Cyclopentolate
Cidomycin	Gentamicin
Cilicaine	Procaine pencillin
Cilicaine-V	Penicillin V
Cillaphen	Penicillin V
Clamoxyl	Amoxycillin
Claradin	Aspirin
Claragine	Aspirin
Claresan	Clofibrate
Clariprin	Aspirin
Cleocin	Clindamycin
Climestrone	Oestrogens-Conjugated
Clinazine	Trifluoperazine
Clinimycin	Tetracycline
Clinovir	Medroxyprogesterone
Clocillin	Cloxacillin
Clomid	Clomiphene
Clomivid	Clomiphene
Clonamol	Paracetamol
Clonopin	Clonazepam
Clont	Metronidazole
Cloralvan	Chloral Hydrate
Clorfen	Chloramphenicol
Cloxypen	Cloxacillin
Cobalparen-Depot	Hydroxocobalamin
Co caps Methyldopa	Methyldopa
Co Caps Penicillin VK	Penicillin V
Co-Caps Tetracycline	Tetracycline
Codicept	Codeine Phosphate
Codlin	Codeine Phosphate
Codral	Aspirin
Cogentin	Benztropine
Cogentinol	Benztropine
Colace	Dioctyl
Colace	Dioctyl Sodium Sulphosuccinate
Colchineos	Colchicine
Colcin	Colchicine

Colfarit	Aspirin
Colgout	Colchicine
Colisone	Prednisone
Collone QA	Cetrimide
Colonorm	Senna
Coloxyl	Dioctyl
Coloxyl	Dioctyl Sodium Sulphosuccinate
Coluric	Colchicine
Combizym	Pancreatin
Comfolax	Dioctyl
Comfolax	Dioctyl Sodium Sulphosuccinate
Compazine	Prochlorperazine
Compocillin VK	Penicillin V
Concordin	Protriptyline
Condanol	Dioctyl
Condanol	Dioctyl Sodium Sulphosuccinate
Conest	Oestrogens-Conjugated
Conestron	Oestrogens-Conjugated
Confortid	Indomethacin
Conjes	Oestrogens-Conjugated
Conotrane	Hydrargaphen
Conova 30	Combined Oral Contraceptives
Constiban	Dioctyl
Constiban	Dioctyl Sodium Sulphosuccinate
Contactisol	Methyl cellulose eye drops
Contenton	Amantadine
Coragoxine	Digoxin
Coramine	Nikethamide
Coraphyllin	Aminophylline
Corathiem	Cinnarizine
Corax	Chlordiazepoxide
Corcillin V	Penicillin V
Cordiaminum	Nikethamide
Cordilox	Verapamil
Coriantin	Chorionic Gonadotrophin
Cormed	Nikethamide
Corophyllin	Aminophylline
Corson	Dexamethasone
Cortancyl	Prednisone
Cor-tar-quin	Coal Tar
Cortico-Gel	A.C.T.H.
Corticotrophin ZN	A.C.T.H.
Cortineff	Fludrocortisone
Cortiron	Deoxycortone Acetate
Cortisumman	Dexamethasone
Coryban-D	Phenylephrine
Cotazym	Pancreatin
Cotazym B	Pancreatin
Coumadine	Warfarin
Cousol	Sulphacetamide eye drops
Cremo-Quin	Clioquinol
Cremorin	Aluminium Hydroxide
Crescormon	Growth Hormone
Crinuryl	Ethacrynic acid
Crodex. C.	Cetrimide
Crystacillin a.s.	Procaine penicillin

Crystapen	Benzyl Penicillin
Crystapen V	Penicillin V
C-Tran	Chlordiazepoxide
Cuemid	Cholestyramine
Cuprenil	Penicillamine
Cuprumine	Penicillamine
C.V.K. (Compocillin VK)	Pencillin V
Cycladiene	Dienoestrol
Cyclogyl	Cyclopentolate
Cyclopar	Tetracycline
Cyclopen	Cyclopentolate
Cyclopezic	Cyclopentolate
Cycloton A.	Cetrimide
Cycloton V.	Cetrimide
Cynomel	Liothyronine
Cyplegin	Cyclopentolate
Cyren-A	Stilboestrol
Cytofol	Folic acid
Cytolen	L. Thyroxine
Cytomel	Liothyronine
Cytosar	Cytarabine
Cytosine Arabinoside	Cytarabine
Cytoxan	Cyclophosphamide
D-Amp	Ampicillin
Dabroson	Prednisone
Dabylen	Diphenhydramine
Dacortin	Prednisone
Dagenan	Sulphapyridine
Daktarin	Miconazole
Dalacin C	Clindamycin
Dametine	Dehydroemetine
Danatrol	Danazol
Danol	Danazol
Dantoin	Phenytoin
Dantrium	Dantrolene
Daonil	Glibenclamide
Dapotum	Fluphenazine
Daraprim	Pyrimethamine
Darocillin	Penicillin V
Darostrep	Streptomycin
Dartal	Thiopropazate
Dartalan	Thiopropazate
Davoxin	Digoxin
D.B.I.	Phenformin
D.B. Retard	Phenformin
D-cillin	Ampicillin
DDAVP	Desmopressin
Decabiotic	Tetracycline
Decacort	Dexamethasone
Decaderm	Dexamethasone
Decadron	Dexamethasone
Deca-Durabol	Nandrolone Decanoate
Deca-Durabolin	Nandrolone Decanoate
Decaesadril	Dexamethasone
Deca Nephrine	Phenylephrine

Decasterolone	Dexamethasone
Declostatin	Demeclocycline
Decofluor	Dexamethasone
Decortin	Prednisone
De Cortisyl	Prednisone
Dectan	Dexamethasone
Decycline	Tetracycline
Deferoxamine	Des-Ferrioxamine
Defiltran	Acetazolamide
Degest	Phenylephrine
Dehepan novum	Hydroxocobalamin
Delatestryl	Testosterone Enanthate
Delalutin	Hydroxyprogesterone
Delcortin	Prednisone
Delestrogen	Oestradiol Valerate
Deltacillin	Penicillin V
Delta cortene	Prednisone
Delta-cortone	Prednisone
Delta Dome	Prednisone
Delta-prenovis	Prednisone
Deltasone	Prednisone
Deltison	Prednisone
Delphicort	Triamcinolone
Dema	Tetracycline
Demerol	Pethidine
De-Methyl-Chlortetracycline	Demeclocycline
Demofax	Chlorhexidine
Demulen	Combined Oral Contraceptives
Demulen 50.	Combined Oral Contraceptives
Dendrid	Idoxuridine
Dentojel	Quinine
Deparkine	Sodium Valproate
Depakene	Sodium Valproate
Depamine	Penicillamine
Depigman	Monobenzone ointment
Depocillin	Procaine Penicillin
Depo Heparin	Heparin
Depo Provera	Medroxyprogesterone
Deprex	Amitriptyline
Derbac soap	Gamma Benzene Hexachloride
Derboc-liquid Co	Malathion
Deripen	Ampicillin
Dermairol	Tretinoin
Dermaline	Dithranol ointment
Dermohex	Hexachlorophane
Dermonistat	Miconazole
Deronil	Dexamethasone
Desacort	Dexamethasone
Desacort-Beta	Betamethasone
Desacortone	Dexamethasone
Desalark	Dexamethasone
Desameton	Dexamethasone
Desentol	Diphenhydramine
Deseril	Methysergide
Desernil	Methysergide

Deseronil	Dexamethasone
Desferal	Desferrioxamine
Desma	Stilboestrol
Desmoid pillen	Methylene Blue
Desquam-X	Benzoyl peroxide
Dethamedin	Dexamethasone
Dexacortal	Dexamethasone
Dexambutol	Ethambutol
Dexamed	Dexamethasone
Dexameth	Dexamethasone
Dexamethadrone	Dexamethasone
Dexa-Scheroson	Dexamethasone
Dexa-Sine	Dexamethasone
Dexinolon	Dexamethasone
Dexmethsone	Dexamethasone
Dexone	Dexamethasone
DF. 118	Dihydrocodeine
D-Feda	Pseudoephedrine
Diabeta	Glibenclamide
Diabetal	Chlorpropamide
Diabetoral	Chlorpropamide
Diabines	Chlorpropamide
Diabinese	Chlorpropamide
Diabex S.R.	Metformin
Diabexyl	Metformin
Diacin	Nicotinic acid
Diacipen V.K.	Penicillin V
Di-Adreson	Prednisone
Dialoxin	Digoxin
Diammaglobuline	Immune Serum globulin
Diamox	Acetazolamide
Diapax	Chlordiazepoxide
Diapid	Lysine Vasopressin
Diarsed	Diphenoxylate
Diarsed	Diphenoxylate with Atropine
Diastatin	Nystatin
Diazol	Acetazolamide
Dibein	Phenformin
Dibenyline	Phenoxybenzamine
Dibenzyline	Phenoxybenzamine
Dibotin	Phenformin
Diconal	Dipipanone
Dicorvin	Stilboestrol
Didoc	Acetazolamide
Diethyl Stilboestrol	Fosfestrol
Difhydan	Phenytoin
Diagacin	Digoxin
Digolan	Digoxin
Digoxine	Digoxin
Di-Hydan	Phenytoin
Dihydral	Diphenhydramine
Dihydramine	Diphenhydramine
Dijex	Aluminium Hydroxide
Dilabid	Phenytoin
Dilantin	Phenytoin
Dilax	Dioctyl

Dilax	Dioctyl Sodium Sulphosuccinate
Dimethazine	Sulphadimidine
Dimethazine & Merzin	Sulphadimidine
Diminsol	Sulphadimidine
Diminsul	Sulphadimidine
Dioctyl	Dioctyl Sodium Sulphosuccinate
Dioctyl Forte	Dioctyl
Dioctyl Medo	Dioctyl
Diodoquin	Di-Iodhydroxyquinoline
Diomedicone	Dioctyl
Diomedicone	Dioctyl Sodium Sulphosuccinate
Diossidone	Phenylbutazone
Dipar	Phenformin
Direma	Hydrochlorthiazide
Direx	Iron Dextran
Direxiode	Di-Iodohydroxyquinoline
Disadine	Povidone Iodine
Disebrin	Heparin
Disonate	Dioctyl
Disonate	Dioctyl Sodium Sulphosuccinate
Dispril	Aspirin
Distamine	Penicillamine
Distaquaine VK	Penicillin V
Distilbene	Stilboestrol
Distraneurin	Chlormethiazole
Dithrolan	Dithranol
Ditoin	Phenytoin
Diucen H	Hydrochlorthiazide
Diuchlor H	Hydrochlorthiazide
Diuramide	Acetazolamide
Diurilix	Chlorothiazide
Divulsan	Phenytoin
Dixarit	Clonidine
D.M.S.O.	Dimethyl Sulphoxide
Doca	Deoxycortone Acetate
Docelan	Hydroxocobalamin
Dociton	Propranolol
Docivit	Hydroxocobalamin
Dolamin	Paracetamol
Dolanex	Paracetamol
Dolantin	Pethidine
Dolipol	Tolbutamide
Doliprane	Paracetamol
Dolophine	Methadone
Dolosal	Pethidine
Domeboro	Aluminium Acetotartrate
Domical	Amitriptyline
Domicillin	Ampicillin
Donopon GP	Metoclopramide
Dopamet	Methyldopa
Dopar	Levodopa
Dopastral	Levodopa
Dopram	Doxapram
Dorbanex	Danthron with Poloxamer 188
Dordane	Danthron
Dormel	Chloral hydrate

Dormwell	Dichloralphenazone
Doryl	Carbachol
Dowlings wart paint	Formaldehyde
Dowmycin E	Erythromycin
Dowpen	Penicillin V
Doxinate	Dioctyl Sodium Sulphosuccinate
Doxtacillin	Ampicillin
Diphentyn	Phenytoin
D-Penamine	Penicillamine
Drenusil	Polythiazide
Drixine	Oxymetazoline
Dryptal	Frusemide
Drize	Chlorpheniramine
D.S.S.	Dioctyl
DTIC-Dome	Dacarbazine
Duapen	Benzathine Penicillin
Dufaston	Dydrogesterone
Dulcepen-G	Benzathine Penicillin
Dumocyclin	Tetracycline
Duna-phorine	Morphine
Duphaston	Dydrogesterone
Durabol	Nandrolone Phenylpropionate
Durabolin	Nandrolone Phenylpropionate
Duracillin a.s.	Procaine penicillin
Duracton	A.C.T.H.
Duretter Kalium	Potassium Supplements
Duroferon	Ferrous Sulphate
Duro-Tuss	Pholcodine
Dygratyl	Dihydrotachysterol
Dyloform	Ethinyloestradiol
Dymadon	Paracetamol
Dymocillin	Benzyl Penicillin
Dyneric	Clomiphene
Ebserpine	Reserpine
Ecobutazone	Phenylbutazone
Economycin	Tetracycline
Econochlor	Chloramphenicol
Econocil VK	Penicillin V
Ecotrin	Aspirin
Ecoval 70	Betamethasone
Edecril	Ethacrynic acid
Edecrin	Ethacrynic acid
Edral	Ethinyloestradiol
Edrol	Ethinyloestradiol
Efacin	Nicotinic acid
Efcortelan	Hydrocortisone Sodium Succinate
Efcortilan	Hydrocortisone Sodium Succinate
Efodine	Povidone Iodine
Efudix	5. Fluorouracil
Egocappol	Salicylic acid
Ekko	Phenytoin
Ekvacillin	Cloxacillin
Elatrol	Amitriptyline
Elavil	Amitriptyline
Elenium	Chlordiazepoxide

Elentol	Gamma Benzene Hexachloride
Eliranol	Promazine
Elmarine	Chlorpromazine
Elmedal	Phenylbutazone
Elmidone	Primidone
Elsprin	Aspirin
Eltroxin	L. Thyroxine
Elyx	Dioctyl Sodium Sulphosuccinate
Elyzol	Metronidazole
Elzyme	Pancreatin
Embequin	Di-Iodohydroxyquinoline.
Emcol	Dioctyl
Emcol	Dioctyl Sodium Sulphosuccinate
Emcinka	Erythromycin
Emeldopa	Levodopa
Emelmycin	Neomycin
Emeside	Ethosuximide
Emoform	Formaldehyde
Emprazil	Pseudoephedrine
E-Mycin	Erythromycin·
Encorton	Prednisone
Endep	Amitriptyline
Endoxan	Cyclophosphamide
Endoxana	Cyclophosphamide
Enduxan	Cyclophosphamide
Enicol	Chloramphenicol
Ensobarb	Phenobarbitone
Enteritan	Clioquinol
Enteroquin	Clioquinol
Entero-Valodon	Clioquinol
Entero-Vioform	Clioquinol
Entizol	Metronidazole
Entrophen	Aspirin
Enzypan	Pancreatin
E-Pam	Diazepam
Epanutin	Phenytoin
Epidione	Troxidone
Epidropal	Allopurinol
Epileo petit-mal	Ethosuximide
Epilim	Sodium Valproate
Epilol	Phenobarbitone
Epinephrin	Adrenaline
Eppy	Adrenaline eye drops
Epsylone	Phenobarbitone
Equigyne	Oestrogens-Conjugated
Eraldin	Practolol
Eratrex	Erythromycin
Erbaprelina	Pyrimethamine
Ercoquin	Hydroxychloroquine
Ercotina	Propantheline
Erftopred	Prednisone
Ergenyl	Sodium Valproate
Ergomat	Ergotamine Tartrate
Ergotart	Ergotamine Tartrate
Eributazone	Phenylbutazone
Eromel	Erythromycin

Eromycin	Erythromycin
Erostin	Erythromycin
Ertonyl	Ethinyloestradiol
Erycen	Erythromycin
Erycinum	Erythromycin
Erydin	Isoprenaline
Erypar	Erythromycin
Erythrocin	Erythromycin
Erythromid	Erythromycin
Erythromyctine	Erythromycin
Erythro-ST.	Erythromycin
Esbaloid	Bethanidine
Esbatal	Bethanidine
Escalol 506	Padimate A
Esidrex	Hydrochlorthiazide
Eskabarb	Phenobarbitone
Eskalith	Lithium
Eskaserp	Reserpine
Eskornade	Phenylpropanolamine
Estigyn	Ethinyloestradiol
Estinyl	Ethinyloestradiol
Estraguard	Dienoestrol
Estralutin	Hydroxyprogesterone
Estratab	Oestrogens-Conjugated
Estratab	Oestradiol Valerate
Estromed	Oestrogens-Conjugated
Estropan	Oestrogens-Conjugated
Estrovis	Quinestrol
Ethibute	Phenylbutazone
Ethophylline	Aminophylline
Ethrilk	Erythromycin
Ethryn	Erythromycin
Ethyll	Ethinyloestradiol
Etibi	Ethambutol
Etin	Ergotamine Tartrate
Etivex	Ethinyloestradiol
Etrenol	Hycanthone
Eubasinum	Sulphapyridine
Eudemine	Diazoxide
Eudorm	Chloral Hydrate
Euglucon	Glibenclamide
Eugynon 30	Combined Oral Contraceptives
Euphyllin	Aminophylline
Euphylline	Aminophylline
Eurax	Crotamiton
Euraxil	Crotamiton
Eusaprim	Co Trimoxazole
Euthyrox	L. Thyroxine
Evacilin	Procaine penicillin
Evex	Oestrogens-Conjugated
Exmigra	Ergotamine Tartrate
Exmigrex	Ergotamine Tartrate
Extencilline	Benzathine Penicillin
Extil	Pseudoephedrine
E-Z Scrub	Hexachlorophane
E-Z Scrub	Povidone Iodine

Fab. A. Vit	Vitamin A
Factorate	Anti-haemophilic globulin
Falcopen V	Penicillin V
Famet	Sulphamethizole
Fansidar	Pyrimethamine
Farlutal	Medroxyprogesterone
Farmacyrol	Dienoestrol
Fasigyn	Tinidazole
Febrigesic	Paracetamol
Febrogesic	Paracetamol
Feevone	Terbutaline
Felsules	Chloral Hydrate
Femacoid	Oestrogens-Conjugated
Femergin	Ergotamine Tartrate
Femest	Oestrogens-Conjugated
Feminone	Ethinyloestradiol
Femogen	Oestrogens-Conjugated
Femogex	Oestradiol Valerate
Femulen	Ethynodiol
Fenantion	Phenytoin
Fenicol	Chloramphenicol
Fenopron	Fenoprofen
Fenox	Phenylephrine
Fenoxcillin	Penicillin V
Fenoxypen	Penicillin V
Feosol	Ferrous sulphate
Feospan	Ferrous Sulphate
Fer-In-Sol	Ferrous Sulphate
Feritard	Ferrous Sulphate
Fermentmycin	Tetracycline
Ferofor	Ferrous sulphate
Ferosan-Tydales	Ferrous Sulphate
Ferro-O$_2$	Ferrous sulphate
Ferro 66	Ferrous sulphate
Ferro-gradumet	Ferrous sulphate
Ferrophor-Dragees	Ferrous sulphate
Fertodur	Cyclofenil
Fespan	Ferrous sulphate
Fibroxin	Digoxin
Filair	Terbutaline
Fisostin	Physostigmine
Fivepen	Benzyl Penicillin
Flebocortid	Hydrocortisone Sodium Succinate
Flagyl	Metronidazole
Flavoquine	Amodiaquine
Flexazone	Phenylbutazone
Flocilline	Procaine penicillin
Floraquin	Di-Iodohydroxyquinoline
Florequin	Di-Iodohydroxyquinoline
Florinef	Fludrocortisone
Florocycline	Tetracycline
Floxapen	Flucloxacillin
Fluazine	Trifluoperazine
Flucort	Fluocinolone
Flufacid	Flufenamic acid
Flumen	Chlorothiazide

Fluonid	Fluocinolone
Fluormone	Dexamethasone
Fluorocort	Dexamethasone
Fluoroplex	5-Fluorouracil
Folacin	Folic acid
Folasic	Folic acid
Folcodan	Pholcodine
Foldine	Folic acid
Folettes	Folic Acid
Foligan	Allopurinol
Follistrel	Norgestrel
Follutein	Chorionic Gonadotrophin
Folsan	Folic acid
Folvite	Folic Acid
Forpen	Benzyl Penicillin
Fortalgesic	Pentazocine
Fortecortin	Dexamethasone
Fortral	Pentazocine
Fortralin	Pentazocine
Fortuss	Dihydrocodeine
Framygen	Framycetin
Francacilline	Procaine penicillin
Franyl	Frusemide
Frusid	Frusemide
Fucidin	Sodium Fusidate
Fucidina	Sodium Fusidate
Fucidine	Sodium Fusidate
Fulcin	Griseofulvin
Fulvicin-U/F	Griseofulvin
Fungalex	Nystatin
Fungilin	Amphotericin B
Fungistatin	Nystatin
Fungizone	Amphotericin B
Furamide	Diloxanide
Fybogel	Ispaghula Husk
Galenomycin	Tetracycline
Gamastan	Immune Serum globulin
Gamatet	Human Antitetanus Immunoglobulin
Gamma	Immune Serum globulin
Gammabyk	Immune Serum globulin
Gammacorten	Dexamethasone
Gammagee	Immune Serum globulin
Gammapovit	Immune Serum globulin
Gammar	Immune Serum globulin
Gamma Veinine	Immune Serum globulin
Gamma-Venin	Immune Serum globulin
Gamophen	Hexachlorophane
Gamulin	Immune Serum globulin
Gamulin T	Human Antitetanus Immunoglobulin
Ganeake	Oestrogens-Conjugated
Ganphen	Promethazine Hydrochloride
Gantrisin	Sulphafurazole
Grantrisan	Sulphafurazole
Gantriscine	Sulphafurazole
Gantrisine	Sulphafurazole

Garamycina	Gentamicin
Garamyan	Gentamicin
Gardenal	Phenobarbitone
Gelfilm ophthalmic	Gelatin eye lamellae
Gelox	Aluminium hydroxide
Genapax	Gentian Violet
Gene-cycline	Tetracycline
Genesis	Oestrogens-Conjugated
Genisol	Coal Tar
Genoxal	Cyclophosphamide
Gentran 40	Dextran 40
Gentalline	Gentamicin
Genticin	Gentamicin
Geomycine	Gentamicin
Gestapuran	Medroxyprogesterone
Gill Liquid	Hexachlorophane
Gilucor nitro	Glyceryl Trinitrate
Glanil	Cinnarizine
Glaucomide	Acetazolamide
Glaupax	Acetazolamide
Glucal	Calcium Gluconate
Gluceptate	Erythromycin
Glucophage	Metformin
Glucopostin	Phenformin
Glutril	Glibenclamide
Glyestrin	Oestrogens-Conjugated
Glynite	Glyceryl trinitrate
Glysennid	Senna
Gonadex	Chorionic Gonadotrophin
Gonadotraphon L.H.	Chorionic Gonadotrophin
Gotimycin	Chloramphenicol
G.P.V.	Penicillin V
Godamed	Aspirin
Grifulvin-V	Griseofulvin
Grisactin	Griseofulvin
Grisefuline	Griseofulvin
Grisovin	Griseofulvin
Gris-Peg	Griseofulvin
G.T.	Tetracycline
Guanar	Diphenhydramine
G.V.S.	Gentian Violet
Gynaflex	Noxythiolin
Gynergen	Ergotamine Tartrate
Gyno-Daktarin	Miconazole
Gynolett	Ethinyloestradiol
Gynorest	Dydrogesterone
Gynovlar 21	Combined Oral Contraceptives
Gynovules	Di-Iodohydroxyquinoline
Haemofort	Ferrous sulphate
Haldol	Haloperidol
Halivite	Vitamin A
Halotestin	Fluoxymesterone
Hämocura	Heparin
Harmogen	Piperazine Oestrone Sulphate
Harvatropin	Chorionic Gonadotrophin

M

Haurymellin	Metformin
Haynon	Chlorpheniramine
Hayphryn	Phenylephrine
Hazol	Oxymetazoline
Heflin	Cephalothin
Helfo-dopa	Levodopa
Hemineurin	Chlormethiazole
Heminevrin	Chlormethiazole
Hemofil	Anti-Haemophilic globulin
Hemostyptanon	Oestriol
Hepagon novum	Hydroxocobalamin
Hepalean	Heparin
Hepathrom	Heparin
Heprinar	Heparin
Heracillin	Flucloxacillin
Herisan	Neomycin
Herpid	Idoxuridine
Herpidu	Idoxuridine
Herplex	Idoxuridine
Herzul	Propranolol
Hexachlorone	Hexachlorophane
Hexacreme	Hexachlorophane
Hexacycline	Tetracycline
Hexadrol	Dexamethasone
Hexaklen	Hexachlorophane
Hexaphenyl	Hexachlorophane
Hexol	Chlorhexidine
Hibernal	Chlorpromazine
Hibiscrub	Chlorhexidine
Hibitan	Chlorhexidine
Hibitane	Chlorhexidine
Hi-pen	Penicillin V
Histadur	Chlorpheniramine
Histadyl E.C.	Codeine Phosphate
Histaids	Chlorpheniramine
Histalix	Diphenhydramine
Histalon	Chlorpheniramine
Histantil	Promethazine Hydrochloride
Histaspan	Chlorpheniramine
Histatil	Promethazine HCL
Histol	Chlorpheniramine
Holin	Oestriol
Homogonal	Menopausal Urinary Gonadotrophin
Homo-tet	Human Antitetanus Immunoglobulin
Honvan	Fosfestrol (diethy stilboestrol)
Honvol	Fosfestrol (diethyl stilboestrol)
Hormofemin	Dienoestrol
Hormomed	Oestriol
Hostacillin	Procaine penicillin
Hostacortin	Prednisone
Hostacyclin	Tetracycline
Humafac	Anti-haemophilic globulin
Humegon	Menopausal Urinary Gonadotrophin
Humorsol	Demecarium Bromide
Humotet	Human Antitetanus Immunogloblin
Hu-Tet	Human Antitetanus Immunoglobulin

Hyasorb	Benzyl Penicillin
Hycor eye drops	Hydrocortisone eye drops
Hydracycline	Tetracycline
Hydrazide	Hydrochlorthiazide
Hydroazol	Acetazolamide
Hydrea	Hydroxyurea
Hydrid	Hydrochlorthiazide
Hydro-Aquid	Hydrochlorthiazide
Hydrocortisone	Hydrocortisone Sodium Succinate
Hydrocortistab	Hydrocortisone eye drops
Hydrodiuretex	Hydrochlorthiazide
Hydromedin	Ethacrynic acid
Hydronsan	Isoniazid
Hydrosaluret	Hydrochlorthiazide
Hydrosaluric	Hydrochlorthiazide
Hydrosone	Hydrocortisone eye drops
Hydroxo	Hydroxocobalamin
Hydroxo-B12	Hydroxocobalamin
Hydroxobase	Hydroxocobalamin
Hydrozide	Hydrochlorthiazide
Hyeloril	Hydrochlorthiazide
Hygicreme	Chlorhexidine
Hygroton	Chlorthalidone
Hylenta	Benzyl Penicillin
Hyperazin	Hydrallazine
Hyperpaxa	Methyldopa
Hyperstat	Diazoxide
Hypertet	Human Antitetanus Immunoglobulin
Hypnolone	Phenobarbitone
Hypnorex	Lithium
Hypomellose	Methylcellulose eye drops
Hyproval PA	Hydroxyprogesterone
Hytakerol	Dihydrotachysterol
Ibacillin-Aqueous	Procaine penicillin
I-Care	Phenylephrine
Ichthammol	Ichthyol
Icipen 300	Penicillin V
Ictorivil	Clonazepam
I do A	Vitamin A
Iduridin	Idoxuridine
Iduviran	Idoxuridine
Igege	Immune Serum globulin
Igroton	Chlorthalidone
Iktorivil	Clonazepam
Iliadin-Mini	Oxymetazoline
Ilosone	Erythromycin
Ilotycin	Erythromycin
Ilozoft	Dioctyl
Ilozoft	Dioctyl Sodium Sulphosuccinate
Imacillin	Amoxycillin
Imbrilon	Indomethacin
Imferdex	Iron Dextran
Imferon	Iron Dextran
Immu-G	Immune Serum globulin
Immuglobin	Immune Serum globulin

Immu-Tetanus	Human Antitetanus immunoglobulin
Imodium	Loperamide
Imperacin	Tetracycline
Impugan	Frusemide
Imural	Azathioprine
Imuran	Azathioprine
Imurek	Azathioprine
Imurel	Azathioprine
Inacid	Indomethacin
Indacin	Indomethacin
Inderal	Propranolol
Indocid	Indomethacin
Indocin	Indomethacin
Indomee	Indomethacin
Infrocin	Indomethacin
Ingelan	Isoprenaline
I.N.H.	Isoniazid
Inimur	Nifuratel
Inocortyl	Prednisone
Inostral	Disodium Cromoglycate
Insilange-D	Tolbutamide
Insomnol	Methylpentynol
Insoral	Phenformin
Instantine	Aspirin
Intal	Disodium Cromoglycate
Intrabutazone	Phenylbutazone
Intracort	Hydrocortisone Sodium Succinate
Intraglobin	Immune Serum globulin
Intraval	Thiopentone
Intrazine	Promazine
Invite-B$_1$	Thiamine
Ioquin	Di-Iodohydroxyquinoline
Ipoglicone	Tolbutamide
Iron Hy-Dex	Iron Dextran
Ironorm	Iron Dextran
Isactid	A.C.T.H.
Ismelin	Guanethidine
Ismelin eye drops	Guanethidine eye drops
isobicina	Isoniazid
Isocillin	Penicillin V
Isodine	Povidone Iodine
Isogel	Ispaghula Husk
Isoglaucon	Clonidine
Iso-Intranefrin	Isoprenaline
Isolin	Isoprenaline
Isonefrine	Phenylephrine
Isophrin	Phenylephrine
Isopropydrin	Isoprenaline
Isoptim	Verapamil
Isopto Alkaline	Methyl cellulose eye drops
Isopto Atropine	Atropine eye drops
Isopto Carpine	Pilocarpine
Isoptocetamide	Sulphacetamide eye drops
Isopto-cetamide	Sulphacetamide eye drops/ointment
Isopto Epinal	Adrenaline eye drops
Isopto-Eserine	Physostigmine

Isopto fluid	Methylcellulose eye drops
Isopto Frin	Phenylephrine
Isopto-Maxidrex	Dexamethasone
Isopto plain	Methylcellulose eye drops
Isopto-tears	Methylcellulose eye drops
Isotamine	Isoniazid
Isotinyl	Isoniazid
Isotropina	Phenylephrine
Isovon	Isoprenaline
Isozid	Isoniazid
Ispaghul	Ispaghula Husk
Ispenoral	Penicillin V
Isuprel	Isoprenaline
Ivepirine	Aspirin
Jacutin	Gamma Benzene Hexachloride
Jatcetin	Chloramphenicol
Jatcillin	Penicillin V
Jatroneural	Trifluoperazine
Jectofer	Iron Sorbitol
Jellin	Fluocinolone
Jetrium	Dextromoramide
Juvacor	Nikethamide
Juvastigmin	Neostigmine
Juvepirine	Aspirin
K-10	Potassium supplement
Kabikinase	Streptokinase
Kadol	Phenylbutazone
Kajos	Mist. Potassium Citrate
Kalacide	Hexachlorophane
Kaleorid	Potassium supplement
Kalilente	Potassium supplement
Kalinor	Potassium supplement
Kalipor	Potassium supplement
Kalitabs	Potassium supplement
Kalium	Potassium Chloride
Kamaver	Chloramphenicol
Kaochlor	Potassium supplements
Kaodene	Codeine Phosphate
Ka-pen	Benzyl Penicillin
Kardonyl	Nikethamide
Kato	Potassium supplement
Katonium	Potassium Chloride
Katorin	Potassium supplements
Kavepenin	Penicillin V
Kay-Cee-L	Potassium supplements
Kay-Ciel	Potassium supplement
Kaywan	Vitamin K,
K Contin	Potassium Chloride
K-Contin	Potassium supplements
Keflodin	Cephaloridine
Kefspor	Cephaloridine
Kelocyanor	Cobaltedetate
Kemadrin	Procyclidine
Kemi	Propranolol
Kemicetine	Chloramphenicol

Kenacort	Triamcinolone
Keralyt	Salicylic acid
Kerecid	Idoxuridine
Kessodanten	Phenytoin
Kessodrate	Chloral Hydrate
Kessomycin	Erythromycin
Kesso-pen	Benzyl Penicillin
Kesso-pen-VK	Penicillin V
Kesso-tetra	Tetracycline
Keteocort	Prednisone
Klarikordal-Retard	Glyceryl trinitrate
K-Lor	Potassium supplement
Kloref	Potassium supplements
Klor-lyte	Potassium supplements
Klorpromex	Chlorpromazine
K-lyte	Mist Potassium Citrate
Koate	Anti haemophilic globulin
Konakion	Vitamin K,
Korazin	Chlorpromazine
Korazine	Chlorpromazine
Korostatin	Nystatin
Korum	Paracetamol
Kryobulin	Anti-haemophilic globulin
K-San	Potassium supplements
Kwell	Gamma Benzene Hexachloride
Kwellada	Gamma Benzene Hexachloride
Kylx	Dioctyl
Lacril	Methylcellulose eye drops
Lamoryl	Griseolfulvin
Lamprene	Clofazimine
Lanacrist	Digoxin
Lanatoxin	Digoxin
Lanceat	Flufenamic acid
Lanchloral	Chloral hydrate
Lanicor	Digoxin
Lanoxin	Digoxin
Lanpen	Penicillin V
Lantuss	Pholcodine
Largactil	Chlorpromazine
Larodopa	Levodopa
Larotid	Amoxycillin
Larozyl	Amitriptyline
Lasan	Dithranol ointment
Lasan Pomade	Dithranol ointment
Lasilix	Frusemide
Lasix	Frusemide
Ledafoline	Folinic acid
Ledclair	Sodium Calcium Edetate
Ledercillin VK	Penicillin V
Ledercort	Triamcinolone
Lederfoline	Folinic Acid
Ledermycin	Demeclocycline
Lederstatin	Demeclocycline
Ledertrexate	Methotrexate
Ledopa	Levodopa

Lemazine	Promethazine Hydrochloride
Lemprometh	Promethazine Hydrochloride
Lemtrex	Tetracycline
Lenazine	Promethazine Hydrochloride
Lenitral	Glyceryl Trinitrate
Lennacol	Chloramphenicol
Lensen	Diphenhydramine
Lentizol	Amitriptyline
Leo k	Potassium Chloride
Leo-K·	Potassium supplements
Lergigan	Promethazine Hydrochloride
Lethidrone	Nalorphine
Letter	L. Thyroxine
Leucovorin	Folinic Acid
Leukomycin	Chloramphenicol
Levate	Amitriptyline
Levaxin	L. Thyroxine
Levius	Aspirin
Levoid	L. Thyroxine
Levopa	Levodopa
Lexacycline	Tetracycline
Lexxor	Hydrochlorthiazide
Libritabs	Chlordiazepoxide
Librium	Chlordiazepoxide
Libuden	Griseofulvin
Limbitrol	Amitriptyline
Linctifed	Pseudoephedrine
Lingraine	Ergotamine Tartrate
Lingran	Ergotamine Tartrate
Lingrene	Ergotamine Tartrate
Linoral	Ethinyloestradiol
Lioresal	Baclofen
Liparlon	Clofibrate
Liprinal	Clofibrate
Liquemin	Heparin
Liquiprin	Paracetamol
Liranol	Promazine
Lisacort	Prednisone
Liskantin	Primidone
Litalir	Hydroxyurea
Lithane	Lithium
Lithicarb	Lithium
Lithionit	Lithium
Lithium duriles	Lithium
Lithium Oligosol	Lithium
Lithocarb	Lithium
Lithonate	Lithium
Lithotabs	Lithium
Litrison	D.L. Methionine
Lixaminol	Aminophylline
L.M.D.	Dextran 40
Lobamine	D.L. Methionine
Localyn	Fluocinolone
Loestrin 20	Combined oral contraceptives
Lomodex 40	Dextran 40
Lomotil	Diphenoxylate

Lomotil	Diphenoxylate with Atropine
Lomudal	Disodium Cromoglycate
Lopresor	Metoprolol
Lopress	Hydrallazine
Loqua	Hydrochlorthiazide
Lorexane	Gamma Benzene Hexachloride
Loridine	Cephaloridine
Lorphen	Chlorpheniramine
L.P.G.	Benzathine Penicillin
L. Polamidon	Methadone
L.P.V.	Penicillin V
Lucosil	Sulphamethizole
Luf-Iso	Isoprenaline
Luminal	Phenobarbitone
Luminaletten	Phenobarbitone
Lutate	Hydroxyprogesterone
Luteocrin	Hydroxyprogesterone
Lutometrodiol	Ethynodiol
Luxazone	Dexamethasone
Lynoral	Ethinyloestradiol
Lyogen	Fluphenazine
Lyophrin	Adrenaline eye drops
Lypressin	Lysine Vasopressin
Lysodren	Mitotane (O^1 P^1 DDD)
Lysoform	Formaldehyde
Lyteca	Paracetamol
Macmiror	Nifuratel
Madopar	Levodopa and decarboxylase inhibitor
Magnoplasm	Magnesium Sulphate
Malaquin	Chloroquine
Malarex	Chloroquine
Malarivon	Chloroquine
Malgesic	Phenylbutazone
Mallorol	Thioridazine
Malocide	Pyrimethamine
Malogen	Testosterone Propionate
Malogen L.A.	Testosterone Enanthate
Malogex	Testosterone Enanthate
Maloprim	Pyrimethamine
Manicol	Mannitol
Maniprex	Lithium
Manoxol	Dioctyl
Manoxol	Dioctyl Sodium Sulphosuccinate
Mantadix	Amantadine
Marboran	Methisazone
Mareline	Amitriptyline
Marevan	Warfarin
Marezine	Cyclizine
Marsone	Prednisone
Marzine	Cyclizine
Matulane	Procarbazine
Maxeran	Metoclopramide
Maximed	Protriptyline
Maxitrol	Neomycin
Maxolon	Metoclopramide

M & B 693	Sulphapyridine
M-B tabs	Methylene Blue
Measurin	Aspirin
Mebadin	Dehydroemetine
Medihaler Ergotamine	Ergotamine Tartrate
Medilium	Chlordiazepoxide
Medomet	Methyldopa
Megacilin	Procaine penicillin
Megacillin	Benzathine Penicillin
Megacillin	Benzyl Penicillin
Megapen	Procaine penicillin
Megaphen	Chlorpromazine
Meginalisk	Betahistine
Meladinine	Methoxsalen
Melitase	Chlorpropamide
Melleretten	Thioridazine
Mellaril	Thioridazine
Melleril	Thioridazine
Mellitol	Tolbutamide
Menest	Oestrogens-Conjugated
Meniace	Betahistine
Menogen	Oestrogens-Conjugated
Menolyn	Ethinyloestradiol
Menotrol	Oestrogens-Conjugated
Meonine	D.L. Methionine
Mephyton	Vitamin K,
Mercaptamine	Cysteamine
Merislon	Betahistine
Merizone	Phenylbutazone
Meronidal	Metronidazole
Meropenin	Penicillin V
Mestinon	Pyridostigmine
Metalcaptase	Penicillamine
Metaprel	Orciprenaline
Metasolon	Dexamethasone
Metem	Aluminium Hydroxide
Methisul	Sulphamethizole
Methnine	D.L. Methionine
Methocel H. G.	Methylcellulose eye drops
Methoplain	Methyldopa
Methopt	Methylcellulose eye drops
Methoxypsoralen	Methoxsalen
Methyl CCNU	Semustine
Meth-zine	Promethazine Hydrochloride
Meticorten	Prednisone
Metiguanide	Metformin
Metindol	Indomethacin
Metoclol	Metoclopramide
Metopirone	Metyrapone
Metral	Phenformin
Mexitil	Mexilitine
Mexocine	Demeclocycline
Mezin	Sulphadimidine
Mezolin	Indomethacin
Miambutol	Ethambutol
Micatin	Miconazole

Microgynon 30	Combined Oral Contraceptives
Microlut	Norgestrel
Microluton	Norgestrel
Micronett	Norethisterone
Micronor	Norethisterone
Micronovum	Norethisterone
Mictrin	Hydrochlorthiazide
Midamor	Amiloride
Midone	Primidone
Midronal	Cinnarizine
Mikalyt	Potassium supplement
Mikro-30	Norgestrel
Millafol	Folic acid
Millicorten	Dexamethasone
Minajel	Aluminium Hydroxide
Minihep	Heparin
Minilix	Aminophylline
Minilyn	Combined Oral Contraceptives
Minim Sulphacetamide	Sulphacetamide eye drops/ointment
Minims Chloramphenicol	Chloramphenicol eye drops
Minims Ophthalmic Drops	Atropine eye drops
Minims Opthalmic Drops	Sulphacetamide eye drops
Minims Ophthalmic Drops	Sulphacetamide eye drops/ointment
Mini PE	Norethisterone
Minirin	Desmopressin
Minisone	Betamethasone
Minovlar	Combined Oral Contraceptives
Minzil	Chlorothiazide
Mio-Carpine-SMP	Pilocarpine
Miostat	Carbachol
Mi-Pilo	Pilocarpine
Miral	Dexamethasone
Miriamycine	Tetracycline
Mistalco	Aluminium Hydroxide
Mistol Mist	Phenylephrine
Mistura C	Carbachol
Mistura-D	Phenylephrine
Mistura P	Pilocarpine
Mobenol	Tolbutamide
Moco	Dexamethasone
Modamide	Amiloride
Modane	Danthron
Modecate	Fluphenazine
Moditen	Fluphenazine
Moebiquin	Di-Iodohydroxyquinoline
Molcer	Dioctyl
Molcer	Dioctyl Sodium Sulphosuccinate
Mol-Iron	Ferrous sulphate
Mona salyl	Aspirin
Monistat	Miconazole
Monphytol	Salicylic acid
Moriperan	Metoclopramide
Moronal	Nystatin
Morplan CHSA	Cetrimide
Motrin	Ibuprofen
MsMed	Oestrogens-Conjugated

Muracine	Tetracycline.
Mustargen	Mustine
Myacyne	Neomycin
Myambutol	Ethambutol
Mycetin-Opthiole	Chloramphenicol eye drops
Mycifradin	Neomycin
Myciguent	Neomycin
Mycinol	Chloramphenicol
Mycostatin	Nystatin
Mydriacyl	Tropicamide
Myriaticum	Tropicamide
Mydrilate	Cyclopentolate
Mynah	Ethambutol & Isoniazid
Myochrysine	Gold
Myocrisin	Gold
Myoplegic	Cyclopentolate
Myriaticum	Tropicamide
Mysoline	Primidone
Mysteclin	Tetracycline
Nack	Chlordiazepoxide
Nadopen-V	Penicillin V
Nadozone	Phenylbutazone
Nafrine	Oxymetazoline
Napamol	Paracetamol
Napamol	Paracetamol
Naprosyn	Naproxen
Narcan	Naloxone
Narex	Phenylephrine
Nasivin	Oxymetazoline
Nasmil	Disodium Chromoglycate
Nastenon	Oxymetholone
Natigoxin	Digoxin
Naturetin	Bendrofluazide
Naturine	Bendrofluazide
Natrophyllin	Aminophylline
Natrophylline	Aminophylline
Natulan	Procarbazine
Navane	Thiothixene
Navidrex	Cyclopenthiazide
Naxen	Naproxen
Naxogin	Nimorazole
Naxogyn	Nimorazole
Nebs	Paracetamol
Neobacrin	Neomycin
Neo Banex	Propantheline
Neo-Benol	Hydroxocobalamin
Neo-Betalin 12	Hydroxocobalamin
Neobiotic	Neomycin
Neobram	Neomycin
Neocin	Neomycin
Neo-Codema	Hydrochlorthiazide
Neocortef	Neomycin
Neo-Cytamen	Hydroxocobalamin
Neo-dibetic	Tolbutamide
Neo-Epinine	Isoprenaline

Neo-Estrone	Oestrogens-Conjugated
Neo-flumen	Hydrochlorthiazide
Neogest	Norgestrel
Neoloid	Castor Oil
Neohombreol	Testosterone Propionate
Neomate	Neomycin
Neo Mercazole	Carbimazole
Neomin	Neomycin
Neo-Morphazole	Carbimazole
Neo Morrhuol	Neomycin
Neonaclex	Bendrofluazide
Neopan	Neomycin
Neopap	Paracetamol
Neo-Pens	Benzyl Penicillin
Neopirine 25	Aspirin
Neophryn	Phenylephrine
Neophyllin	Aminophylline
Neopt	Neomycin
Neo-serp	Reserpine
Neosporin	Neomycin
Neosulf	Neomycin
Neoteben	Isoniazid
Neo-tetrine	Tetracycline
Neo-Thyreostat	Carbimazole
Neo-tric	Metronidazole
Neo-Zoline	Phenylbutazone
Nepenthe	Morphine
Nephril	Polythiazide
Nesdonal	Thiopentone
Neurolithium	Lithium
Nevimycin	Chloramphenicol
Nevrol	Paracetamol
Nez	Phenylephrine
Nezeril	Oxymetazoline
Niac	Nicotinic acid
Nicangin	Nicotinic acid
Nichisedan	Flufenamic acid
Nico-400	Nicotinic acid
Nicobid	Nicotinic acid
Nicolar	Nicotinic acid
Niconacid	Nicotinic acid
Niconyl	Isoniazid
Nico-span	Nicotinic acid
Nicotinex	Nicotinic acid
Nicyl	Nicotinic acid
Nida	Metronidazole
Niferex	Iron Dextran
Nigloid	Tolbutamide
Nigracap	Chloral hydrate
Nilstat	Nystatin
Ninol	D.L. Methionine
Niratron	Chlorpheniramine
Nisone	Prednisone
Nitoman	Tetrabenazine
Nitora	Glyceryl trinitrate
Nitrangin	Glyceryl trinitrate

Novophenyl	Phenylbutazone
Novopoxide	Chlordiazepoxide
Novopropamide	Chlorpropamide
Novoridazine	Thioridazine
Novorythro	Erythromycin
Novosoxazole	Sulphafurazole
Novosprin	Aspirin
Novostrep	Streptomycin
Novotetra	Tetracycline
Novotriptyn	Amitriptyline
Noxyflex	Noxythiolin
N.S.B.	Noxythiolin
Nucleoton	Pancreatin
Nulogyl	Nimorazole
Nuseals Aspirin	Aspirin
Nutracillin	Penicillin V
Nutrizym	Pancreatin
Nydrazid	Isoniazid
Nystan	Nystatin
Nystatin-Dome	Nystatin
Nystavescent	Nystatin
Oblivon	Methylpentynol
Oculotect	Vitamin A
Ocusol	Sulphacetamide eye drops/ointment
Octyl Softener	Dioctyl
Octyl Softener	Dioctyl Sodium Sulphosuccinate
Oekolp	Stilboestrol
Oestrilin	Oestrogens-Conjugated
Oestro-Feminal	Oestrogens-Cojugated
Oestromon	Stilboestrol
Oestropak Morning	Oestrogens-Conjugated
Ogen	Piperazine Oestrone Sulphate
Oleomycetin	Chloramphenicol
Omatropina Lux	Homatropine
Omca	Fluphenazine
Omnes	Nifuratel
Omnipen	Ampicillin
Onazine	Chlorpromazine
Ondogyne	Cyclofenil
Ondonid	Cyclofenil
One Alpha	1 α hydroxycholecalciferol
Opclor	Chloramphenicol
O'P'DDD	Mitotane
Ophthalmadine	Idoxuridine
Ophthalmicum	Hydrocortisone eye drops
Op-thal-min	Zinc sulphate
Ophthoolor	Chloramphenicol
Oppazone	Phenylbutazone
Op-sulfa	Sulphacetamide eye drops/ointment
Optamide	Sulphacetamide eye drops/ointment
Optiole S	Sulphacetamide eye drops/ointment
Opulets atropine	Atropine eye drops
Opulets Chloramphenicol	Chloramphenicol eye drops
Opulets-sulphacetamide	Sulphacetamide eye drops/ointment
Oracilline	Penicillin V

Oradexon	Dexamethasone
Orahex	Hexachlorophane
Oramide	Tolbutamide
Orapen	Penicillin V
Orasone	Prednisone
Oratestin	Fluoxymesterone
Ora-Testryl	Fluoxymesterone
Orazinc	Zinc Sulphate
Orbenin	Cloxacillin
Orbenine	Cloxacillin
Orbinamon	Thiothixene
Oretic	Hydrochlorthiazide
Oreton Propionate	Testosterone propionate
Orgadrone	Dexamethasone
Orgastyptin	Oestriol
Oribetic	Tolbutamide
Orinase	Tolbutamide
Orlest 21	Combined oral contraceptives
Oroxine	L. Thyroxine
Orpyrin	Flufenamic acid
Ortho-norvin $\frac{1}{50}$	Combined Oral Contraceptives
Orvepen	Penicillin V
Osmitrol	Mannitol
Osmolax	Ispaghula Husk
Osmosol	Mannitol
Osnervan	Procyclidine
Osopto Homatropine	Homatropine
Ospen	Penicillin V
Otobiotic	Neomycin Polymyxin
Otopol	Polymyxin
Otosporin	Neomycin
Ototrips	Polymyxin
Otriven	Xylometazoline
Otrivine	Xylometazoline
Otrix	Xylometazoline
Ovesterin	Oestriol
Ovestin	Oestriol
Ovran	Combined Oral Contraceptives
Ovran 30	Combined Oral Contraceptives
Ovranette	Combined Oral Contraceptives
Ovrette	Norgestrel
Ovulen	Combined Oral Contraceptives
Ovulen 50	Combined Oral Contraceptives
Ovysmen	Combined Oral Contraceptives
Oxobemin	Hydroxocobalamin
Oxsoralen	Methoxsalen
Oxy-5 Acne	Benzoyl peroxide
Oxydon	Tetracycline
Oxymycin	Tetracycline
P-50	Benzyl Penicillin
Pabafilm	Padimate A
Pabestrol	Stilboestrol
Pacemol	Paracetamol
Pacinol	Fluphenazine
Paclin VK	Penicillin V

Paediathrocin	Erythromycin
Paedo-sed	Dichloralphenazone
Palamkotta	Senna
Palfium	Dextromoramide
Palliacol	Aluminium Hydroxide
Paludrine	Proguanil
Paludrinol	Proguanil
Paludrinol	Proguanil
P.A.M.	Procaine Penicillin with aluminum sterate
Pamol	Paracetamol
Panado	Paracetamol
Panadol	Paracetamol
Panafcort	Prednisone
Panar	Pancreatin
Panasorb	Paracetamol
Panazid	Isoniazid
Panazone	Phenylbutazone
Pancillen	Penicillin V
Pancodone	Oxycodone
Pancrex	Pancreatin
Pancrex V	Pancreatin
Pandel	Paracetamol
Panheparin	Heparin
Pankreon	Pancreatin
Panmycin	Tetracycline
Panodil	Paracetamol
Panoxyl	Benzoyl peroxide
Panteric	Pancreatin
Pantheline	Propantheline
Pantovernil	Chloramphenicol
Panuric	Probenecid
Panwarfin	Warfarin
Paracet	Paracetamol
Paracodin	Dihydrocodeine
Paracort	Prednisone
Paragesic	Pseudoephedrine
Paral	Paraldehyde
Parasin	Paracetamol
Paraxin	Chloramphenicol
Par Estro	Oestrogens-Congugated
Paretest	Testosterone Propionate
Pargitan	Benzhexol
Parkidopa	Levodopa
Parlodel	Bromocriptine
Parmenison	Prednisone
Parmol	Paracetamol
Pasetocin	Amoxycillin
Paspertin	Metoclopramide
Paveral	Codeine Phosphate
Paxel	Diazepam
P.C.	Cetrimide
P.E.B.A.	Phenobarbitone
Pectolin	Pholcodine
Pedameth	D.L. Methionine
Pediamycin	Erythromycin
Pediaphen	Paracetamol

Pen A	Ampicillin
Penapar VK	Penicillin V
Pen-Bristol	Ampicillin
Penbritin	Ampicillin
Penbritine	Ampicillin
Penbrock	Ampicillin
Pen-cilin-V	Penicillin V
Pencitabs	Benzyl Penicillin
Peneran	Benzyl Penicillin
Penicline	Ampicillin
Penidural	Benzathine Penicillin
Penilente L.A.	Benzathine Penicillin
Penioral	Benzyl Penicillin
Peniset	Benzyl Penicillin
Peni-vee	Penicillin V
Pensal	Benzyl Penicillin
Pensyn	Ampicillin
Pentamycetin	Chloramphenicol
Pentazine	Trifluoperazine
Pentazyme	Pancreatin
Pentids	Benzyl Penicillin
Pentids-P a.s.	Procaine Penicillin
Pentothal	Thiopentone
Pentrane	Hydrargaphen
Pentrex	Ampicillin
Pentrexyl	Ampicillin
Pen-Vee	Penicillin V
Pen-Vee-K	Penicillin V
Peragit	Benzhexol
Percorten	Deoxy Cortone Acetate
Percutacrine	L. Thyroxine
Pergonal	Menopausal Urinary Gonadotrophin
Perfadex	Dextran 40
Perfudex	Dextran 40
Permapen	Benzathine Penicillin
Permitil	Fluphenazine
Peroidin	Potassium Perchlorate
Persadox	Benzoyl peroxide
Persantin	Dipyridamole
Persantine	Dipyridamole
Perzadox	Benzoyl peroxide
Petercillin	Ampicillin
Peter Kal	Potassium supplement
Peterphyllin	Aminophylline
Pethoid	Pethidine
Petnidan	Ethosuximide
Pevidine	Povidone Iodine
Pexobiotic	Tetracycline
Pfiklor	Potassium supplement
Pfipen V	Penicillin V
Pfizer-E	Erythromycin
Pfizerpen a.s.	Procaine penicillin
Pfizerpen VK	Penicillin V
Pharmacillin	Benzyl Penicillin
Phasal	Lithium
Phenaemal	Phenobarbitone

Phenaemaletten	Phenobarbitone
Phenased	Phenobarbitone
Phen Bar	Phenobarbitone
Phenbutazol	Phenylbutazone
Phendex	Paracetamol
Phenephrin	Phenylephrine
Phenergan	Promethazine Hydrochloride
Phenhydan	Phenytoin
Pheno-caps	Phenobarbitone
Phenomet	Phenobarbitone
Phentoin	Phenytoin
Phenybute	Phenylbutazone
Phenylbutazone	Phenylbutazone
Phiasol AS	Padimate A
Phiso-med	Hexachlorophane
Pholcolin	Pholcodine
Pholevan	Pholcodine
Pholtrate	Pholcodine
Pholtussin	Pholcodine
Phosmycine	Tetracycline
Phospholine Iodide	Ecothiopate
Phyldrox	Aminophylline
Phyllocontin	Aminophylline
Phylodrox	Aminophylline
Physeptone	Methadone
Phytadon	Pethidine
Phytodermine	Salicylic acid
Phytomenadione	Vitamin K
Pict's solution	Formaldehyde
Pilocar	Pilocarpine
Pilocarpina Lux	Pilocarpine
Pilopt	Pilocarpine
Pima	Potassium Iodide
Piranex	Chlorpheniramine
Piriton	Chlorpheniramine
PK-Merz	Amantadine
Placemol	Paracetamol
Plaquenil	Hydroxychloroquine
Plaquinol	Hydroxychloroquine
Plegomazine	Chlorpromazine
Pluryl	Bendrofluazide
Polmiror	Nifuratel
Polmix	Polymyxin
Pologal picis	Coal Tar
Polycillin	Ampicillin
Polycycline	Tetracycline
Polyfax	Polymyxin
Polymox	Amoxycillin
Posalfilin	Podophyllin paint
Potassion	Potassium supplement
Povidine K	Povidone Iodine
Pramidex	Tolbutamide
Praecirheumin	Phenylbutazone
Pragmatar	Salicylic acid
Prazine	Promazine
Predalon	Chorionic Gonadotrophin

Predeltin	Prednisone
Prednicen M	Prednisone
Predni-F	Dexamethasone
Prednilone	Prednisone
Prednilonga	Prednisone
Predniment	Prednisone
Predni-tablinen	Prednisone
Prednital	Prednisone
Pregnesin	Chorionic Gonadotrophin
Pregnyl	Chorionic Gonadotrophin
Premarin	Oestrogens-Conjugated
Premaspin	Aspirin
Presinol	Methyldopa
Presomen	Oestrogens-Conjugated
Presone	Prednisone
Priadel	Lithium
Primogonyl	Chorionic Gonadotrophin
Primogyn	Ethinyloestradiol
Primogyn C.	Ethinyloestradiol
Primogyn Depot	Oestradiol Valerate
Primogyn M.	Ethinyloestradiol
Primolut-Depot	Hydroxyprogesterone
Primoteston Depot	Testosterone Enanthate
Primperan	Metoclopramide
Primolut M	Norethisterone
Principen	Ampicillin
Prioderm	Malathion
Priscol	Tolazoline
Priscoline	Tolazoline
Pro-Actidil	Triprolidine
Pro-Actidilon	Triprolidine
Pro-Banthine	Propantheline
Probecid	Probenecid
Proben	Probenecid
Probexin	Probenecid
Procalm	Chlorpromazine
Procapan	Procainamide
Procillin	Procaine penicillin
Proclon	Chlorpromazine
Procytox	Cyclophosphamide
Prodigox	Digoxin
Prodixamon	Propantheline
Prodol	Aspirin
Profilate	Anti haemophilic globulin
Progan	Promethazine Hydrochloride
Progesterone-Retard	Hydroxyprogesterone
Proglicem	Diazoxide
Progynon	Ethinyloestradiol
Progynon C	Ethinyloestradiol
Progynon-Depot	Oestradiol Valerate
Progynon M	Ethinyloestradiol
Progynova	Oestradiol Valerate
Proklar-M	Sulphamethizole
Proladone	Oxycodone
Prolixin	Fluphenazine

Proluton Depot	Hydroxyprogesterone
Promachel	Chlorpromazine
Promachlor	Chlorpromazine
Promacid	Chlorpromazine
Promanyl	Promazine
Promapar	Chlorpromazine
Promapar	Chlorpromazine
Promarchel	Chlorpromazine
Promarchlor	Chlorpromazine
Promarit	Oestrogens-Conjugated
Promazettes	Promazine
Promecid	Chlorpromazine
Promethapar	Promethazine Hydrochloride
Promezerine	Promazine
Promosol	Chlorpromazine
Pronestyl	Procainamide
Propiocine	Erythromycin
Propadrine	Phenylpropanolamine
Propred	Prednisone
Prostacton	L. Thyroxine
Prostaphlin A	Cloxacillin
Prostigmin	Neostigmine
Protactyl	Promazine
Protensin	Chlordiazepoxide
Proternal	Isoprenaline
Pro-Tet	Human Antitetanus Immunoglobulin
Prothazine	Promethazine Hydrochloride
Protran	Chlorpromazine
Pro-Tran	Promazine
Protren	Chlorpromazine
Proval	Paracetamol
Provera	Medroxyprogesterone
Provilax	Dioctyl
Provilax	Dioctyl Sodium Sulphosuccinate
Proviodine	Povidone Iodine
Provoprin-500	Aspirin
Proxen	Naproxen
Psoriderm	Coal Tar
Psorox	Coal tar
Pularin	Heparin
PV Carpine	Pilocarpine
PVF K	Penicillin V
P.V.K.	Penicillin V
P.V.O.	Penicillin V
Pyknolepsinum	Ethosuximide
Pyoredol	Phenytoin
Pyralen	Paracetamol
Pyrogallic Acid	Pyrogallol
QID amp	Ampicillin
Q.I.D. mycin	Erythromycin
Q.I.D. pen VK	Penicillin V
Q.I.D. tet	Tetracycline
Quadcin	Tetracycline
Quadnite	Promethazine Hydrochloride
Quadracyclin	Tetracycline

Quantalan	Cholestyramine
Quatrax	Tetracycline
Quellada	Gamma Benzene Hexachloride
Quensyl	Hydroxychloroquine
Questran	Cholestyramine
Quilonum	Lithium
Quinate	Quinine
Quinbisan	Quinine
Quinsan	Quinine
Rastinon	Tolbutamide
Raurine	Reserpine
Rau-Sed	Reserpine
Reacthin	A.C.T.H.
Reasec	Diphenoxylate + atropine
Recifruit	Castor oil
Recolip	Colfibrate
Rectalad-Aminophylline	Aminophylline
Rectocalcium	Calcium gluconate
Rectodelt	Prednisone
Rectules	Chloral Hydrate
Reddoxydrin	Aminophylline
Refobacin	Gentamicin
Regelan N	Clofibrate
Regitin	Phentolamine
Regitine	Phentolamine
Reglan	Metoclopramide
Regonol	Pyridostigmine
Regulex	Dioctyl
Regulex	Dioctyl Sodium Sulphosuccinate
Rekawan	Potassium supplement
Relanium	Diazepam
Relaxil	Chlordiazepoxide
Remsed	Promethazine Hydrochloride
Renese	Polythiazide
Repamol	Paracetamol
Resedrex	Reserpine
Resercrine	Reserpine
Resedrex	Reserpine
Reserpanca	Reserpine
Reserpoid	Reserpine
Resochin	Chloroquine
Resoferix	Ferrous sulphate
Ressec	Diphenoxylate with Atropine
Restin elixir	Paracetamol
Restwel	Dichloralphenazone
Retardin	Diphenoxylate
Retardin	Diphenoxylate with Atropine
Retcin	Erythromycin
Retet	Tetracycline
Retin-A	Tretinoin
Retinoic Acid	Tretinion
Reumajust A	Flufenamic acid
Rexamycin	Tetracycline
Rheomacrodex	Dextran 40
Rhindecon	Phenylpropanolamine

Rhodiglobin	Immune Serum globulin
Rhonal	Aspirin
Rhythmodan	Disopyramide
Rifadin	Rifampicin
Rifinah	Rifampicin Plus I.N.A.H.
Rikodeine	Dihydrocodeine
Rimactane	Rifampicin
Rimactazid	Rifampicin Plus I.N.A.H.
Rimifon	Isoniazid
Rinderon	Betamethasone
Rinurel	Phenylpropanolamine
Riocyclin	Tetracycline
Rivotril	Clonazepam
Ro-ampen	Ampicillin
Robicillin VK	Pencillin V
Robimycin	Erythromycin
Robitet	Tetracycline
Rocilin	Penicillin V
Ro-cillin VK	Penicillin V
Rocycline	Tetracycline
Rogitine	Phentolamine
Roin	Cinnarizine
Roscopenin	Penicillin V
Rosolid	Chlordiazepoxide
Rotensept	Chlorhexidine
Rougoxin	Digoxin
Rounox	Paracetamol
Rovamycin	Spiramycin
Rubesol-LA	Hydroxocobalamin
Rufol	Sulphamethizole
Rum K	Potassium supplement
Ruthmol	Potassium Chloride
Rynacrom	Disodium Cromoglycate
Ryser	Reserpine
Rythmodan	Disopyramide
Rythrocaps	Erythromycin
Saal-F	Flufenamic acid
Salactol	Salicylic acid
Salicylate	Aspirin
Salimol	Sulphamethizole
Salisan	Chlorothiazide
Saluren	Chlorothiazide
Salures	Bendrofluazide
Saluric	Chlorothiazide
Salzone	Paracetamol
Sanatrichom	Metronidazole
Sanclomycine	Tetracycline
Sandocal	Calcium gluconate
Sando K	Potassium Chloride
Sando-K	Potassium supplements
Sandomigran	Pizotifen
Sandomigrin	Pizotifen
Sandril	Reserpine
Sansert	Methysergide
Sapoderm	Hexachlorophane

Saroten	Amitriptyline
Saventrine	Isoprenaline
Sawacillin	Amoxycillin
Sawasone	Dexamethasone
Scabanca	Benzyl Benzoate
Scherofluron	Fludrocortisone
Scheroson F	Hydrocortisone eye drops
Scopolamine	Hyoscine
S-Dimidine	Sulphadimidine
Sebaveen Shampoo	Salicylic acid
Sebizon	Sulphacetamide eye drops/ ointment
Seboderm	Cetrimide
Seclopyrine	Aspirin
Sedabar	Phenobarbitone
Sedaraupin	Reserpine
Seda-Tablinen	Phenobarbitone
Sed Lingtus	Pholcodine
Sednaco	Pholcodine
Sednine	Pholcodine
Seguril	Frusemide
Selectomycin	Spiramycin
Seloken	Metoprolol
Sembrina	Methyldopa
Senade	Senna
Sendoxan	Cyclophosphamide
Sennokott	Senna
Sennosides	Senna
Senokot	Senna
Senpurgin	Senna
Septipulmon	Sulphapyridine
Septra	Co Trimoxazole
Septran	Co Trimoxazole
Septrin	Co Trimoxazole
Sequestrene Na$_2$ Ca	Sodium Calcium Edetate
Serazone	Chlorpromazine
Serc	Betahistine
Serenace	Haloperidol
Serenack	Diazepam
Serfin	Reserpine
Serozone	Chlorpromazine
Serpacil	Reserpine
Serpasil	Reserpine
Serpate	Reserpine
Serpax	Reserpine
Serpiloid	Reserpine
Serpone	Reserpine
Sertina	Reserpine
Servisone	Prednisone
Sevinol	Fluphenazine
Sexovid	Cyclofenil
Sifacycline	Tetracycline
Siguent Hycor (eye)	Hydrocortisone eye drops
Silquat C100	Cetrimide
Simplene	Adrenaline eye drops
Simplotan	Tinidazole

Sinemet	Levodopa and Decarboxylase inhibitor
Sintomicetine	Chloramphenicol
Siponol O	Dioctyl Sodium Sulphosuccinate
Siponol-O-100	Dioctyl
Siqualone	Fluphenazine
Siragan	Chloroquine
SK-ampicillin	Ampicillin
S.K.-Apap	Paracetamol
S.K. Erythromycin	Erythromycin
Skleromexe	Clofibrate
SK-Oestrogens	Oestrogens-Conjugated
S.K. Soxazole	Sulphafurazole
Slow-Fe	Ferrous sulphate
Slow K	Potassium Chloride
Slow K	Potassium supplements
S.-Methizole	Sulphamethizole
SMP Homatropine	Homatropine
Sobelin	Clindamycin
Sobiodopa	Levodopa
Sodium Sulamyd	Sulphacetamide eye drops/ointment
Sodothiol	Sodium Thiosulphate
Soframycin	Framycetin
Solantyl	Phenytoin
Solatene	Vitamin A
Solazine	Trifluoperazine
Solcetas	Aspirin
Solfoton	Phenobarbitone
Solium	Chlordiazepoxide
Soliwax	Dioctyl
Soliwax	Dioctyl Sodium Sulphosuccinate
Solnicol	Chloramphenicol
Soloxsalen	Methoxsalen
Solprin	Aspirin
Solu-A	Vitamin A
Solu-Cortef	Hydrocortisone Sodium Succinate
Solu-Diazine	Sulphadiazine
Solu-Glyc	Hydrocortisone Sodium Succinate
Solu-Glye	Hydrocortisone Sodium Succinate
Solusal	Aspirin
Solutedarol	Triamcinolone
Solvejod	Potassium Iodide
Solvezink	Zinc Sulphate
Somacton	Growth Hormone
Somophyllin	Aminophylline
Sone	Prednisone
Sorbifer	Ferrous sulphate
Sosegon	Pentazocine
Sosol	Sulphafurazole
Soufre Oligosol	Sodium Thiosulphate
Soxamide	Sulphafurazole
Soxomide	Sulphafurazole
Soy-Dome	Hexachlorophane
Spagulax	Ispaghula Husk
Spaneph	Ephedrine
Span K	Potassium supplements
Sparine	Promazine

Specilline G	Benzyl Penicillin
Speciodopa	Levodopa
Spectraban	Padimate A
Spersacarpine	Pilocarpine
Spersadex	Dexamethasone
Spersanicol	Chloramphenicol eye drops
Spersatropine	Atropine eye drop
Sporiline	Tolnaftate
SSKI	Potassium Iodide
ST-52	Fosfestrol (diethyl Stilboestrol)
Stabillin VK	Penicillin V
Stabinol	Chlorpropamide
Stanilo	Spectinomycin
Staphobristol	Cloxacillin
Staphybiotic	Cloxacillin
Staphylex	Flucloxacillin
Steclin	Tetracycline
Stecsolin	Tetracycline
Stelazine	Trifluoperazine
Stemetil	Prochlorperazine
Stental	Phenobarbitone
Sterandryl	Testosterone Propionate
Sterets H	Chlorhexidine
Steridermis	Hexachlorophane
Sterogyl-15	Vitamin D
Sterop Sulphacetamide Sodium Drops	Sulphacetamide eye drops
Ster-zac	Hexachlorophane
Stesolid	Diazepam
Stibilium	Stilboestrol
Stie-Lasan	Dithranol ointment
Stilbetin	Stilboestrol
Stilbol	Stilboestrol
Stilphostrol	Fosfestrol (diethyl Stilboestrol)
Stomiline	Aluminium Hydroxide
Stovarsol	Acetarsol
Stoxil	Idoxuridine
Strepolin	Streptomycin
Streptase	Streptokinase
Strept-evanules	Streptomycin
Streptosol	Streptomycin
Stugeron	Cinnarizine
Succinat A	Chloramphenicol
Sudabid	Pseudoephedrine
Sudafed	Pseudoephedrine
Sulagen	Sulphafurazole
Sulf-10	Sulphacetamide eye drops/ointment
Sulfacalyrn	Sulphacetamide eye drops/ointment
Sulfadine	Sulphadimidine
Sulfagan	Sulphafurazole
Sulfalar	Sulphafurazole
Sulfametin	Sulphamethizole
Sulfapred	Sulphacetamide eye drops/ointment
Sulfasan	Sulphafurazole

Sulfagan	Sulphafurazole
Sulfazole	Sulphafurazole
Sulfisan	Sulphafurazole
Sulfisin	Sulphafurazole
Suflizole	Sulphafurazole
Sulmycin	Gentamicin
Sulphacetamido I.Q.	Sulphacetamide eye drops
Sulphacetamide I.Q.	Sulphacetamide eye drops/oint.
Sulphadine	Sulphadimidine
Sulphamethazine	Sulphadimidine
Sulphamezathine	Sulphadimidine
Sultanol	Salbutamol
Sultrin	Triple Sulpha
Sunflo Oil	Sun Flower seed oil
Supasa	Aspirin
Supen	Ampicillin
Suppolosal	Pethidine
Supramycin N	Tetracycline
Suractin	Ampicillin
Surgiderm	Hexachlorophane
Surika	Flufenamic acid
Suscardia	Isoprenaline
Suspenin	Procaine penicillin
Sustamycin	Tetracycline
Suxinutin	Ethosuximide
S.V.C.	Acetarsol
Svedocyklin	Tetracycline
Symmetrel	Amantadine
Synalar	Fluocinolone
Synamol	Fluocinolone
Synandone	Fluocinolone
Synapause	Oestriol
Syncorta	Deoxycortone Acetate
Syncortyl	Deoxycortone Acetate
Syndopa	Levodopa
Synemol	Fluocinolone
Synmiol	Idoxuridine
Synocthen	Tetracosactrin
Synpenin	Ampicillin
Synstigmin	Neostigmine
Synthecillin	Ampicillin
Synthroid	L. Thyroxine
Syntopressin	Lysine Vasopressin
Sytobex-H	Hydroxocobalamin
TAB 39	Oestrogens-Conjugated
Talwin	Pentazocine
Tapar	Paracetamol
Taractan	Chlorprothixene
Tarasan	Chlorprothixene
Tarcortin	Coal tar
Tardocillin	Benzathine Penicillin
Tauredon	Gold
Tazone	Phenylbutazone
Tb-Phlogin	Isoniazid
Teevex	Crotamiton

Tegopen	Cloxacillin
Tegretol	Carbamazepine
Teldrin	Chlorpheniramine
Teledrin	Chlorpheniramine
Tementil	Prochlorperazine
Temlo	Paracetamol
Tempra	Paracetamol
Tenicridine	Mepacrine
Tenserp	Reserpine
Tensilon	Edrophonium Chloride
Tensium	Diazepam
Teofyllamin	Aminophylline
Tepanil	Phenylpropanolamine
Tercolix	Codeine Phosphate
Terfluzin	Trifluoperazine
Termidor	Paracetamol
Terramycin	Tetracycline
Tertroxin	Liothyronine
Testate	Testosterone Enanthate
Testex	Testosterone Propionate
Testine	Testosterone Propionate
Testostroval-PA	Testosterone Enanthate
Testoviron	Testosterone Propionate
Testoviron-Depot	Testosterone Enanthate
Tetabullin	Human Antitetanus Immunoglobulin
Tetagam	Human Antitetanus Immunoglobulin
Tetaglobuline	Human Antitetanus Immunoglobulin
Tetanobulin	Human Antitetanus Immunoglobulin
Tetanol	Tetanus Toxoid
Teta-Tabs	Thiamine
Tetatoxoid	Tetanus Toxoid
Tetavax	Tetanus Toxoid
Tetnor	Phenylbutazone
Tetrabid	Tetracycline
Tetrachel	Tetracycline
Tetracyn	Tetracycline
Tetradecin	Tetracycline
Tetral	Tetracycline
Tetralean	Tetracycline
Tetramykoin	Tetracycline
Tetrex	Tetracycline
Tetrex PMT	Tetracycline
Tetrosol	Tetracycline
Therapen	Benzyl Penicillin
Therapen i.m.	Procaine Penicillin
Thianeuron	Thiamine
Thioril	Thioridazine
Thiosulfil	Sulphamethizole
Thiuretic	Hydrochlorthiazide
Thoradex	Chlorpromazine
Thorazine	Chlorpromazine
Thrombophob	Heparin
Thrombo-Vetren	Heparin
Thyratabs	L. Thyroxine
Thyrine	L. Thyroxine
Thyronorman	Potassium Perchlorate

Thyroxevan	L. Thyroxine
Thyroxinal	L. Thyroxine
Thyroxinique	L. Thyroxine
Tibinide	Isoniazid
Ticelgesic	Paracetamol
Ticinil	Phenylbutazone
Ticipect	Diphenhydramine
Tifomycine	Chloramphenicol
Tifosyl	Thiotepa
Tikacillin	Penicillin V
T-Immun	Tetanus Toxoid
Tinacidin	Tolnaftate
Tinactin	Tolnaftate
Tinaderm	Tolnaftate
Toin Unicelles	Phenytoin
Tolbutol	Tolbutamide
Tolbutone	Tolbutamide
Toniron	Ferrous sulphate
Tonoftal	Tolnaftate
Topmycin	Chlortetracycline
Torecan	Thiethylperazine
Tosmilen	Demecarium Bromide
Totacillin	Ampicillin
Totapen	Ampicillin
Totolin	Phenylpropanolamine
Totomycin	Tetracycline
Transannon	Oestrogens-Conjugated
Trapanal	Thiopentone
Trasicor	Oxprenolol
Tremin	Benzhexol
Tresochin	Chloroquine
Triagin	Glyceryl Trinitrate
Triamcort	Triamcinolone
Trib	Co Trimoxazole
Trichazol	Metronidazole
Trichomonacide	Acetarsol
Tricloryl	Triclofos
Triclos	Triclofos
Tricodein	Codeine Phosphate
Tricodeine	Codeine Phosphate
Tridione	Troxidone
Trifluoper-Ez-Ets	Trifluoperazine
Triflurin	Trifluoperazine
Trihexy	Benzhexol
Trikacide	Metronidazole
Trikamon	Metronidazole
Trilene	Trichlorethylene
Trilium	Chlordiazepoxide
Trimedone	Troxidone
Trimetoprim-Sulfa	Co Trimoxazole
Trinuride	Pheneturide
Tri Iodothyronine	Liothyronine
Triodurin	Oestriol
Triogesic	Phenylpropanolamine
Triominic	Phenylpropanolamine
Triophen 10	Aspirin

Triotussic	Phenylpropanolamine
Triovex	Oestriol
Triptil	Protriptyline
Triptafen	Amitriptyline
Tri thyrone	Liothyronine
Trixyl	Benzhexol
Trobicin	Spectinomycin
Trocosone	Oestrogens-Conjugated
Trolovol	Penicillamine
Tropium	Chlordiazepoxide
Troymycetin	Chloramphenicol
Truxal	Chlorprothixene
Truxalettem	Chlorprothixene
Trypsogen	Pancreatin
Tryptanol	Amitriptyline
Tryptizol	Amitriptyline
Tuscodin	Dihydrocodeine
Tussaphed	Pseudoephedrine
Tussinol	Pholcodine
Tussokon	Pholcodine
Tylenol	Paracetamol
Ultandren	Fluoxymesterone
Ultracorten	Prednisone
Ultradine	Povidone Iodine
Uniflu	Phenylephrine
Unihepa	D.L. Methionine
Unimycin	Tetracycline
Unisoil	Castor oil
Uranap	D.L. Methionine
Uracid	D.L. Methionine
Urecid	Probenecid
Urekene	Sodium Valproate
Uridon	Chlorthalidone
Urocydal	Sulphamethizole
Urogan	Sulphafurazole
Urolene Blue	Methylene Blue
Urolex	Sulphamethizole
Urolin	Sulphamethizole
Urolucosil	Sulphamethizole
Urosan lotion	Padimate A
Urosin	Allopurinol
Uroz	Sulphamethizole
Urozide	Hydrochlorthiazide
Urtilone	Prednisone
U.S. 67	Sulphafurazole
U. tet	Tetracycline
Uticillin VK	Penicillin V
Utrasul	Sulphamethizole
Uricone	Mexenone
Uvistat	Mexenone
Vaam-DHQ	Di-Iodohydroxyquinoline
Vagestrol	Stilboestrol
Valadol	Paracetamol
Valisone	Betamethasone

Valium	Diazepam
Valoid	Cyclizine
Vanair	Benzoyl Peroxide
Vapo-N-Iso	Isoprenaline
Vasitrin	Glyceryl Trinitrate
Vasolan	Verapamil
Vasosulf	Sulphacetamide eye drops
Vasosulf	Sulphacetamide eye drops/ointment
Vasotherm	Nicotinic acid
V-Cillin	Penicillin V
V-Cillin K	Penicillin V
V-Cil-K	Penicillin V
VC-K500	Penicillin V
Veekay	Penicillin V
Veetids	Penicillin V
Veldopa	Levodopa
Venocort	Hydrocortisone Sodium Succinate
Ventolin	Salbutamol
Veracur	Formaldehyde
Vericap PLL	Podophyllin paint
Verin	Thiamine
Versotrane	Hydrargaphen
Vertigon	Prochlorperazine
Vesagex	Cetrimide
Vetren	Heparin
Via-Quil	Chlordiazepoxide
Viarox	Beclomethasone Dipropionate
Vibeden	Hydroxocobalamin
Vibex	Thiamine
Vibrocil	Phenylephrine
Vi Dom A	Vitamin A
Vidopen	Ampicillin
Vikacillin	Penicillin V
Vioform	Clioquinol
Viokase	Pancreatin
Vio-Serpine	Reserpine
Vira-A	Vidarabine
Viraxacillin	Procaine Penicillin
Viraxacillin V	Penicillin V
Virofral	Amantadine
Virormone	Testosterone Propionate
Virungent	Idoxuridine
Vi-Siblin	Ispaghula Husk
Vitobun	Thiamine
Vivactil	Protriptyline
Vivol	Diazepam
Vogan	Vitamin A
Volon	Triamcinolone
Wampocap	Nicotinic acid
Waran	Warfarin
Warfilone	Warfarin
Warnerin	Warfarin
Waxsol	Dioctyl
Waxsol	Dioctyl Sodium Sulphosuccinate
Wellconal	Dipipanone

Welldorm	Dichloralphenazone
Wescopen	Benzyl Penicillin
Wescopred	Prednisone
Wescotol	Tolbutamide
Wescozone	Phenylbutazone
Westadone	Methadone
Whitfields ointment	Benzoic Acid ointment
Winoxin	Digoxin
Winpred	Prednisone
Wintracin	Tetracycline
Win-V-K	Penicillin V
Wycillin	Procaine Penicillin
Xylocard	Lignocaine
Yadalan	Chlorothiazide
Zalpon	Hexachlorophane
Zarontin	Ethosuximide
Zentropil	Phenytoin
Zeste	Oestrogens-Conjugated
Zincfrin	Zinc Sulphate
Zincomed	Zinc Sulphate
Zinkaps-220	Zinc Sulphate
Zipan	Promethazine Hydrochloride
Zoline	Tolazoline
Zyklolat	Cyclopentolate
Zyloprim	Allopurinol
Zyloric	Allopurinol
Zypanar	Pancreatin